The Vital Shoulder Complex

An Illustrated Guide to Assessment, Treatment, and Rehabilitation

The Vital Shoulder Complex

An Illustrated Guide to Assessment,
Treatment, and Rehabilitation

John Gibbons

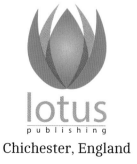

lotus
publishing

Chichester, England

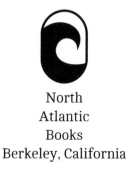

North
Atlantic
Books

Berkeley, California

First published in 2019 by
Lotus Publishing
Apple Tree Cottage, Inlands Road, Nutbourne, Chichester, PO18 8RJ, and
North Atlantic Books
Berkeley, California

Illustrations Amanda Williams
Photographs Ian Taylor
Text Design Medlar Publishing Solutions Pvt Ltd., India
Cover Design Wendy Craig
Printed and Bound in India by Replika Press

The Vital Shoulder Complex: An Illustrated Guide to Assessment, Treatment, and Rehabilitation is sponsored and published by the Society for the Study of Native Arts and Sciences (dba North Atlantic Books), an educational nonprofit based in Berkeley, California, that collaborates with partners to develop cross-cultural perspectives; nurture holistic views of art, science, the humanities, and healing; and seed personal and global transformation by publishing work on the relationship of body, spirit, and nature.

North Atlantic Books' publications are available through most bookstores. For further information, visit our website at www.northatlanticbooks.com or call 800-733-3000.

Medical Disclaimer
The following information is intended for general information purposes only. Individuals should always consult their health care provider before administering any suggestions made in this book. Any application of the material set forth in the following pages is at the reader's discretion and is his or her sole responsibility.

British Library Cataloging-in-Publication Data
A CIP record for this book is available from the British Library
ISBN 978 1 905367 93 1 (Lotus Publishing)
ISBN 978 1 62317 417 0 (North Atlantic Books)

Library of Congress Cataloging-in-Publication Data
Names: Gibbons, John, 1968- author.
Title: The vital shoulder complex : an illustrated guide to
     assessment, treatment, and rehabilitation / John Gibbons.
Description: Berkeley, California : North Atlantic Books;
     Nutbourne, Chichester : Lotus Publishing, 2019. |
     Includes bibliographical references and index.
Identifiers: LCCN 2018056270 (print) | LCCN 2018057623
     (ebook) | ISBN 9781623174187 (e-book) |
     ISBN 9781623174170 (North Atlantic Books : pbk.) |
     ISBN 9781905367931 (Lotus Publishing : pbk.)
Subjects: | MESH: Shoulder Joint—physiopathology |
     Shoulder Joint—injuries | Joint Diseases—diagnosis |
     Joint Diseases—rehabilitation
Classification: LCC RD557.5 (ebook) | LCC RD557.5 (print)
     | NLM WE 810 | DDC 617.5/72044—dc23
LC record available at https://lccn.loc.gov/2018056270

Contents

Preface

At one time I thought that this book would be my first publication rather than my fifth. I have been lecturing the Shoulder Joint Master class at the University of Oxford for many years now and it has been by far one of my most popular courses for physical therapists. I consider its popularity to be due in part to the fact that many therapists and even patients/athletes that come into the clinic struggle with this particular area of the body. As you read through the pages of this book, you will see that I have included many factors that can affect or relate to the shoulder complex: for example, did you know that the gall bladder or liver can present pain to the shoulder region? If not, then I hope you find the 'differential diagnosis' chapter useful. Many therapists believe that all shoulder and arm pain is coming from the cervical spine and they focus all their effort on this area and completely neglect the shoulder complex. The fact that this entire book is about the shoulder complex indicates my own view of its importance.

I have a sort of 'case study' in my friend Howard Weller, with whom I frequently exercise before classes or clinic. I mention Howard because he has had both shoulder joints replaced and he has just turned 50. Ignoring medical advice to 'lift nothing' he continues to exercise and, if I am honest, I have to say he has had serious gains in strength and size since the shoulders have been replaced. I enjoy the regular training sessions, so thank you Howard!

The subject is, of course, complex in both name and nature – even more so in the active, living body – and in the chapter on the pelvis and the gluteal muscles I discuss a couple of case studies of patients who presented to my clinic with shoulder pain. I have also included many chapters on the assessment procedures for the shoulder complex that I use in my own clinic and with various treatment strategies through muscle energy techniques, soft tissue release using active and passive movements as well as taping techniques. The final chapter is about rehabilitative exercises that you can recommend to your patients (and athletes) to take home after treatment.

Acknowledgments

All my thanks go to Jon Hutchings of Lotus Publishing for having the faith and confidence in me to continue with the dream of writing – without you all of my books, including this one, would not have been written and subsequently published.

My thanks to Ian Taylor, who spent a vast amount of time and effort taking and editing the many photographs contained within this book, and who has done an amazing job.

To Stephanie Pickering (editor), without her patience and input this book would definitely not read as well as it does!

Amanda Williams for her amazing illustrations even though many times she probably has no idea of what it is I am asking for and this probably goes for all of my books!

To my mother, Margaret Gibbons, and to my sister Amanda Williams and her husband Philip, and to their children Victoria (who will be 19 this year) and James (who is approaching 22), I thank you all for 'just being there' as I know the last year has been terrible not just for myself but for everybody involved in my life.

Denise Thomas, my fiancé and the model in the book, who has stuck with me through thick and thin, especially through 2017, when I lost my son to a tragic motorcycle accident. I truly, truly wanted to thank you from the bottom of my heart for all of your continued support, love and especially inspiration.

Since the passing of my son, I have begun to realize my purpose in life, and that is to educate as many therapists throughout the world as I can, to try to help them achieve great things in their lives. I hope to do that through my lectures and books. I therefore personally want to thank you, the readers, as without your continual support I definitely would not be able to do what I do.

Dedication

To my amazing son Thomas Rhys Gibbons, who sadly left my world at 10.51 p.m. on the 28 February 2017, at the age of 17 years and 17 days. Rest in peace my little Tom-Tom – you will be truly missed. We will meet again and that's for sure, but not yet as I have too much to achieve with my life first and sadly you have made me realize that!

List of abbreviations

AC joint/ACJ	acromioclavicular joint
ACL	anterior cruciate ligament
AHC	anterior horn cell
AROM	active range of motion
ASIS	anterior superior iliac spine
CSP	cervical spine
DDD	degenerative disc disease
EMG	electromyogram
GH	glenohumeral joint
GIRD	glenohumeral internal rotation dysfunction
Gmax	gluteus maximus
GTO	Golgi tendon organ
HVT	high velocity thrust
IGHL	inferior glenohumeral ligament
ITB	iliotibial band
LOAF muscles	lateral lumbricals (first and second), opponens pollicis, abductor pollicis brevis, flexor pollicis brevis
MET	muscle energy technique
MGHL	middle glenohumeral ligament
MRI	magnetic resonance imaging
OA	osteoarthritis
PHC	posterior horn cell
PIR	post-isometric relaxation
PROM	passive range of motion
PSIS	posterior superior iliac spine
QL	quadratus lumborum
RI	reciprocal inhibition
ROM	range of motion
SAB	subacromial bursa
SALT and Pepper muscles	subscapularis, anterior deltoid, latissimus dorsi and teres major plus pectoralis major
SAS	subacromial space
SC joint/SCJ	sternoclavicular joint
SGHL	superior glenohumeral ligament
SCM	sternocleidomastoid
SIJ	sacroiliac joint
SITS muscles	supraspinatus, infraspinatus, teres minor and subscapularis
SLAP lesion	superior labral (tear from) anterior (to) posterior
SRP	symptom-reducing protocol
SSMP	shoulder symptom modification procedure
ST joint	scapulothoracic joint
STJ	subtalar joint
TFL	tensor fasciae latae
THL	transverse humeral ligament
TOS	thoracic outlet syndrome
TP	transverse process
TRX	total body resistance exercise
TVA	transversus abdominis
UCS	upper crossed syndrome
US	ultrasound

Introduction

I have many goals for writing this text but the main one is simply that you, the reader, whether you are a physical therapist, a medical doctor, or a patient or athlete suffering with chronic shoulder pain, will achieve a better understanding of what actually goes on within the shoulder region, and better understand both why a patient might be having this pain and more importantly, what you can do about it.

This is the fifth book I have written and published and I never thought when I started back in 2010 that these books would be as successful as they are. I have taught thousands of physical therapists in countries such as China, Singapore, Dubai, India, Serbia, Portugal, Ireland and of course the UK and it gives me enormous pleasure that they have been found to be useful by those I have taught or who have read my books and articles. Writing and lecturing is by far the most inspirational thing that I do in my life: not only does it give me pleasure but I believe that I am changing peoples lives and making them better physical therapists – and this has the added benefit of improving the overall well-being of the patients they are treating.

The text includes many case studies throughout, and these cases are actual patients and athletes that have visited my clinic at the University of Oxford. I hope you find them of interest and that you can relate the studies here to your thoughts about your own patients and that maybe, just maybe, you will have a light bulb moment – if so then I have achieved my ambition by being able to help you!

In terms of shoulder-related injuries, some of the readers of this book may not be trained in any form of physical therapy but simply want to know a little bit about shoulder function and injuries and so on. I would like here to mention one particular injury (of many) I sustained and this was to the acromioclavicular joint (ACJ). This joint is an interesting structure. The injury happened in December 2015 when I went mountain biking with my son to a place in Merthyr Tydfil, in the valleys of South Wales. It is a fantastic place for off road downhill biking! We had been there a couple of times before but this time was different, because rather than renting bikes, I decided to use our own bikes as I was trying to save some money. On the third trip downhill my rear brake had ceased to function properly so suddenly I only had a front brake to slow down my descent. Anyway, before I knew it I went too fast around a corner and braked hard and now felt myself travelling in mid air thinking to myself 'this is going to hurt …'. I landed on my right scapula and head (glad I had a full face helmet on!) and immediately felt the right AC joint separate. While I lay there my son cycled back to see me and the first thing he said was 'come on dad, get up and let's do it again!' Feeling very sorry for myself I said 'I need an X-ray!' Driving home was very awkward to say the least. Finally, 2 hours later, and an X-ray showed a separation (grade II). I thought I would be back doing my triceps dips, pull ups, bench and shoulder presses within a month – how wrong I was! Even now, 2 years later, I am still struggling to do a bodyweight dip because I would say that the AC joint in its simplistic form is a type of mechanical *strut*, *hinge* or a *linkage* that permits movement and the ligaments that support this structure have now been damaged. So when I teach or see patients with an AC joint separation I normally say to them, whatever time you think it will take you to get back to normal function, you need to at least treble the timescale. That to me is a little more realistic.

You can probably guess that for the majority of patients this is unwelcome news – they do not want to hear that it will take many months, or even a year or so, for their injury to heal, especially when they thought it would recover in a matter of weeks.

The body is naturally a self-healer; it has been designed to do just that. However, certain parts of the body do not heal easily. One structure in particular, the anterior cruciate ligament (ACL) of the knee, is probably the easiest injury to mention in this context because once this has been fully torn the body finds it near impossible to repair and most of these tears will require surgical intervention. The reason I mentioned the ACL is just a reminder that the practitioner cannot fix everything and everybody and sometimes we need some guidance and assistance from other professionals, I hope when the time is needed you remember that and have the confidence to seek help.

While reading this book you will come across many photographs. As you and I have found in the past, it is very difficult to understand a fascinating yet highly complex subject such as the shoulder, the underlying complexities associated with the cervical spine and the subsequent exiting nerve pathways with only static pictures to illustrate the anatomy and the various assessments, treatment and rehabilitative techniques that I am trying to portray and demonstrate. My overall goal in writing this text with all the associated pictures, figures and case studies is to assist you the to have a far better understanding of what has been written about the shoulder complex. I hope I achieve that goal but more importantly, that you actually *enjoy* reading this book and in time you might recommend this book to your friends. Some of you will already be a subscriber on my YouTube channel and I currently have hundreds of videos on all aspects of manual therapy and sports medicine-related subjects that you are able to access for FREE and some of these videos will include most (if not all) of the multitude of techniques shown throughout this text.

In the meantime I hope you enjoy reading this book, which I have personally written for you!

John Gibbons

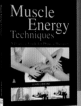
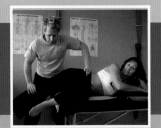
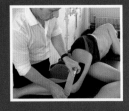
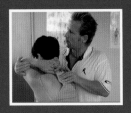

1

Functional anatomy of the shoulder complex

There are currently numerous medical textbooks about this subject on the shelves of bookstores throughout the world. If I am honest, though, I have to say I find many of these a difficult read, often both dull and written in a complex way that is hard to follow. I sometimes struggle with the (often too small) print, there are not enough color pictures and so on … It may be that is just me; however, I have taught many thousands of students and a majority of those I ask agree with what I am saying. I am therefore aiming to write this particular text in such a way that all therapists of physical therapy, or even patients that have pain in the shoulder or neck region, can actually read this book and truly understand what it is I am trying to write about.

Before I continue discussing all the areas of the shoulder region as well as all of its associated structures I need to clarify a few basics. First, the shoulder joint is actually called the glenohumeral joint (gleno – glenoid – is the socket and humeral is the humerus – the long bone of the upper arm). This particular area might well be the main source of shoulder pain for patients visiting the doctor or the physical therapist. However, and as you will read in later chapters, there are numerous other joints of the shoulder region as well as other associated structures that can also be the source (causative factor) for the presenting symptoms for shoulder pain. Therefore the term *shoulder complex* will be more appropriate in this text.

The major goal for the shoulder complex is to simply and functionally place and position the *fingers of the hand*; for example, we need our shoulder complex to place our hand above our head, to reach the top shelf of the cupboard for a glass, to scratch our backs when we have

an itch, or to reach across the body to put on our seatbelt in the car.

The shoulder is unique in its make-up because the majority of the ligaments (with the exception of the coracoacromial ligament) and the capsule are not particularly strong when compared to other joints in the body. This is because the shoulder has to sacrifice a stability role to allow greater mobility. This places extra pressure on the associated muscles of the rotator cuff and these muscles now have a sort of dual function to provide the required mobility as well as maintaining overall stability for the joint.

My goal for this chapter is to relate the underlying anatomy of the shoulder complex to simple day-to-day functions, hence the concept *functional anatomy*.

Let me try and explain what I mean by the above statement: rather than stating things in the usual way, such as this 'bony landmark' is the 'superior angle' of the 'scapula', and this bony landmark is the greater tubercle of the 'humerus' and so on, my overall plan throughout is to try and make understanding anatomy, assessments, and even treatments and rehabilitative exercises of this fascinating area a bit more exciting, or at least a little bit more interesting if that is at all possible. So I would like to look at anatomy in a slightly different way than one might expect. For example, the bony area that is commonly known as the superior angle of the scapula, as well as the superior medial border of the scapula, allows for the attachment of the levator scapulae muscle, and when this muscle contracts it can assist in elevation of the scapula (shoulder girdle elevation); the muscle in question can also assist the side bending motion of the cervical spine (lateral flexion); this is possible because of its attachments to the transverse processes of the cervical spine from the levels of C1–4. When the cervical spine is in a state of protraction or forward head posture, the levator scapulae will be contracting eccentrically to maintain this position, hence the patient potentially having discomfort bilaterally to the superior angle due to the increased stress directly caused from the unnatural forward head position. When we come to treat the levator scapulae, one might want to stretch it; however, if for some reason the cervical spine is in a state of protraction then this muscle is already in a lengthened (eccentrically contracted) position and the goal in this case might be to try and change the position of the cervical spine and also the position of the shoulder girdle by promoting specific movements to offload this muscle.

The idea of the above discussion is to get you to think about alternative ways of understanding functional anatomy so that it hopefully makes more sense and in time it will become easier for you to remember certain snippets from the text. I hope my book in particular has the ability to help you when the time is needed, especially when you are in front of your patients and taking them through a musculoskeletal assessment, with a subsequent treatment plan. The last thing I (as a practitioner of manual therapy) would want you to do with patients is to simply rub where the patient says it hurts. Always keep in mind the following statement by Dr Ida Rolf: 'Where the pain is, the problem is not'!

I would be delighted to think colleagues and students of physical therapy might really enjoy reading this book especially because of the way I have tried to explain the anatomical components of the shoulder complexity and the way this specific region of the upper limb interacts with so many (if not all) of the other areas of the musculoskeletal system. However, before we get to that point we still have to cover certain anatomical components of the shoulder complex to truly understand 'functional anatomy'. Let us start with the study of bones.

■ Osteology – the study of bones

Scapula

The scapula (shoulder blade) is a flat, triangular shaped bone that gets its Latin name because it has the appearance of a *trowel* or *shovel*. The scapula is also called *omo* (from the Greek word *omos*, meaning shoulder). There are many bony landmarks that provide the necessary attachments

for the soft tissues (muscles, tendons and ligaments, etc.) that are located on this unique bone (figure 1.1a–c).

Angles

There are three angles that are associated with the scapula: superior, inferior and lateral.

The *superior angle* is smooth and relatively rounded; it is covered by the upper trapezius muscles and provides for some of the fiber attachment for the levator scapulae muscle. The superior angle is approximately in line with the second thoracic vertebra (T2).

The meeting of the medial and lateral borders forms the *inferior angle*; it is the lowest anatomical region of the scapula and is thicker and rougher compared to the superior angle. Some of the fibers of the latissimus dorsi muscle cross and attach to the inferior angle and this area also provides the necessary attachment for the teres major muscle. The inferior angle is approximately in line with the seventh thoracic vertebra (T7).

The *lateral angle* is also known as the head of the scapula; it is by far the largest part of the scapula and naturally forms the cavity called the glenoid fossa. The surface is covered in hyaline or articular cartilage and the outer raised edge has a rim of fibrocartilage that is called the glenoid labrum. Superior to the glenoid fossa is a small attachment site called the supraglenoid tubercle and this bony landmark allows the attachment of the long head of the biceps brachii muscle. Inferior to the glenoid fossa is a small landmark called the infraglenoid tubercle and this allows the attachment for the long head of the triceps brachii muscle.

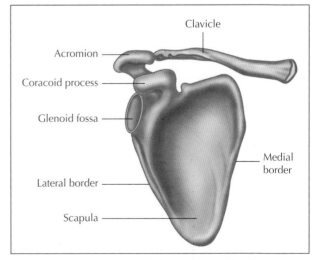

Figure 1.1a: *Anterior view of the anatomical landmarks located on the scapula*

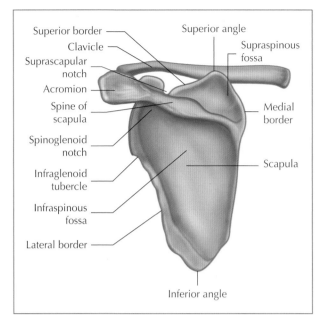

Figure 1.1b: *Posterior view of the anatomical landmarks located on the scapula*

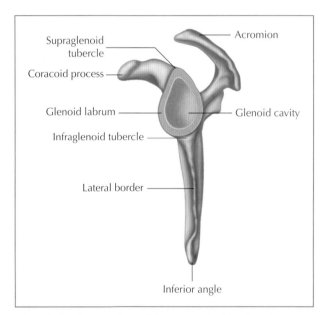

Figure 1.1c: *Lateral view of the anatomical landmarks located on the scapula*

Borders

The scapula has three borders: superior, medial (or vertebral), and lateral (or axillary).

The *superior border* runs from the superior angle to the base of the coracoid process and is the shortest and thinnest of the three borders. There is an area on the superior border called the suprascapular notch and between this notch and the base of the coracoid process there is a ligament called the superior transverse scapula ligament. There is a natural space formed inferior to

the ligament, called a *foramen*, and this space allows the passage of the suprascapular nerve. This specific nerve innervates the muscles of the supraspinatus and infraspinatus and originates from the cervical levels of C5 and C6 from the brachial (arm) plexus.

The *medial or vertebral border* is the longest of all the three borders and is formed between the superior and inferior angles of the scapula. This border has four muscle attachments: starting from the highest point we have the levator scapulae; next in line is the rhomboid minor to the middle part of the border, and then rhomboid major to the lower part, with the serratus anterior muscle having a long attachment onto the anterior edge of the medial border.

The base of the glenoid fossa initially forms the starting point for the *lateral or axillary border* and it travels to the inferior angle of the scapula and is the thickest of the three borders. In terms of muscle attachments: starting at the highest point is the triceps long head and this muscle attaches to the infraglenoid tubercle, which is located inferior to the glenoid fossa but is still located on the lateral border. Next is the teres minor, and lastly the teres major; and attaching to the anterior surface and along the lateral border is the subscapularis muscle.

Spine of scapula

The spine of the scapula is located approximately at the level of the third thoracic vertebra (T3). It is a ridge of bone that has its root origin from the medial border and it travels laterally and ends at the acromion process. Superiorly (above) the spine contains the supraspinous fossa where the supraspinatus muscle attaches. Inferiorly to the spine there is a large mass called the infraspinous fossa and this is where the infraspinatus muscle attaches. The trapezius has an attachment to the superior lip of the spine and the deltoid muscle directly has an attachment to the inferior lip of the spine of the scapula. Between the supraspinous fossa and the infraspinous fossa there is a foramen called the spinoglenoid notch that allows for the passage of the suprascapular nerve to innervate the infraspinatus muscle.

Acromion

The acromion is a continuation from the spine of the scapula; it has an articulation with the distal clavicle and this joint is known as the acromioclavicular (AC) joint. The acromion or the actual *acromion process* forms the roof over the glenohumeral joint and it has been known to have three distinct shapes, type I (flat), type II (curved) and type III (hooked), as described by Bigliani et al. (1986).

Depending on this specific shape of the acromion process it could possibly relate to specific tears of the rotator cuff muscles and in particular the supraspinatus muscle. The more the process goes from being flat to curved or hooked the higher the incidence of rotator cuff pathology. The acromion allows for the attachment of the trapezius and deltoid muscles.

Coracoid process

This unique projection is named for its resemblance to a *raven's beak*; it provides stability for the shoulder along with the acromion. There are three muscles that attach to the coracoid process: pectoralis minor, biceps brachii short head and the coracobrachialis. There are also many ligaments that attach, as well as the trapezoid and conoid, which together make up the coracoclavicular ligament; there are also the coracoacromial and coracohumeral ligaments, which attach directly to the acromion and humerus respectively.

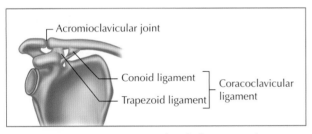

Figure 1.2: *Ligaments associated with the coracoid process*

Humerus

This long bone connects the scapula to the elbow and naturally connects the two bones of the lower arm, the radius and the ulna. The proximal (upper) part of the humerus is formed by a head that is rounded, and has two separate necks; one is known as the anatomical (true) neck and the other is known as the surgical neck because the latter area is the common site for a fracture and is a familiar place for surgical intervention if required.

There are two bony landmarks that are called tubercles or tuberosities. The greater tubercle allows for the attachment of the supraspinatus and slightly posterior/inferior to the greater tubercle is the attachment site of infraspinatus and the teres minor muscles. The lesser tubercle allows the attachment of the subscapularis muscle. Between these two bony landmarks is an area that is sometimes called the intertubercular (inter- between, tubercular – tubercle) sulcus (depression or fossa) or is simply known as the bicipital groove. It is called the biceps (bicipital) groove because the long head of the biceps travels through this depression between the two tubercles. The long head of biceps is also held in position by a ligament called the transverse humeral ligament and if this ligament happens to tear then the biceps long head tendon is potentially able to flick out of its natural groove and cause a snapping type of shoulder complaint.

Located on the medial proximal shaft of the humerus is the area that the muscles of the pectoralis major, teres major and latissimus dorsi attach and when I was personally taught anatomy, my lecturer mentioned to the class that there is an easier way to remember the muscle attachments for this specific place of the humerus by saying the following: there is a 'lady,' which he related to the long head of the biceps tendon, and she is lying between two 'majors' (pectoralis major and teres major)

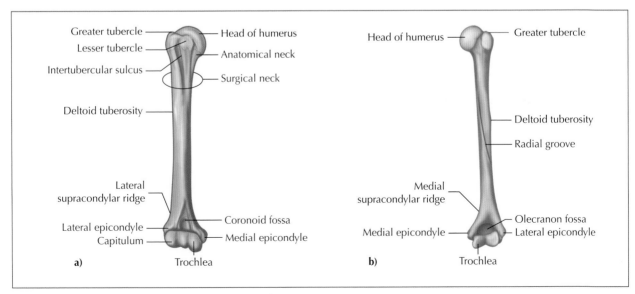

Figure 1.3a & b: *Anatomical landmarks located on the humerus*

and at her feet is the latissimus dorsi muscle. I have never forgotten this as my anatomy lecturer had all types of snippets that made learning more interesting. I especially liked this visualization as I was once in the British army so the concept of the *majors* put a smile on my face.

Lower down the shaft and near the lateral side of the humerus there is a roughened triangular area called the deltoid tuberosity and this, as you can probably guess, is for the attachment of the deltoid muscle.

Note: A word of caution. Many patients that have presented to my clinic with shoulder pain actually point to this area of the deltoid tuberosity and say they think it is their 'deltoid' causing them the pain but I can probably guarantee that this is not the actual case, for, as you will read throughout this book, the deltoid tuberosity is a common site for referred pain.

CASE STUDY

An American professor came to my clinic with pain to the area of the deltoid tuberosity. The pain had come on a few days earlier when he was out walking his dog one morning, with his hands in his pockets. The dog saw a rabbit and quickly gave chase, and this action wrenched the professor's right arm out of his pocket and he immediately felt pain and started to rub the area of the humerus that the deltoid inserts to (deltoid tuberosity). When I carried out the assessment, I kept it relatively simple and found that passive motion of external rotation (I performed the movement for my patient) caused discomfort to the area of the deltoid tuberosity and so did resisted internal rotation of the humerus (I asked the patient to resist against my pressure). I diagnosed a partial thickness tear (strain) to his subscapularis muscle. An MRI confirmed this a few days later when the professor visited his consultant in the US. I told the patient that because the subscapularis is part of the rotator cuff muscle group and is an integral part of the joint capsule and ligaments, these muscles of the cuff and the capsule have a tendency to refer to the area of the deltoid tuberosity. (The techniques I used to assess the patient will be covered in this text.)

Clavicle

The clavicle or collarbone is classified as a long bone and is the only long bone in the body that lies horizontally. In Latin it is named the 'little key' because of the similarity

of a key in a lock and the rotatory motion of the clavicle along its axis when the shoulder joint abducts. Connecting with the scapula it makes up the shoulder girdle or pectoral girdle and its function is to provide a strut-like support between the scapula and the sternum. It is the most commonly fractured bone in the body and this normally happens by falling onto outstretched arms or through direct contact. Medially there is an articulation with the manubrium of the sternum and the proximal end of the clavicle is generally rounded and that is called the sternoclavicular joint (SC joint or SCJ). On its lateral or distal end, which is more flat in appearance, there is an articulation with the acromion of the scapula and that is called the acromioclavicular joint (AC joint or ACJ).

There are many muscles and ligaments that directly attach to the clavicle and these are the pectoralis major, upper trapezius, anterior fibers of deltoid, sternocleidomastoid, subclavius and sternohyoid muscles. There are also the coracoclavicular ligaments individually known as the trapezoid and conoid and they both attach to the distal end of the clavicle.

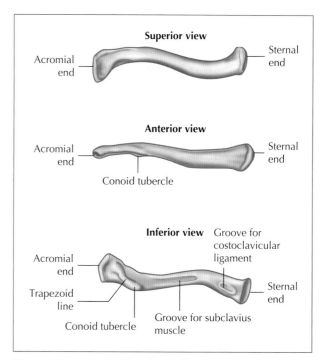

Figure 1.4: *Anatomical landmarks located on the clavicle*

■ Arthrology – the study of joints

The shoulder complex is made up of four unique and individual joints and these are the glenohumeral (GH), sternoclavicular (SC), acromioclavicular (AC) and the scapulothoracic (ST) joints.

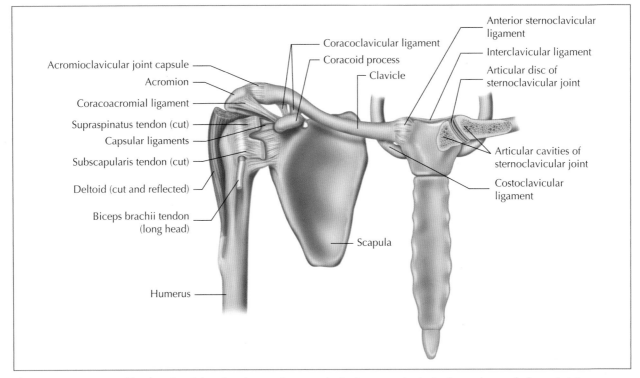

Figure 1.5: *Anatomical landmarks of the glenohumeral, sternoclavicular, acromioclavicular and scapulothoracic joints*

Glenohumeral joint

The glenohumeral (GH) joint is classified as a typical ball and socket synovial joint and is located between the rounded proximal convex head of the humerus and the concave surface of the glenoid cavity or fossa (depression) of the scapula. It is possibly best described as a golf ball (humeral head) sitting on a tee (glenoid fossa) – if you play or watch golf you will understand the concept. This joint has a superb range of mobility; however, having this range of motion does come at a price by sacrificing and reducing the GH joints' inherent stability mechanisms. Because of the natural instability of the GH joint it has to rely on other passive and dynamic structures to assist: passive stabilizers are the glenoid labrum, joint capsule and the associated ligaments; the dynamic stabilizers are made up from the muscles of the rotator cuff as well as the long head of the biceps brachii muscle.

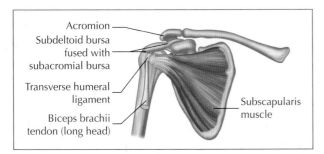

Figure 1.6: *Anatomical landmarks for the glenohumeral joint*

Glenoid labrum and the joint capsule/ligaments

The glenoid labrum has been considered to be a redundant fold of dense fibrous connective tissue with a small amount of fibrocartilage. The labrum has been designed in such a unique way that it enhances the shape of the glenoid fossa by approximately 50%. The labrum has an attachment to the specific bands of the glenohumeral ligaments and also to the tendon of the long head of the biceps brachii muscle. The joint capsule is an interesting structure because overall it is so lax (relatively speaking) compared to all other joint capsules of the body and this is because of the naturally large excursions of specific movements that the glenohumeral joint has to go through – remember the shoulder joint will sacrifice stability for mobility.

The capsule, however, has reinforcements to assist its function of stability and these are provided by the integration and blending of the rotator cuff muscle group, and secondly by the glenohumeral ligaments. The glenohumeral ligaments are thickenings of the joint capsule; they comprise the superior glenohumeral ligament (SGHL), the middle glenohumeral ligament (MGHL) and the inferior glenohumeral ligament (IGHL); they attach from the anterior and inferior part of the glenoid as well as the labrum and attach to the anatomical neck of the humeral head. Thirdly, the

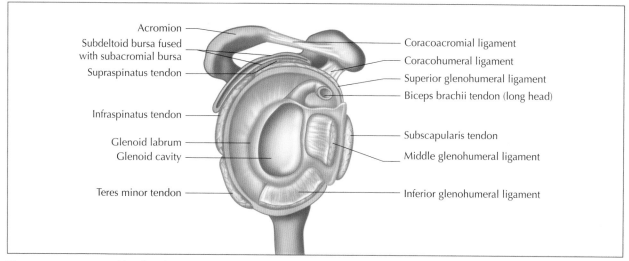

Figure 1.7: *Anatomical landmarks for the glenoid labrum and ligaments*

coracohumeral ligament also enhances and promotes the overall stabilization mechanisms for the joint capsule. It is considered that the IGHL is the most important stabilizer of them all, especially to prevent anterior-inferior shoulder dislocation, and this soft tissue is the most frequently injured structure during dislocations. The ligament actually consists of three parts, an *anterior band*, a *posterior band* and an *inferior axillary pouch.* The anterior band (also called the superior band of the inferior ligament) and the posterior band collectively have a similar appearance and function to a structure that is called a hammock. I am sure we have all at some point tried lying in one of these, sometimes with funny consequences (i.e., you have fallen out of one!).

The inner component of the joint capsule is lined with a synovial membrane and subsequently lubricated by synovial fluid. It reaches to the tendon of the long head of biceps synovial sheath as this biceps tendon penetrates the capsule. In relationship to specific movements of the glenohumeral joint and the capsule, external rotation will tighten the anterior capsule; horizontal flexion tightens the posterior capsule; the superior capsule is continually taut while the arm is resting by your side when you are standing; and the inferior capsule (least supported) is stretched maximally in full shoulder flexion and abduction.

The overall passive stability of the glenohumeral joint inherently comes from the static passive structures of the glenoid labrum, the joint capsule, the glenohumeral ligaments and the natural shape and position of the two opposing bony surfaces as well as the dynamic stabilizing muscles of the rotator cuff, long head of biceps tendon and rotator muscles of the scapula. Unfortunately, as mentioned earlier, the joint capsule is so lax that

potentially 1–3 cm can separate the glenohumeral joint if a traction force is applied in a certain direction.

Anterior stability of the shoulder is more of a concern than posterior stability. Why? It is because the majority of dislocations and subluxations happen in an anterior-inferior position. In terms of function for the shoulder ligaments, the superior glenohumeral ligament and the coracohumeral stabilize the humeral head in an inferior direction and during 45–60 degrees of abduction the middle glenohumeral ligament and the subscapularis tendon provide anterior stability, while at the same time the smallest ligament of them all, the superior glenohumeral ligament, slackens. The inferior glenohumeral ligament provides the greatest stability in an anterior-inferior direction.

Sternoclavicular joint

The sternoclavicular (SC) joint is typically classified as a synovial plane articulation that actually comprises two saddle shaped surfaces; one is located at the medial/proximal end of the clavicle and one at the notch formed by the manubrium, which is the superior part of the sternum. The SC joint is the only bony attachment of the appendicular skeleton to the axial skeleton. The clavicle does not directly contact the manubrium as a fibrocartilaginous disc separates the joint space. This disk increases the congruency between the two associated bones of the clavicle and sternum and divides the SC joint into two separate joint cavities. The disc also functions to absorb any force that is directed to it along the clavicle from its lateral end. A fibrous joint capsule and the following three ligaments provide the stability of the SC joint; the sternoclavicular, costoclavicular and interclavicular ligaments (figure 1.8).

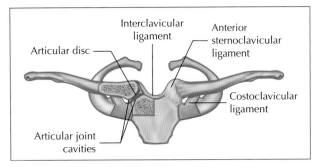

Figure 1.8: *Sternoclavicular joint and associated ligaments*

Acromioclavicular joint

The acromioclavicular (AC) joint is also classified as a synovial plane joint even though it is basically a pseudo (false) joint. It is located between the concave shape of the acromion part of the scapula and the distal convex end of the clavicle. Its primary function is to allow the arm to be raised above the head as the AC joint will allow additional motion of the scapula on the thorax as one performs overhead types of movement. Up to the age of two years the AC joint is initially a fibrocartilaginous union with no joint space present. At approximately three years of age the joint space develops into two separate joint cavities and a small disc is formed that becomes a meniscoid by the time of the second decade. To increase the stability of the joint, the AC joint has a superior and inferior ligament as well as the coracoclavicular ligaments, which are known individually as the trapezoid (lateral) and conoid (medial)

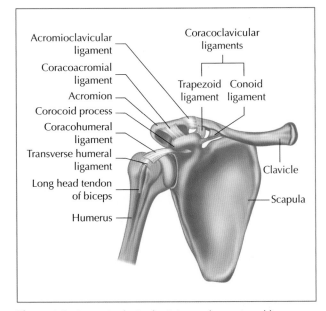

Figure 1.9: *Acromioclavicular joint and associated ligaments*

ligaments. These ligaments attach the scapula firmly to the clavicle (figure 1.9) and prevent any excessive rotation.

Scapulothoracic joint or scapulocostal joint

This articulation between the scapula and thorax is classified as a pseudo (false) joint because it lacks the following structures: joint capsule, synovial membrane and synovial fluid, and also lacks ligamentous support. However, the scapulothoracic (ST) joint, true or not, is an integral part of the shoulder complex. The ST joint is formed by the convex shape of the posterior thoracic cage and the concave surface of the anterior aspect of the scapula and the main function of the ST joint is to basically *suspend* the humerus in *space* and to assist the overall position for optimal alignment that improves the functional support of the glenohumeral (GH) joint.

■ Neutral position of the scapula and the scapular plane or scaption

The scapula is ideally situated between the second and seventh thoracic vertebrae (T2–7) and is located approximately 2 inches (5 cm) from the vertebral or medial border of the scapula to the spinous processes of the thoracic spine. The scapula generally sits around 30 degrees off the frontal axis, with the glenoid fossa facing anteriorly; this position is known as the *scapular plane* and motion in this specific plane is generally referred to as *scaption* (figure 1.10). The scapular plane or scaption is considered to be the most functional position for the shoulder complex as this neutral position will assist in reducing impingement type of syndromes within the shoulder complex and in particular to the glenohumeral joint.

■ Scapulothoracic motion

Osar 2012 discusses 12 cardinal motions of the ST joint: protraction, retraction, elevation, depression, upward rotation, downward rotation, internal rotation, external rotation, posterior tilting, anterior tilting, adduction and abduction.

- *Protraction.* Movement of the entire shoulder complex along the transverse plane of motion in an anterior direction. The protractors of the shoulder include serratus anterior, pectoralis major and minor.

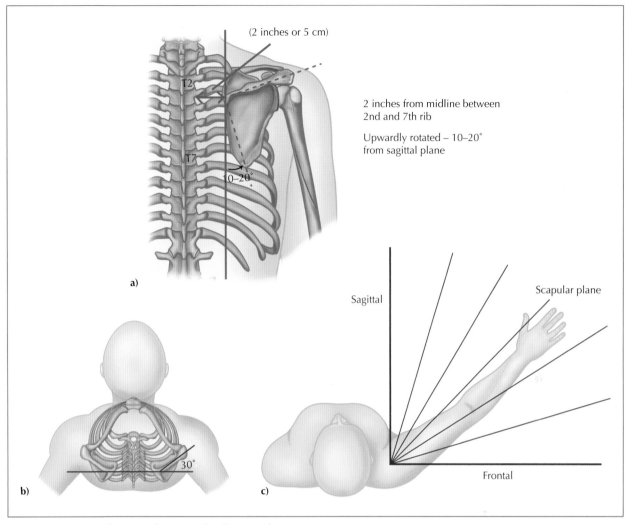

Figure 1.10a–c: *a & b. Neutral position for the scapula, c. scaption*

- *Retraction.* Movement of the entire shoulder complex along the transverse plane of motion in a posterior direction. The retractors of the shoulder include the rhomboids, middle, upper and lower trapezius and the latissimus dorsi.
- *Elevation.* Raising of the scapula in a superior direction along the ribcage. The elevators of the scapula include the upper trapezius, levator scapula and rhomboids.
- *Depression.* Lowering of the scapula in an inferior direction along the ribcage. The scapula depressors include the lower trapezius, latissimus dorsi, pectoralis minor, lower fibers of the pectoralis major and lower fibers of the serratus anterior.
- *Upward rotation.* Rotation in an upward direction along the ribcage so that the glenoid fossa points towards the ceiling. The upward rotators of the scapula include the upper and lower trapezius and the serratus anterior.
- *Downward rotation.* Rotation of the scapula in a downward rotation along the frontal motion so that the glenoid fossa points toward the floor. The downward rotators of the scapula include the pectoralis minor, levator scapulae and the rhomboids.
- *Internal rotation.* This occurs when the scapula tilts anteriorly along a vertical axis. This motion is primarily a function of the pectoralis complex.
- *External rotation.* External scapular rotation occurs when the anteromedial aspect of the scapula approximates the thoracic cage along a vertical axis. All three divisions of the trapezius and serratus anterior are primarily responsible for this motion.
- *Posterior tilting.* Posterior tilting is movement along a sagittal axis where the superior angle moves away from the thorax and the inferior angle of the scapula approximates the thorax. The lower trapezius and lower fibers of the serratus anterior are mostly responsible for posterior tilting of the scapula.
- *Anterior tilting.* Anterior tilting is movement along a sagittal axis where the superior angle approximates

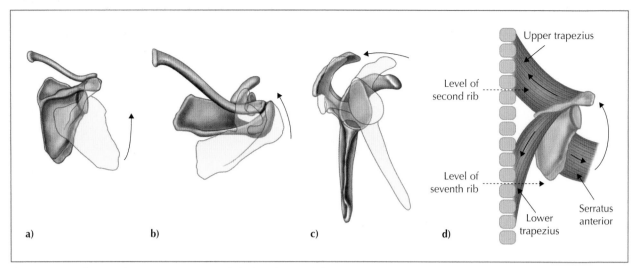

Figure 1.11a–d: *Scapular motion: a: upward (light color) and downward rotation; b: internal (light color) and external rotation; c: anterior and posterior (light color) tilting; d: scapular force couples. The serratus anterior and the upper and lower trapezius work together to produce upward rotation and control downward rotation*

the thorax and the inferior angle moves away from the thorax. Pectoralis minor and the short head of the biceps muscle are mostly responsible for anterior tilting of the scapula.

- *Adduction.* This refers to the scapulae approximating each other or moving closer toward the midline of the body. The adductors of the scapula include the middle trapezius and rhomboids.

- *Abduction.* This refers to the scapulae moving away from each other or moving away from the midline of the body. The abductors of the scapula include the serratus anterior and pectoralis minor.

2

Muscles and motion of the shoulder complex

As I have previously written, referring to gait and the walking cycle, 'we all take the simple motion of walking for granted.' Everything is connected both anatomically and functionally, from the initial contact of our foot and ankle with the ground to the relationship this has to the upper limb of the shoulder complex, and even the effect on the motion of the cervical spine. Everything anatomically needs to be functioning correctly and in harmony for us to perform the everyday movement of walking.

One could say the same of the shoulder complex. Do you not think we often take movements of the shoulder for granted? People who have never had a shoulder issue, past or present, however, may not be able to relate to what I am saying.

A PERSONAL CASE STUDY FROM THE AUTHOR

I have sustained two full dislocations of the right glenohumeral joint. One of these happened when I was kayaking over a waterfall in North Wales with some Royal Marine Commandos (seemed like a good idea at the time!) and the second was when I was canoeing in Canada. The first time the doctor relocated the humerus (under general anesthetic) and it was obvious that there was a neurological complication as well as all the usual soft tissue damage that is present with a full anterior dislocation. As a result of the sustained trauma, I ended up with damage to the axillary nerve – so much so that my deltoid and teres minor muscles (innervated by the

axillary nerve) did not activate normally until the nerve eventually regenerated many months later. I naturally had difficulty lifting my arm above my head. Surprisingly, the motion caused no actual pain but I had weakness because of the sustained nerve injury. I was pleased to find that any overhead motions slowly improved over the following few months. In the second dislocation the shoulder joint actually relocated itself during a specific motion, which was pretty lucky.

I have also sprained my right acromioclavicular joint (ACJ) a few times, and this has happened many times over the years (mountain biking, kayaking and skiing among other activities), so now I am left with a step deformity of the right AC joint. This does not really bother me much (unless I do a lot of overhead motions); but because of my job as a lecturer in sports medicine, and especially knowing the life I used to lead, I perfectly understand the consequences of my extreme activities.

Another complaint I would like to briefly mention, is that I have an excessive and permanent winging of the right scapula (figure 2.1). I think this is the result of trauma to the long thoracic nerve (C5/6/7), sustained during that first shoulder dislocation many years ago. Some therapists say it is related to a weakness of the serratus anterior muscle, since it is this muscle that controls the scapula position and if it is weak or inhibited then the scapula gives the appearance of winging. In my particular case, however, I would disagree because I have spent 20 plus years trying to activate the serratus anterior muscle, with no joy, and I would suggest that the winging position is a neurological issue to the long thoracic nerve (innervation

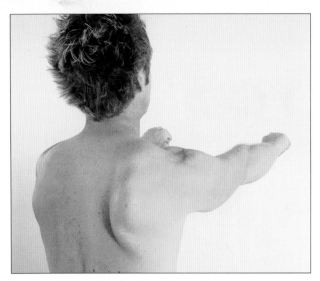

Figure 2.1: *Scapula winging of the author*

to the serratus anterior muscle from the levels of C5/6/7) rather than being from a simple muscle weakness.

■ Myology – the study of muscles

Rotator cuff

The rotator cuff comprises four muscles commonly known as the SITS muscles: the supraspinatus, infraspinatus, teres minor and subscapularis. Each muscle serves a specific purpose to the function of the glenohumeral joint; however, their role collectively is to depress and stabilize the humeral head within the glenoid fossa. The rotator cuff has been likened to a sleeve of a shirt cuff. The following analogy seems to make more sense to me. Picture yourself driving a manual (gear) car and when you go to change

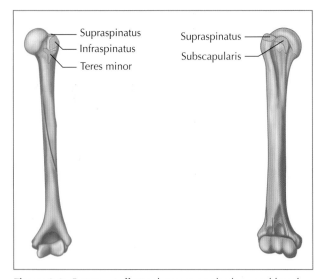

Figure 2.2: *Rotator cuff attachments on the humeral head*

gear you place your hand with open fingers around the gear stick. Think of the gear stick as the head of the humerus and the fingers that are splayed around it as the muscles of the rotator cuff. Let us for a moment imagine this concept; visualize actual *webs* between all the spaces of each of the fingers so that so they are all interconnected. I personally think that this best describes the rotator cuff muscle group because at the end of the day there are four individual muscles and they can all influence each other due to their specific individual attachment sites onto the humeral head and cuff as well as all four muscles (fingers) being interconnected (imaginary webs).

Let us now take a more detailed look at the rotator cuff muscle group.

Supraspinatus

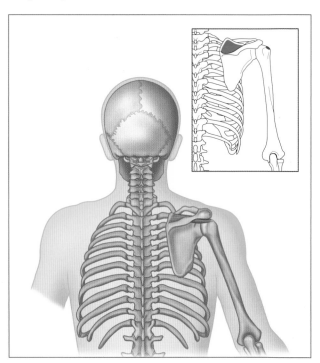

Figure 2.3: *Supraspinatus*

Origin: Supraspinous fossa, above the spine of the scapula.

Insertion: Greater tubercle at the top of humerus and the capsule of shoulder joint.

Nerve: Suprascapular nerve (C5, C6), from the upper trunk of the brachial plexus.

Think about the word 'supraspinatus' just for a second. *Supra* means above and *spinatus* relates to the spine of the scapula so this muscle attaches from an area above the spine of the scapula called the supraspinous fossa and travels laterally under the roof of the shoulder (acromion) to attach to the greater tubercle or tuberosity of the humerus. The action of this muscle is unique and is what I call the *fine tuner* of the shoulder joint. The muscle is probably responsible for, or at least part involved in, the majority of patients that present with shoulder pain, even though the pain is typically only the symptomology and generally not the underlying causative factor. This idea is pithily expressed by Dr Ida Rolf, who states, 'where the pain is, the problem is not.' This is exactly the case for the shoulder complex: a patient or athlete might present to the clinic complaining of a supraspinatus tendinopathy or something similarly related but the actual causative factor/s of the pain might be coming from a distant site, as you will read later in this book.

Function of the supraspinatus

The general consensus (even though it has been debated over the years) relating to the current evidence for the contraction of the supraspinatus is that it serves to initiate the motion of shoulder abduction in the frontal plane for the first 10–15 degrees while at the same time also being responsible for externally rotating the humerus. The larger deltoid muscle needs the fine-tuning capabilities of the supraspinatus to create a specific angle of the humerus for shoulder abduction to continue (figure 2.4). The supraspinatus attaches to the greater tubercle of the humerus and the contraction of this muscle approximates the head of the humerus into the glenoid fossa and basically seats the humeral head within the joint and hence starts the initial motion of abduction. While the

supraspinatus is in a state of contraction, this movement pattern is naturally permitted because of the convex shape of the humeral head gliding inferiorly down the concave shape of the glenoid fossa. If the movement of abduction was only performed by the larger deltoid muscle and not with the co-activation of the supraspinatus muscle because it is either weakened, inhibited or torn then the activation of the deltoid alone would cause a superior glide of the humerus and subsequently this would cause a jamming of the humeral head within the subacromial space and one of two things would happen, a subacromial type of impingement ensues, e.g., tendinopathy or bursitis and/ or a limited range of motion that will mimic a type of adhesive capsulitis or a frozen shoulder. Either way, the deltoid muscle needs the co-contraction of supraspinatus and vice versa, the supraspinatus needs the assistance of the deltoid. I have been known when lecturing to call the deltoid the gross muscle activator and the supraspinatus the fine-tuner/controller for the motion of shoulder joint abduction and I like what I say, as I believe it is a true comment.

I believe that once the supraspinatus has initiated the motion of abduction it then exerts an external rotation force to the humerus. I consider it does this motion (external rotation) to assist the continual contraction of the deltoid muscle. While the supraspinatus controls part of the external rotation of the humerus, it needs some assistance as it cannot do all the hard work on its own. This is where the infraspinatus muscle is now recruited. The infraspinatus greatly assists the supraspinatus during shoulder motion, especially when the shoulder

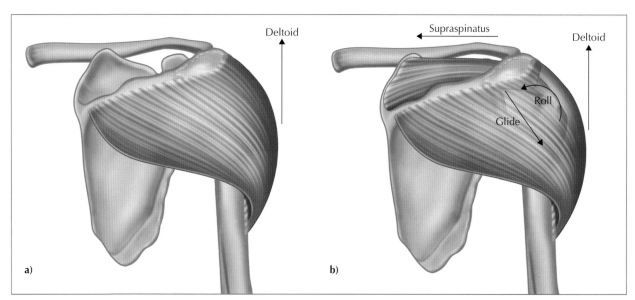

Figure 2.4a & b: *Abduction angle of the deltoid. a: The vertical direction of force from the contraction of the deltoid. b: With a slight angle caused by the supraspinatus, the deltoid can now continue abduction*

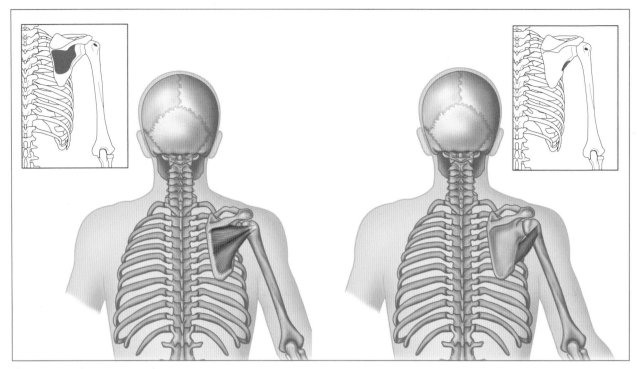

Figure 2.5: *Infraspinatus and teres minor*

approximates 60–90 degrees of abduction. The importance for the specific range of motion is mainly because the humerus needs to be rotating in an external rotation direction between these specific degrees of motion as this will cause the greater tubercle of the humeral head to rotate *away* from the ever approaching acromion process; subsequently, this external rotation will reduce the likelihood of impingement-type syndromes.

The supraspinatus also acts to prevent the humeral head from subluxating. This possibility is due to the rounded shape of the convex head of the humerus, which causes the humeral bone to have a tendency to roll downwards and outwards. The supraspinatus attachment onto the greater tuberosity of the humerus will greatly assist in preventing these two potentially subluxing motions.

Supraspinatus and adduction of the glenohumeral joint

We now come to an interesting concept, which is the following; at 90 degrees and beyond of shoulder abduction of the GH joint the supraspinatus muscle actually becomes an *adductor* rather than retaining its initial role as an *abductor*. Put simply, the supraspinatus muscle changes it role from abduction to adduction. Why is this? It is because the humeral head from approximately 90 degrees and beyond is required to depress and become stable within the glenoid fossa; this is also accomplished by the

co-activation of the subscapularis muscle (as you will read shortly). Earlier studies showed the supraspinatus was only involved in the initiation of abduction with its maximum activation at 100 degrees; however, this has been disproven and the supraspinatus is shown to be active throughout the full range of abduction.

Infraspinatus and teres minor

Infraspinatus

Origin: Infraspinous fossa, below the spine of the scapula.

Insertion: Greater tubercle at the top of humerus and the capsule of shoulder joint.

Nerve: Suprascapular nerve (C5, C6), from the upper trunk of the brachial plexus.

Teres minor

Origin: Lateral/axillary border of the scapula.

Insertion: Posterior inferior aspect of the greater tubercle at the top of humerus and the capsule of the shoulder joint.

Nerve: Axillary nerve (C5, C6), from the upper trunk and posterior cord of the brachial plexus.

As the name implies, the infraspinatus attaches below (*infra*) the spine of the scapula to the area known as the infraspinous fossa and travels laterally to the posterior aspect of the greater tubercle or tuberosity, just below the insertion point of supraspinatus. The teres minor attaches from the axillary or lateral border of the scapula and travels laterally and superiorly to the greater tubercle, just below the insertion point of the infraspinatus muscle. The infraspinatus and teres minor work in harmony (even though they have separate nerve innervations) to externally rotate the humerus especially during abduction between 60–90 degrees. These muscles collectively work together to assist in rotating the greater tubercle of the humerus externally, posteriorly and inferiorly – so much so that an extra space is created for the passage of the supraspinatus tendon and subacromial bursa to glide within the subacromial space. If there were a weakness or inhibition of these two muscles then the likelihood of an impingement syndrome would increase because the humeral head would maintain a position of internal rotation and the greater tubercle of the humerus could potentially be compressed underneath the acromion process. These two muscles also aid the head of the humerus to depress within the glenoid fossa during overhead movements by counteracting the superior pull of the deltoid muscle.

Subscapularis

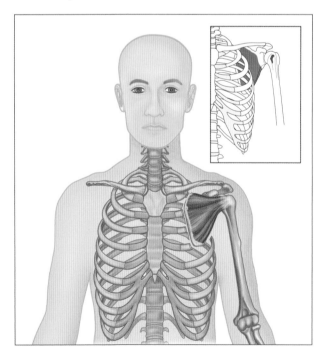

Figure 2.6: *Subscapularis*

Origin: Subscapular fossa (anterior surface of scapula).

Insertion: Lesser tubercle at the top of the humerus and the capsule of shoulder joint.

Nerve: Upper and lower subscapular nerves (C5, C6, C7), from the posterior cord of the brachial plexus.

The subscapularis muscle attaches from the anterior surface of the scapula, specifically called the subscapular fossa, and inserts onto the lesser tubercle or tuberosity of the humerus. This muscle is responsible for internal rotation of the glenohumeral joint as well as being able to depress, stabilize and adduct the humeral head within the glenoid fossa during overhead movements. The subscapularis in one way is antagonistic (opposite) as well synergistic (helper or assister) to the muscles of the infraspinatus, teres minor and posterior deltoid because the subscapularis has a posterior pull on the humerus while the other muscles have an anterior pull, but they all work collectively or synergistically to *centralize* the humeral head within the glenoid fossa. Weakness or inhibition of the subscapularis potentially allows the humeral head to displace anteriorly because the other larger internal rotators, latissimus dorsi and teres major, take over the role for the internal rotation and subsequently this can cause the humerus to be forced into an anterior glide position due to the fact that the subscapularis has lost its ability to control the posterior glide motion of the humeral head. If this situation arises then an impingement type of syndrome or even a bicipital tendinopathy of the long head of the biceps brachii muscle can follow.

Other muscles of the shoulder complex

There are a multitude of other muscles, apart from the rotator cuff that have attachments in one way or another that directly or indirectly influence the functionality of the shoulder complex. These muscles are related to where they have their specific attachment points as listed below.

Thoracoscapular muscles
Pectoralis minor (figure 2.7) and the serratus anterior (figure 2.8) are the only two muscles that attach directly from the thorax to the scapula.

Pectoralis minor

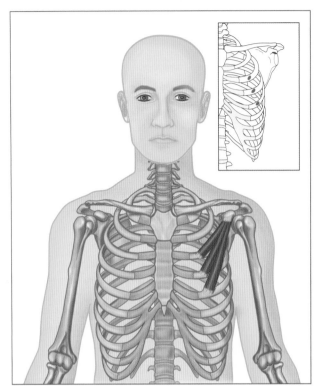

Figure 2.7: *Pectoralis minor*

Origin: Ribs 3–5.

Insertion: Coracoid process of scapula.

Nerve: Medial pectoral nerve (C8, T1) and arises from the medial cord of the brachial plexus.

The pectoralis minor attaches from the ribs (3–5) and inserts to the beak like projection called the coracoid process of the scapula; it is the main muscle that is responsible for causing anterior tilting of the scapula. If this muscle is hypertonic or in a state of facilitation, then it can typically lead on to creating the forward shoulder position. The normal function of this muscle is to protract, depress and downwardly rotate the scapula. This muscle has an accessory role in assisting respiration (attachment to ribs 3–5) and dysfunctional breathing patterns have been considered to be one of the major causes for hypertonicity or overcontracture of the pectoralis minor. Also, the neurovascular bundle of the brachial plexus (C5–T1) and the subclavian artery pass directly underneath the pectoralis minor so a sustained contraction of this muscle can give rise to a condition called thoracic outlet syndrome (TOS). This condition will be discussed in a later chapter in this book.

Serratus anterior

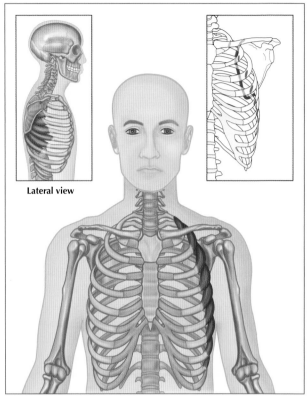

Lateral view

Figure 2.8: *Serratus anterior*

Origin: Ribs 1–8/9.

Insertion: Anterior surface of the medial border of the scapula.

Nerve: Long thoracic nerve (C5, C6, C7).

Out of all the muscles that attach to the shoulder complex, the serratus anterior is considered to be the main stabilizing muscle of the scapula. This muscle attaches from the first 8/9 ribs to the inner part of the scapula and its function is to protract, abduct and upwardly rotate the scapula. However, its main function is to stabilize the scapula against the thoracic cage and weakness of this muscle (lower fibers in particular) can be seen by an increased elevation of the scapula on overhead movements such as abduction and flexion and a dysfunctional movement pattern called *winging* of the scapula could be seen, especially as the arm is returning back from the overhead position. Damage to the long thoracic nerve (C5–7), can potentially cause a permanent winging.

Thoracohumeral muscles
Pectoralis major

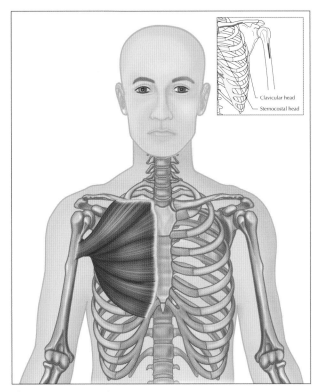

Figure 2.9: *Pectoralis major*

Origin: *Clavicular head* – medial half or two-thirds of front of clavicle. *Sternocostal portion* – sternum and adjacent upper six costal cartilages.

Insertion: Lateral lip of the intertubercular sulcus (bicipital groove) of the humerus.

Nerve: *Nerve to upper fibers* – lateral pectoral nerve (C5, C6, C7). *Nerve to lower fibers* – lateral and medial pectoral nerves (C6, C7, C8, T1).

The pectoralis major is the only muscle that connects from the anterior aspect of the thorax to the humerus. The function of the pectoralis major collectively is to medially rotate and horizontally adduct (flex) the humerus. The *clavicular portion* flexes (from extension) and medially rotates the shoulder joint, and horizontally adducts the humerus towards the opposite shoulder. The *sternocostal portion* obliquely adducts the humerus towards the opposite hip from an abducted position as well as extending (from flexion) and medially rotates the humerus. If the arm is fixed then the pectoralis major and pectoralis minor will assist in pulling the trunk to the fixed humerus (pull up motion) and is one of the main climbing muscles by pulling the body up to the arms that are now fixed.

Scapulohumeral muscles

These muscles that attach from the scapula to the humerus are the rotator cuff (already explained), the teres major, coracobrachialis and all the specific fibers of the deltoid muscle.

Teres major

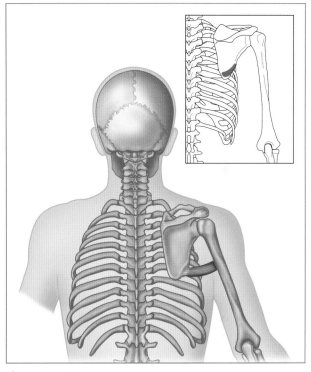

Figure 2.10: *Teres major*

Origin: Inferior angle and lateral border of the scapula.

Insertion: Medial lip of the intertubercular sulcus of the upper humerus.

Nerve: Lower subscapular nerve (C5, C6), arises from the posterior cord of the brachial plexus.

The word *teres* actually means *round* so this is a large round muscle compared to the smaller round muscle of teres minor that is an integral part of the rotator cuff. This muscle works synergistically with the latissimus dorsi in relation to adduction, extension and medial rotation of the humerus (glenohumeral joint).

Coracobrachialis

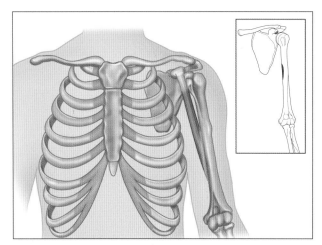

Figure 2.11: *Coracobrachialis*

Origin: Coracoid process of the scapula.

Insertion: Medial middle surface of the humerus.

Nerve: Musculocutaneous nerve (C5, C6) arises from the anterior divisions of the upper and middle trunks of the brachial plexus.

The coracobrachialis, as the name suggests, attaches from the coracoid to the brachii (arm). This muscle is a weak flexor and adductor of the humerus and if this muscle becomes hypertonic the scapula could develop an anterior tilt giving the appearance of a forward rounded shoulder.

Deltoid

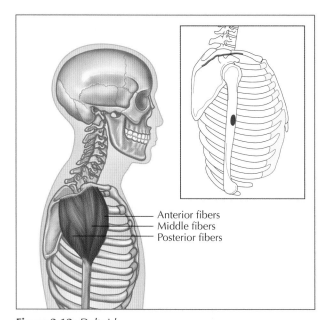

Anterior fibers
Middle fibers
Posterior fibers

Figure 2.12: *Deltoid*

Origin: Clavicle, acromion process and spine of the scapula.

Insertion: Deltoid tuberosity on the middle of the shaft of the humerus.

Nerve: Axillary nerve (C5, C6).

The deltoid muscle has three sets of fibers and the anterior fibers are responsible for flexion, horizontal flexion or horizontal adduction and medial rotation of the glenohumeral joint (GH). The middle fibers assist the supraspinatus muscle for the movement of abduction and the posterior fibers extend, horizontally extend or horizontally abduct and laterally rotate the GH. If the infraspinatus and teres minor become weakened or inhibited then the posterior fibers of the deltoid becomes the prime mover; if that is the case then there is now a potential for the humeral head to be forced anteriorly, causing an anterior humeral glide syndrome by pulling the humeral head forward within the glenoid fossa.

Spinohumeral muscles
Latissimus dorsi

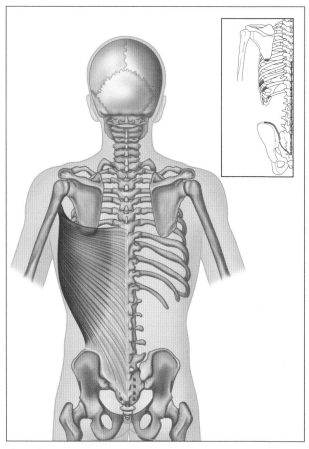

Figure 2.13: *Latissimus dorsi*

Origin: A broad sheet of tendon which is attached to the spinous processes of the lower six thoracic vertebrae and all the lumbar and sacral vertebrae, (T7–S5). Posterior part of iliac crest as well as the lower three or four ribs and the inferior angle of the scapula.

Insertion: Twists to insert in the intertubercular sulcus (bicipital groove) of the humerus, just below the shoulder joint.

Nerve: Thoracodorsal nerve (C6, C7, C8), from the posterior cord of the brachial plexus.

The latissimus dorsi muscle has many functions, from the GH joint perspective, this muscle will extend, internally rotate and adduct. It is the only muscle out of all the muscles of the shoulder complex that attaches from the vertebral column to the humerus. The latissimus dorsi muscle can also assist in forced respiration by lifting the lower ribs because of the lower attachment sites to the lower three or four ribs.

There are oblique fibers of the latissimus dorsi that assist the lower trapezius and serratus anterior muscle by controlling the inferior and lateral motion of the scapula around the thorax cage because these fibers cross and attach to the inferior angle of the scapula. This muscle is also part of the posterior oblique sling (outer core system) that connects with the thoracolumbar fascia and contralateral gluteus maximus (Gmax) (figure 2.14). These groups of muscles and fascia are part of the outer core myofascial sling system that plays an integral part of sacroiliac joint (SIJ) stability through force closure mechanisms.

This muscle is also thought of to be one of the primary stabilizers for the SIJ, lumbar and thorax as well as being able to accelerate and decelerate rotatory motions for the trunk and spine. If the latissimus dorsi muscle is overactive or hypertonic because of a potentially weakened or inhibited Gmax on the contralateral side (opposite), then the latissimus dorsi now becomes the stabilizing structure for the SI joint because the Gmax cannot fulfil its role anymore. In doing so the shoulder biomechanics are altered because of the specific attachments sites of the latissimus dorsi to the humerus and the scapula. This process can cause an anterior tilting and depression of the scapula, resulting in an overactive levator scapulae and upper trapezius muscles. Over time, these repeated dysfunctional patterns would naturally cause the patient to present with pain to the area of the neck and shoulder.

The latissimus has an attachment to the inferior angle of the scapula so this muscle will assist the rhomboids and levator scapulae to depress and downwardly rotate the scapula.

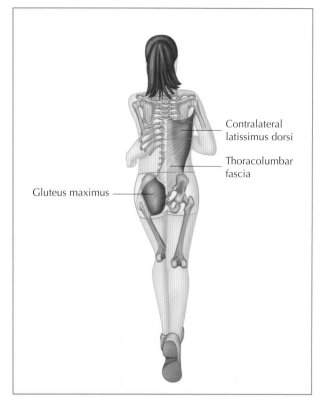

Contralateral latissimus dorsi

Thoracolumbar fascia

Gluteus maximus

Figure 2.14: *Posterior oblique sling*

Spinoscapular muscles
Trapezius

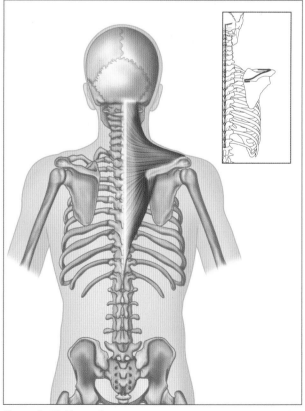

Figure 2.15: *Trapezius*

Origin: Base of skull (occipital bone). Spinous processes of seventh cervical vertebra (C7) and all thoracic vertebrae (T1–12).

Insertion: Lateral third of clavicle. Acromion process. Spine of scapula.

Nerve: Accessory XI nerve. Ventral ramus of cervical nerves (C2, C3, C4).

Levator scapulae

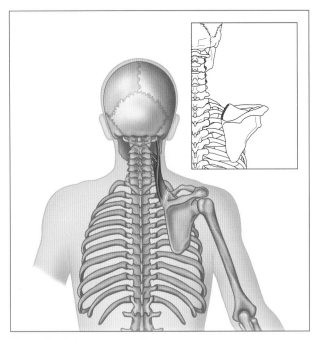

Figure 2.16: *Levator scapulae*

Origin: Transverse processes of the first three or four cervical vertebrae (C1–4).

Insertion: Upper medial or vertebral border and superior angle of the scapula.

Nerve: Dorsal scapular nerve (C4, C5) and cervical plexus (C3, C4).

The trapezius muscle and the upper fibers in particular will elevate the scapula and assist in lateral flexion of the cervical spine. The upper fibers of the trapezius are thought of as synergists with the levator scapulae muscle as they perform a similar role; however, in certain circumstances they are antagonists (opposite); for example, the levator scapulae will rotate the cervical spine to the ipsilateral side (same side), whereby the upper fibers of the trapezius assist in rotating the cervical spine to the contralateral side (opposite side). The upper trapezius works in harmony with the lower fibers of the trapezius as well as the serratus anterior to upwardly rotate the scapula, while the levator scapulae works in harmony with the pectoralis minor and rhomboids to downwardly rotate the scapula. The middle fibers of the trapezius work in unison with the rhomboids minor and major to retract the scapula.

Rhomboids minor and major

Origin: *Rhomboid minor* – C7 and T1 spinous process.
Rhomboid major – T2–5 spinous process.

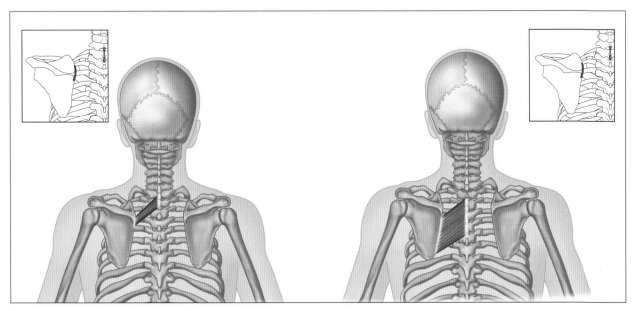

Figure 2.17: *Rhomboids minor and major*

Insertion: Medial or vertebral border of the scapula.

Nerve: Dorsal scapular nerve (C4, C5).

Scapuloradial muscles
Biceps brachii

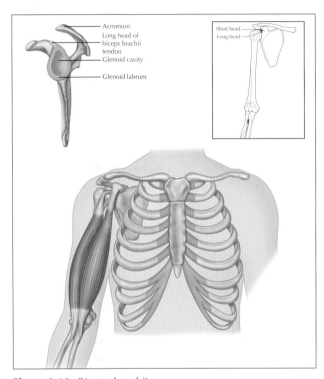

Figure 2.18: *Biceps brachii*

Origin: The long head attaches from the supraglenoid tubercle and the short head attaches from the coracoid process.

Insertion: Radial tuberosity and bicipital aponeurosis of the deep investing fascia of the forearm.

Nerve: Musculocutaneous nerve (C5, C6).

The biceps brachii is what I call a *food* muscle. Let me give you an example: when you go to pick up an apple, you will initially grip the fruit with your fingers; then the first motion is to supinate the forearm (main action of the biceps), and as you bring the apple towards your mouth the elbow and shoulder now flexes, so the biceps is partly responsible for all three motions. The biceps is unique because it also has many functions in addition to the ones I mentioned above. Its attachment is from the glenoid labrum on the supraglenoid tubercle of the scapula, just above the glenoid fossa, and it passes through the joint capsule and descends inferiorly though the bicipital groove or intertubercular sulcus, which is located between the greater and lesser tuberosity or tubercle. The biceps long head is kept within the groove by the transverse humeral

ligament. On occasion this ligament can tear, and if this happens a snapping type of syndrome ensues, due to the long head flicking in and out of the groove. The long head conjoins with the biceps short head (that has descended inferiorly from the coracoid process of the scapula) to form the muscle belly and it continues to form a tendon, which now attaches to a specific tuberosity located on the radius called the radial tuberosity as well as to a fascial (connective) sheet of tissue called the bicipital aponeurosis.

The biceps long head works in harmony with the four rotator cuff muscles because on its anatomical location, it assists in anterior stabilization of the humerus. Altered biomechanics of the shoulder complex – for example, positional changes like internal rotation of the humerus or anterior tilting of the scapula – can cause an overuse inflammatory condition of the long head of the biceps and this is called bicipital tenosynovitis. The biceps long head can sustain an avulsion injury from its tendinous attachment to the supraglenoid tubercle and this is also part of the glenoid labrum. If the tendon does tear away from the labrum then it is commonly known as a SLAP (superior labrum, anterior to posterior) lesion.

The biceps long head is also implicated as part of the process that is responsible or at least is involved in the maintaining factors for the condition called adhesive capsulitis (frozen shoulder).

Scapula-ulna muscles
Triceps brachii

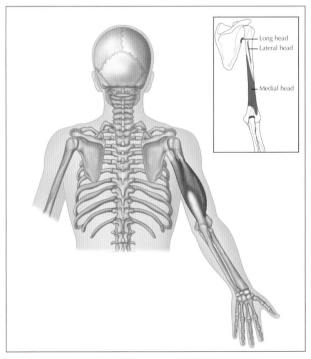

Figure 2.19: *Triceps brachii*

Origin: Long head attaches from the infraglenoid tubercle and the lateral and medial heads attach on the shaft of the humerus.

Insertion: Olecranon process of the ulna.

Nerve: Radial nerve (C5, C6, C7, C8, T1).

The triceps, as the name suggests, is a three-headed muscle and the long head is of particular importance in relation to motion of the shoulder complex. The long head works in unison with the ipsilateral (same side) latissimus dorsi and teres major to adduct and extend the shoulder. The triceps brachii tendon also has an attachment to the posterior capsule and that has to provide some stabilizing influence mechanisms for the glenohumeral joint.

Combined motion: scapulohumeral rhythm (2:1)

To perform the overhead motion of flexion in the sagittal plane and abduction in the frontal plane the shoulder complex needs the precise integration of all of the following joints to work in complete harmony: glenohumeral (GH), scapulothoracic (ST), acromioclavicular (AC) and sternoclavicular (SC).

I use a simple quote to clarify this: 'If any *one* of these *four* joints malfunction then dysfunction will occur!'

Scapulohumeral rhythm in its simplest form is the movement between the joints of the GH and ST with an end range of approximately 160–180 degrees and this is considered normal motion for both flexion and abduction. Basically, scapulohumeral rhythm states that when the humerus abducts the scapula will upwardly rotate at a 2:1 ratio.

Original findings that examined the mechanics and role of the scapula in shoulder function have progressed over time. However, the earliest studies examining two-dimensional scapular motion with the use of radiographs, dating back to Inman et al. (1944), also found an overall 2:1 relationship between glenohumeral elevation and scapular upward rotation, which has remained the classic description of the so-called scapulohumeral rhythm.

For example at 180 degrees of abduction, 120 degrees is mainly coming from motion of the GH joint and the remaining 60 degrees is coming from the upward rotation

of the ST joint. This means at 90 degrees of abduction the shoulder (GH) would have abducted 60 degrees and the scapula (ST) would have rotated 30 degrees, hence the 2:1 ratio – in other words there are 2 degrees of motion from the GH joint for every 1 degree of motion from the ST joint.

Rundqvist et al. (2003) reported scapular dyskinesis (altered motion) in 68–100% of patients with shoulder injuries (including glenohumeral instability, rotator cuff abnormalities and labral tears).

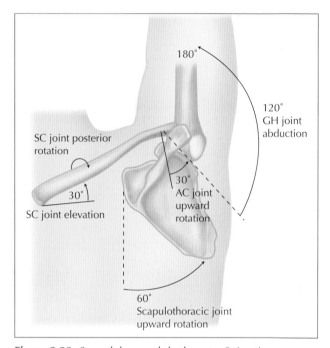

Figure 2.20: *Scapulohumeral rhythm at a 2:1 ratio*

The problem I have now is that I need to add another dimension to this concept. The first 30 degrees of abduction there is little movement from the scapula as motion is predominantly from the GH and then abduction continues at a 2:1 ratio. At 90 degrees of arm abduction, I have already explained that the GH has abducted 60 degrees and the scapula would have rotated 30 degrees at the ST joint; however, the clavicle will have elevated 15 degrees and then starts to rotate posteriorly and these movements are allowed from the sternoclavicular (SC) and acromioclavicular (AC) joints. From 90 to 180 degrees of arm abduction, the GH joint abducts the humerus another 60 degrees (total is 120 degrees) and the scapula upwardly rotates the remaining 30 degrees; however, similar to before, the clavicle now elevates another 15 degrees and posteriorly rotates between 30 and 50 degrees at the SC and AC joint. One could add in another 2:1 rhythm here and call it scapuloclavicular rhythm – this means for every 2 degrees of scapula rotation there is 1 degree of clavicle elevation.

Another note to mention is that the humerus will also need to laterally rotate during full abduction to between 35 and 40 degrees to prevent the greater tubercle approximating the acromion process and the scapula will need to posteriorly tip 30 degrees to allow the scapula full upward rotation of 60 degrees, especially for flexion in the sagittal plane.

The above paragraphs are somewhat daunting, but to put it more simply, the total range of motion for abduction of the glenohumeral joint is 120 degrees. The scapula component is 60 degrees and approximately 50% of this movement is required from specific motion of the clavicle at the SC and AC joints to allow the scapula to upwardly rotate these 60 degrees. Any further degree of upward rotation/elevation is accomplished by posterior rotation of the clavicle. This means that the two smaller joints (SC and AC) will need to be assessed if there are any dysfunctional patterns seen during overhead motion.

Thoracic spine involvement

I also need to add another concept to the above because what I have mentioned is not 100% correct. For full flexion and abduction to occur to 180 degrees of the shoulder complex the last 10–15 degrees is actually coming from extension of the *thoracic spine*. So, basically, 60 degrees is still from scapula rotation, 105 degrees from glenohumeral abduction and 15 degrees from thoracic extension. This area of the spine is very important in terms of restoring end range mobility to the shoulder complex for full flexion and abduction. These movements can be improved by using mobilization and especially manipulative techniques to the thoracic region and these will be discussed in further chapters.

Scapulohumeral rhythm and the rotator cuff

Now let us look at the function of the rotator cuff during this scapulohumeral movement. This is a very interesting topic because experts in the field of sports medicine do not always agree upon what I mention in the following text!

It is generally accepted that in the initiation of abduction for the GH joint approximately the first 10–15 degrees is by the supraspinatus muscle, and then the middle fibers of the deltoid take over, with some ongoing activation of the supraspinatus muscle. At approximately 30 degrees of shoulder abduction (from the GH joint) the scapula will start to upwardly rotate by the contraction of the

upper and lower trapezius as well as the serratus anterior. Naturally, as the abduction motion is continuing there will come a time during the movement – and that is generally considered to be roughly between 60 and 90 degrees (painful arc sign) – that the greater tuberosity of the humerus approximates the acromion process; this approximation can/will potentially compress the soft tissue structures that lie within the subacromial space and hence cause an impingement type of syndrome. To prevent this impingement of the soft tissues from happening the infraspinatus and teres minor muscles are recruited and on contraction they assist by laterally rotating the humerus and the greater tubercle away from acromion process, while shoulder abduction is still continuing.

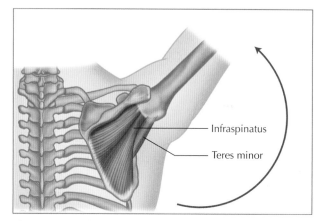

Figure 2.21: *Infraspinatus and teres minor externally rotate the humerus*

As the humerus is continuing its abduction motion (with lateral rotation) with the combination of the scapula upwardly rotating, the subscapularis and supraspinatus now have an *adducting* motion to the humerus. This

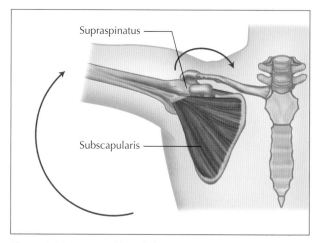

Figure 2.22: *Humeral head depression by supraspinatus and subscapularis during 90–180 degrees of abduction*

effect of adduction will assist the pulling down motion (adducting) or inferiorly gliding of the humeral head deep within the glenoid fossa to prevent impingement and provide overall stability. The reverse will happen on the movement of adduction (this is when one brings the arm back down to the side of the body).

Remember, and just to clarify the above, when one performs the movements of abduction and flexion, it requires precise interaction of each of the four joint articulations (mentioned earlier) as well as the ability of the muscles and soft tissues to be specifically in balance, as they all contribute towards the blueprint of the shoulder complex. It is quite obvious when looking at patients and athletes performing overhead motions that it requires more than just simply looking at the mechanics of the GH joint. One also needs to consider the other three joints, AC, SC and ST, also remembering the relationship of the thoracic spine, since all are integral to the stability and motion for any movements of the arm above the head.

From a clinical perspective for the therapist, external rotation of the glenohumeral joint is naturally a requirement to allow full motion of abduction in the frontal plane because the greater tuberosity has to clear the acromion and coracoacromial ligament to prevent impingement. In pathological conditions of the shoulder such as capsulitis, therefore, stretches to improve lateral rotation and strengthening exercises for the infraspinatus and teres minor (the muscles responsible for the external motion) should be addressed early on in the treatment protocol. Because the scapula allows one third of the overall motion of the shoulder it should be addressed in

every patient that presents with shoulder pathology. It has been demonstrated that the serratus anterior in particular is very important in stabilizing the scapula against the thoracic wall during any overhead serving motions and fatigue to this muscle may be responsible for altered biomechanics to the shoulder complex and subsequent impingement syndromes.

Perry (1988) explained that the most important upward rotators are the trapezius and serratus anterior and although these muscles are of equal size electromyographic (EMG) studies showed that during swimming the serratus anterior works at 75% of its maximum and the trapezius works from 34% to 42% of its maximum. She stated that a 75% workload cannot be maintained during prolonged swimming and training and rehabilitation must include increased emphasis on all the scapular muscles.

Hammer (1991) mentions that swimmers often overdevelop their pectoral and anterior cervical muscles, resulting in slumping posture and weak scapular retractors and adductors (rhomboids, middle trapezius and upper fibers of the latissimus dorsi) and lateral rotators. Weak scapular musculature may result in failure to position the glenoid in time under the humeral head during the recovery phase (abduction and external rotation) of swimming. This may result in acromial impingement of the humeral head structures due to failure of the humeral head to clear the acromion completely. The overdevelopment of internal shoulder rotators compared to external rotators is a possible cause of tendinitis (swimmer's shoulder).

3

Posture, myofascial slings and the inner/outer core

Before we look at the role of the sling systems and the relationship of the inner and outer core muscles to the shoulder girdle complex, I want to discuss *posture*. This particular word is used all the time with patients, athletes and even physical therapists. They say things like 'do you think I have good posture' or 'I know my posture is really poor' or 'is that why I am in so much pain because of my posture?' So lets look at this *postural* concept.

■ Posture

Definition: *Posture* is the attitude or position of the body, as discussed by Thomas (1997).

According to Martin (2002), posture should fulfill three functions:

1. maintain the alignment of the body's segments in any position: supine, prone, sitting, all fours, and standing
2. anticipate change to allow engagement in voluntary, goal-directed movements, such as reaching and stepping
3. react to unexpected perturbations or disturbances in balance.

From the above three functions, it can be seen that posture is an active as well as a static state, and that it is synonymous with balance. Optimal posture must be maintained at all times, not only when holding static positions (e.g., sitting and standing) but also during functional movements in day-to-day activities.

If optimal posture and postural control are to be encouraged during exercise performance, the principles of good static posture must be fully appreciated. Once these are understood, poor posture can then be identified and corrective strategies adopted accordingly and subsequently implemented.

- *Good posture* is the state of muscular and skeletal balance that protects the supporting structures of the body against injury or progressive deformity, irrespective of the attitude (e.g., erect, lying, squatting, or stooping) in which these structures are working or resting.
- *Poor posture* is a faulty relationship of the various parts of the body, producing increased strain on the supporting structures, and resulting in less efficient balance of the body over its base of support.

Regarding shoulder and neck pain, the posture of the patient must be considered and evaluated because when the patient stands in an erect position the scapula has a natural resting position (as you will read later on) and the position of the scapula directly influences the natural alignment of the shoulder joint and in particular the position of the glenoid fossa, which has a specific alignment with the center of gravity. In the round shouldered patient with an increased thoracic kyphosis the scapula position is now altered – it rotates forward and downward and subsequently changes the position of the acromion and glenoid fossa, increasing the chances for an impingement syndrome. If you look at figure 3.1a you will see the patient is able to lift their arms past their ears because the thoracic kyphosis is normal; however, in figure 3.1b there is a limited end range of motion because of the increased thoracic kyphosis.

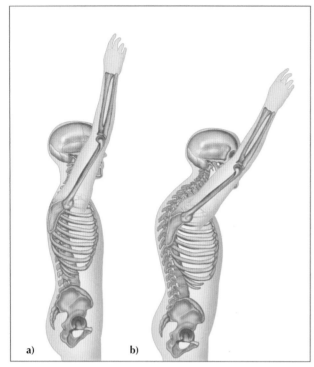

Figure 3.1a & b: *a: Normal range of motion and arms pass the ears; b: limited range of motion due to increased thoracic kyphosis*

Poor posture

Poor posture may be the result of many different contributing factors. One of these is heredity; one needs to be able to evaluate the parents' body type to find out whether this might be the underlying cause and this is relatively difficult in terms of treatment. Another factor can be trauma suffered by the body, or a disease process from inflammatory joint pathologies such as ankylosing spondylitis, or even some form of structural deformity within the musculoskeletal system. This might possibly be through faulty mechanical loading resulting from our daily habits, especially if these began in childhood. A slumped or stooped posture is typically seen in young adults and if uncorrected this daily feeling will eventually become normal for them. For some people sitting has become a regular position, maintained for long periods of time (possibly eight or more hours), and a great many people in today's society are losing the battle against gravity and altering their center of gravity (COG). With correct posture, your postural muscles are fairly inactive and energy efficient, only responding to disruptions in balance in order to maintain an upright position. As you move away from an ideal alignment,

however, postural muscle activity increases, leading to a higher energy expenditure as well as an increase in pain syndromes.

Pain spasm cycle

Ischemia will be a primary source of pain in the initial stages of poor posture. The blood flow through a muscle is inversely proportional to the level of contraction or activity, reaching almost zero at 50–60% of contraction. Some studies have indicated that the body is not able to maintain homeostasis with a sustained isometric contraction of over 10%.

Consider the following example: the weight of the head is approximately 7% of total body weight (shoulders and arms are around 14%). This means that for a person weighing 176 lb (80 kg), the head will weigh around 11–13 lb (5–6 kg). If the head and shoulders move forward, out of ideal alignment, the activation of the neck extensors will increase dramatically, resulting in restricted blood flow. Previous authors have stated that for every inch of forward head posture, the weight of the head on the spine can increase by approximately 10 lb (4.5 kg). For example, if the weight of the head is normally 10 lb (4.5 kg), it will now potentially weigh 20 lb (9 kg) for just a 1 inch (2.5 cm) increase in forward head posture, 30 lb (13.5 kg) for a 2 inch (5 cm) increase, and an unbelievable 40 lb (18 kg) if the head translates 3 inches (7.5 cm), as shown in figure 3.2a.

This prolonged isometric contraction will force the muscles into anaerobic metabolism and increase lactic acid and other irritating metabolite accumulation. If adequate rest is not given, a reflex contraction of the already ischemic muscles may be initiated. This person will have now entered the pain spasm cycle (figure 3.2b).

The neuromuscular system is made up of slow-twitch and fast-twitch muscle fibers, each having a different role in the body's function. Slow-twitch fibers (type I) are active in sustained low-level activity such as maintaining correct posture whereas fast-twitch fibers (type II) are used for powerful, gross movements. Muscles can also be broken down into two further categories: tonic (or postural) and phasic.

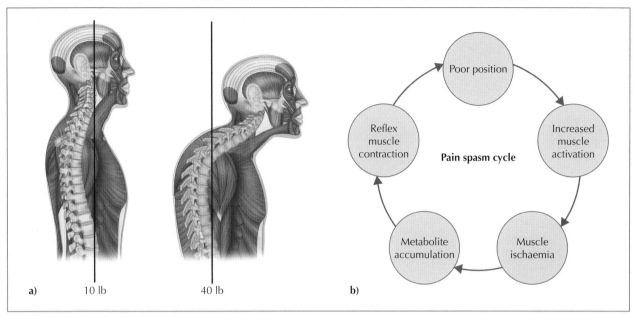

Figure 3.2a & b: *a: The result of a forward head posture; b: pain spasm cycle*

Tonic (postural) and phasic muscles (figure 3.3a&b)

Janda (1987) identified two groups of muscles on the basis of their evolution and development. Functionally, muscles can be classified as tonic or phasic. The tonic system consists of the flexors, which develop later to become the dominant structure. Umphred et al. (2001) identified that the tonic muscles are involved in repetitive or rhythmic activity and are activated in flexor synergies, whereas the phasic system consists of the extensors and emerges shortly after birth. The phasic muscles work eccentrically against the force of gravity and are involved in extensor synergies. The division of muscles into predominantly phasic and predominantly postural for the shoulder complex and cervical spine is given in Table 3.1.

Previous authors have suggested that muscles which have a stabilizing function (postural) have a natural tendency to shorten when stressed, and that other muscles which play a more active/moving role (phasic) have a tendency to lengthen and can subsequently become inhibited (Table 3.2). The muscles that tend to shorten (e.g., pectorals) have a primary postural role and are related to the potential inhibition weakness of the antagonistic muscles of the rhomboids (which you will read about later).

There are some exceptions to the rule, which states that certain muscles follow the pattern of becoming shortened while others become lengthened – some muscles are capable of modifying their structure. For example, some authors suggest that the scalene muscles are postural in nature, while others suggest that they are phasic. We know from specific testing, depending on what dysfunction is present within the muscle framework, that the scalenes

Table 3.1: Phasic and postural muscles of the body of the upper limb

Predominantly postural muscles	Predominantly phasic muscles
Pectoralis major	Rhomboids
Pectoralis minor	Lower trapezius
Levator scapulae	Mid trapezius
Upper trapezius	Serratus anterior
Biceps brachii	Triceps brachii
Infraspinatus	
Subscapularis	
Scalenes	Neck flexors:
Sternocleidomastoid	Supra- and infrahyoid/ longus colli
Suboccipitals	

Table 3.2: Lengthening and shortening of muscles

	Postural	Phasic
Function	Posture	Movement
Muscle type	Type I	Type II
Fatigue	Late	Early
Reaction	Shortening	Lengthening

can be found to be held in a shortened position and tight, but at other times they can be observed to be lengthened and weakened.

There is a distinction between postural and phasic muscles; however, many muscles can display characteristics of both and contain a mixture of type I and type II fibers. The hamstring muscles, for example, have a postural stabilizing function, yet are polyarticular (cross more than one joint) and are notoriously prone to shortening.

Postural/tonic muscles

Also known as tonic muscles, the postural muscles have an antigravity role and are therefore heavily involved in the maintenance of posture. Slow-twitch fibers are

more suited to maintaining posture: they are capable of sustained contraction but generally become shortened and subsequently tight.

Postural muscles are slow-twitch dominant because of their resistance to fatigue, and are innervated by a smaller motor neuron. They therefore have a lower excitability threshold, which means the nerve impulse will reach the postural muscle before the phasic muscle. With this sequence of innervation, the postural muscle will inhibit the phasic (antagonist) muscle, thus reducing its contractile potential and activation.

Phasic muscles

Movement is the main function of phasic muscles. These muscles, which are often more superficial than postural

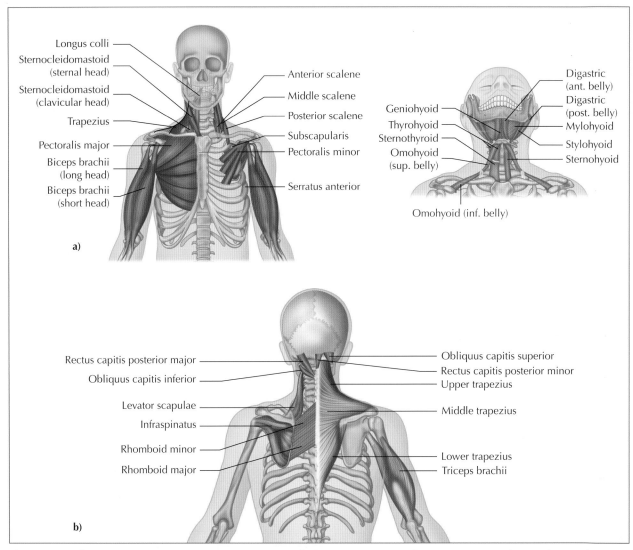

Figure 3.3a & b: *Postural and phasic muscles of the upper limb: a: anterior view; b: posterior view. The purple muscles are predominantly postural, and the green muscles predominantly phasic*

muscles and tend to be polyarticular, are composed of predominantly type II fibers and are under voluntary reflex control.

A shortened, tight postural muscle often results in inhibition of the associated phasic muscle, whose function becomes weakened as a result. The relationship between a tightness-prone muscle and an associated weakness-prone muscle is one way. As the tightness-prone muscle becomes tighter and subsequently stronger, this causes an inhibition of the weakness-prone muscle, resulting in its lengthening and consequent weakening. Think about how this might affect the relationship, for example, between the iliopsoas and the gluteal muscles, or between the pectoralis major/minor and the rhomboids.

■ Muscle activity before and after stretching

Let us take a look at some electromyographic (EMG) studies of trunk muscle activity before and after stretching hypertonic muscles, in this case the erector spinae. In Table 3.3 the hypertonic erector spinae are indicated as being active during trunk flexion. After stretching, these muscles are suppressed both in trunk flexion (which allows greater activation of the rectus abdominis) and in trunk extension (dorsal raise).

Effects of muscle imbalance

The research results of Janda (1983) indicate that tight or overactive muscles not only hinder the agonist through Sherrington's law of reciprocal inhibition as stated by Sherrington (1907) but also become active in movements that they are not normally associated with. This is the

reason why, when trying to correct a musculoskeletal imbalance, you would encourage *lengthening* of an overactive muscle by using a muscle energy technique (MET), prior to attempting to *strengthen* a weak elongated muscle (METs will be explained in Chapter 9).

Think about the following words before you continue reading:

'A *tight* muscle will pull the joint into a dysfunctional position and the *weak* muscle will allow this to happen.'

One possible way to address this, therefore, is to simply apply the following rule:

'Lengthen the short before you strengthen the weak.' For example, we would lengthen the shortened pectoral muscles prior to strengthening the weakened rhomboids.

If muscle imbalances are not addressed, the body will be forced into a compensatory position, which increases the stress placed on the musculoskeletal system, eventually leading to tissue breakdown, irritation, and injury. You are now in a vicious circle of musculoskeletal deterioration as the tonic muscles shorten and the phasic muscles lengthen (Table 3.4).

Muscle imbalances are ultimately reflected in posture. As mentioned earlier, postural muscles are innervated by a smaller motor neuron and therefore have a lower excitability threshold. Since the nerve impulse reaches the postural muscle before the phasic muscle, the postural muscle will inhibit the phasic (antagonist) muscle, thus reducing the contractile potential and activation.

When muscles are subject to faulty or repetitive loading, the postural muscles shorten and the phasic muscles

Table 3.3: EMG recordings of muscle activity (Source: Hammer 1999)

Muscle	1st recording			2nd recording		
Rectus abdominis						
Erector spinae						

weaken, thus altering their length–tension relationship. Consequently, posture is directly affected because the surrounding muscles displace the soft tissues and the skeleton.

Table 3.4: The vicious circle of musculoskeletal deterioration

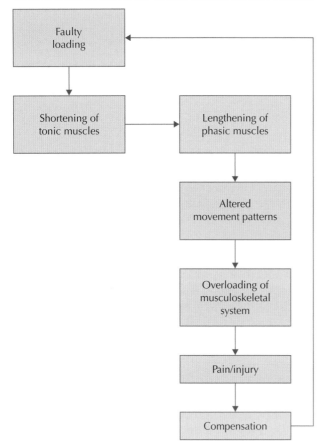

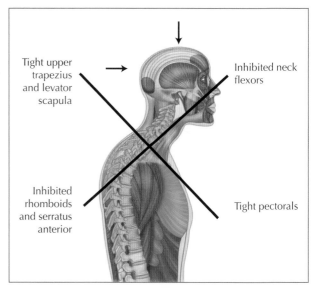

Figure 3.4: *Upper crossed syndrome*

postural changes are seen in UCS, including forward head posture, increased cervical lordosis and thoracic kyphosis, elevated and protracted shoulders, and rotation or abduction and winging of the scapulae. These postural changes decrease glenohumeral stability as the glenoid fossa becomes more vertical due to serratus anterior weakness leading to abduction, rotation, and winging of the scapulae. This loss of stability requires the levator scapula and upper trapezius to increase activation to maintain glenohumeral centration.

Upper crossed syndrome (UCS)

Janda (1988) discussed the upper crossed syndrome (UCS), also referred to as the proximal or shoulder girdle crossed syndrome (figure 3.3). In UCS, tightness of the upper trapezius and levator scapula crosses with tightness of the pectoralis major and minor. Weakness of the deep cervical flexors ventrally crosses with weakness of the rhomboids, middle and lower trapezius. This pattern of imbalance creates joint dysfunction, particularly at the atlanto-occipital joint (OA), cervical spine of C4–5 cervicothoracic joint (CTJ), scapulothoracic articulation, glenohumeral joint, and thoracic spine to the segment of T4–5.

Janda noted that these focal areas of stress, especially to the spine, correspond to transitional zones in which neighboring vertebrae change in morphology. Specific

Muscle tightness

Janda (1987) felt that muscle tightness is the key factor in muscle imbalance. In general, muscles prone to tightness are one third stronger than muscles prone to inhibition. Muscle tightness creates a cascade of events that lead to injury. Tightness of a muscle reflexively inhibits its antagonist, creating muscle imbalance. This muscle imbalance leads to joint dysfunction because of unbalanced forces. Joint dysfunction creates poor movement patterns and compensations, leading to early fatigue. Finally, overstress of activated muscles and poor stabilization lead to injury.

Janda (1993) believed that there are three important factors in muscle tightness: muscle length, irritability threshold, and altered recruitment. Muscles that are tight are usually shorter than normal and display an altered length–tension relationship. Muscle tightness leads to a lowered activation threshold or lowered irritability threshold, which means that the muscle is readily activated with movement. Movement typically takes the path of least resistance and so tight and facilitated muscles are often the first to be recruited in movement patterns. Tight muscles typically maintain their strength, but in extreme cases they can weaken.

■ Core muscle relationships

Inner core unit (local system)

Definition: Static stability is the ability to remain in one position for a long time without losing good structural alignment, as mentioned by Chek (2009).

Static stability is also often referred to as postural stability, although this might be somewhat misleading, since, as Martin (2002) states: 'posture is more than just maintaining a position of the body such as standing. Posture is active, whether it is in sustaining an existing posture or moving from one posture to another.'

The inner core unit (figure 3.5) consists of:

* transversus abdominis (TVA)
* multifidus

* diaphragm
* muscles of the pelvic floor.

Only the TVA and multifidus will be covered in this book, as these muscles are specifically related to postural and phasic imbalances and are easily palpated by the physical therapist.

Since the diaphragm and muscles of the pelvic floor are difficult to palpate, they will not be discussed here.

Transversus abdominis

The transversus abdominis (TVA) is the deepest of the abdominal muscles. It originates at the iliac crest, inguinal ligament, lumbar fascia, and associated cartilage of the inferior six ribs, and attaches to the xiphoid process, linea alba, and pubis.

The main action of the TVA is to compress the abdomen via a 'drawing-in' of the abdominal wall. This drawing-in is observable as a movement of the umbilicus (belly button) toward the spine. The muscle neither flexes nor extends the spine. Kendall et al. (2010) also state that 'this muscle has no action in lateral flexion except that it acts to

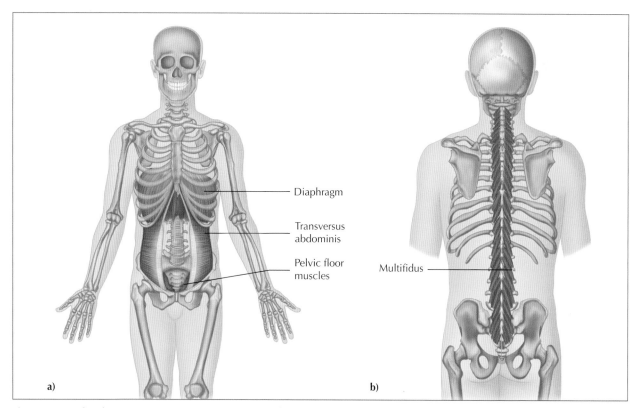

Diaphragm

Transversus abdominis

Pelvic floor muscles

Multifidus

a)

b)

Figure 3.5a & b: *The inner core unit: a: anterior view; b: posterior view*

… stabilize the linea alba, thereby permitting better action by anterolateral trunk muscles [internal and external obliques].'

The TVA appears to be the key muscle of the inner unit. Richardson et al. (1999) found that in people without back pain, the TVA fired 30 milliseconds prior to shoulder movements and 110 milliseconds before leg movements. This corroborates the key role of the TVA in providing the stability necessary to perform movements of the appendicular skeleton. As the TVA contracts during inspiration it pulls the central tendon inferiorly and flattens, thereby increasing the vertical length of the thoracic cavity and compressing the lumbar multifidus.

Multifidus

The multifidus is the most medial of the lumbar back muscles, and its fibers converge near the lumbar spinous processes to an attachment known as the *mammillary process*. The fibers radiate inferiorly, passing to the transverse processes (TPs) of the vertebrae that lie two, three, four, and five levels below. As well as some fibers uniting distally with the sacrotuberous ligament, those fibers that extend below the level of the last lumbar vertebra (L5) anchor to the ilium and the sacrum.

The multifidus is considered to be a series of smaller muscles, which are further divided into *superficial* and *deep* components. There is more muscle mass of the multifidus near the base of the sacrum than at the apex, especially filling the space between the PSISs rather than the ILAs.

The role of the multifidus in producing an extension force is essential to the stability of the lumbar spine, as well as functioning to resist forward flexion of the lumbar spine and the shear forces that are placed upon it. The multifidus muscle also functions to take pressure off the intervertebral discs, so that the body weight is evenly distributed throughout the whole vertebral column. The superficial muscle component acts to keep the vertebral column relatively straight, while the fibers of the deep muscle component contribute to the overall stability of the spine.

Richardson et al. (1999) identified the lumbar multifidus and the TVA as the key stabilizers of the lumbar spine. Both muscles link in with the thoracolumbar fascia to provide what Richardson and colleagues refer to as 'a natural, deep muscle corset to protect the back from injury.'

More recently, Richardson et al. (2002) investigated how these muscles impact the sacroiliac joint (SIJ) using echo-Doppler (a diagnostic ultrasound device that can show if specific muscles are contracting). They were able to demonstrate that when the TVA and multifidus co-contract, the stiffness of the SIJ increases, thereby proving that these muscles are essential to compressing the SIJ and stabilizing the joint under load (force closure) and also that it is critical that this compression occurs at just the right time.

Myofascial outer core (global system)

The force closure muscles of the outer core unit consist of four integrated myofascial sling systems (figures 3.6–3.9):

- posterior (deep) longitudinal sling
- lateral sling
- anterior oblique sling
- posterior oblique sling.

These myofascial slings provide force closure and subsequent stability for the pelvic girdle; failure of any of these slings to secure pelvic and trunk stability, or even weakness in the slings, can lead to pain and dysfunction throughout the whole of the kinetic chain and this includes the shoulder complex and cervical spine. Although the muscles of the outer core unit can be trained individually, effective force closure requires specific coactivation and release of these myofascial slings for optimal function and performance.

The integrated myofascial sling system represents many forces and is composed of several muscles. A muscle may participate in more than one sling, and the slings may overlap and interconnect, depending on the task in hand. There are several slings of myofascial systems in the outer unit and the hypothesis is that the slings have no beginning or end, but rather connect as necessary to assist in the transference of forces. It is possible that the slings are all part of one interconnected myofascial system, and a sling that is identified during any particular motion could merely be a result of the activation of selective parts of the whole sling (Lee 2004).

The identification and treatment of a specific muscle dysfunction (such as weakness, inappropriate recruitment, or tightness) is important when restoring force closure for understanding why parts of a sling may be restricted in motion or lacking in support. Note the following points:

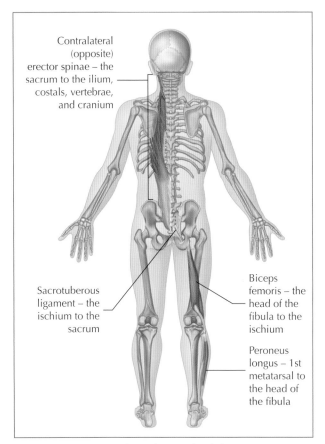

Contralateral (opposite) erector spinae – the sacrum to the ilium, costals, vertebrae, and cranium

Sacrotuberous ligament – the ischium to the sacrum

Biceps femoris – the head of the fibula to the ischium

Peroneus longus – 1st metatarsal to the head of the fibula

Figure 3.6: *Posterior (deep) longitudinal sling*

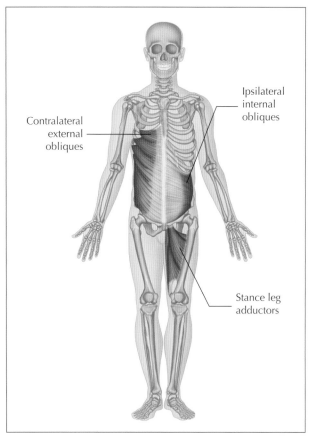

Contralateral external obliques

Ipsilateral internal obliques

Stance leg adductors

Figure 3.8: *Anterior oblique sling*

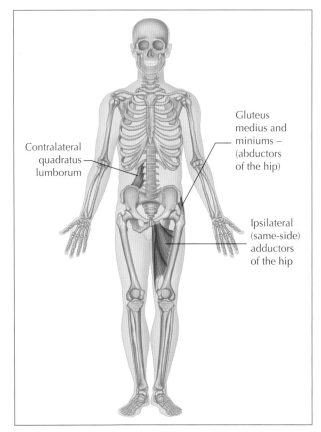

Contralateral quadratus lumborum

Gluteus medius and miniums – (abductors of the hip)

Ipsilateral (same-side) adductors of the hip

Figure 3.7: *Lateral sling*

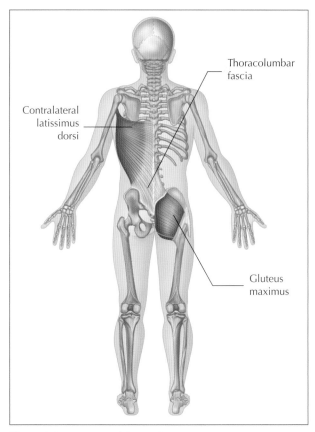

Thoracolumbar fascia

Contralateral latissimus dorsi

Gluteus maximus

Figure 3.9: *Posterior oblique sling*

- The four systems of the *outer core unit* are dependent upon the *inner core unit* for the joint stiffness and stability necessary for creating an effective force generation platform.
- Failure of the inner unit to work in the presence of outer unit demand often results in muscle imbalance, joint injury, and poor performance.
- The outer unit cannot be effectively conditioned by the use of modern resistance machines, as the specific training provided by these types of machine generally does not relate to day-to-day functional movements.
- Conditioning of the outer core unit should include specific exercises that require functional integration of both the inner and outer units, through using controlled movement patterns that relate to any given patient's day-to-day working or sporting environment.

In the next chapter I will try and link and naturally discuss the walking cycle (gait cycle) and the relationship and the effects to the shoulder complex; if you have a good understanding of the information regarding the myofascial sling systems, then, hopefully, it should make perfect sense how these slings are now incorporated into an efficient walking cycle and how it affects the whole of the kinetic chain, from the initial contact with the ground to the natural swinging of the arms to improve propulsion. I truly hope that as you read that particular chapter, the pieces of the jigsaw puzzle will slowly begin to form a recognizable picture. My goal is for you to come back to each specific chapter time and time again, to try to understand and digest what I have written. More importantly, however, I want you to be able to use this information in your own clinical setting to be a more effective therapist, especially when you personally assess and treat your own athletes and patients.

4

Walking and its relationship to the shoulder complex

Despite the fact that this particular topic is discussed in my previous books I include it here, as you will need to understand what actually happens when we walk and run, particularly as it relates to the shoulder. I can guarantee that any dysfunction within the lower kinetic chain, and in particular the area of the knee, hip, pelvis and sacroiliac (SI) joint, will have overall consequences for the function and stability of the upper kinetic chain. You need to be able to step back and look at and assess your patients globally rather than simply looking locally, at where the patient says it hurts.

Imagine this: you are looking for a new pair of trainers – perhaps you have decided to take up running, or you are already a runner and are feeling pain in the lower back or knee and you think it might be as a result of your trainers. The salesperson might ask you to try a pair on and run for a few minutes on a treadmill. They will probably observe your running style from the back. They might even take a video recording and play it back slow time on a screen. They will normally discuss your particular running style (neutral runner or an over pronator, etc.) and recommend trainers according to how you contact the ground while running. This hopefully will have the desired effect of either reducing your knee or back pain or if you are new to running, then at least you are going to start to run with the correct equipment.

I am not here to teach you how to assess patients on a treadmill or using a camera to watch their gait. Rather, I am here to help you understand the links of each of the components of the musculoskeletal chain and whether or not you feel a piece is missing in the overall jigsaw puzzle

that might require further investigation. I was at a medical conference and the surgeon said the best diagnostic tool we have is the 'patient's finger' as we ask them to *point* to where it hurts and then we treat the area of pain. This might be the case for a knee or ankle surgeon but is not enough for the therapist who has now become a therapy-detective and is trying their best to find lots of clues to eventually solve the case. If we only attend to the area of pain, we will probably NEVER solve the case!

We generally take walking (and even running come to that) for granted – it is something that we just *do* … that is, until we suffer pain somewhere in our body, and then the simple action of walking or running becomes very painful. In this section I want to discuss what exactly takes place when we walk and more importantly, how it relates to the kinetic chain of the shoulder complex, and how can we influence it.

Human gait is a very complicated, coordinated series of movements. The gait (walking) cycle is divided into two main phases: the *stance* phase and the *swing* phase. Each cycle begins at initial contact (also known as *heel-strike*) of the leading leg in a stance phase, proceeds through a swing phase, and ends with the next contact of the ground with that same leg. The stance phase is subdivided into *heel-strike*, *mid-stance*, and *propulsion* phases.

The stance phase is the weight-bearing component of each cycle; it is initiated by heel-strike and ends with toe-off from the same foot. The swing phase is initiated with toe-off and ends with heel-strike. It has been estimated that the stance phase accounts for approximately 60% of a single gait cycle, and the swing phase for approximately 40%, as shown in figure 4.1.

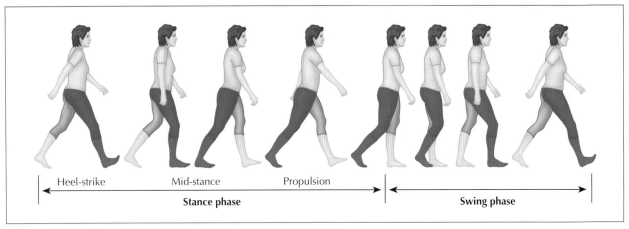

Figure 4.1: *Stance and swing phases of the gait cycle*

■ Heel-strike

If you think about the position of your body just before you contact the ground with your right leg during the contact phase of the stance phase, the right hip is in a position of flexion, the knee is extended, the ankle is dorsiflexed, and the foot is in a position of supination, as shown in figure 4.2. The tibialis anterior muscle, with the help of the tibialis posterior, works to maintain the ankle/foot in a position of dorsiflexion and inversion.

In normal gait, the foot strikes the ground at the beginning of the heel-strike in a supinated position of approximately 2 degrees. A normal foot will then move through 5–6 degrees of pronation at the subtalar joint (STJ) to a position of approximately 3–4 degrees

of pronation, as this will allow the foot to function as a 'mobile adaptor.'

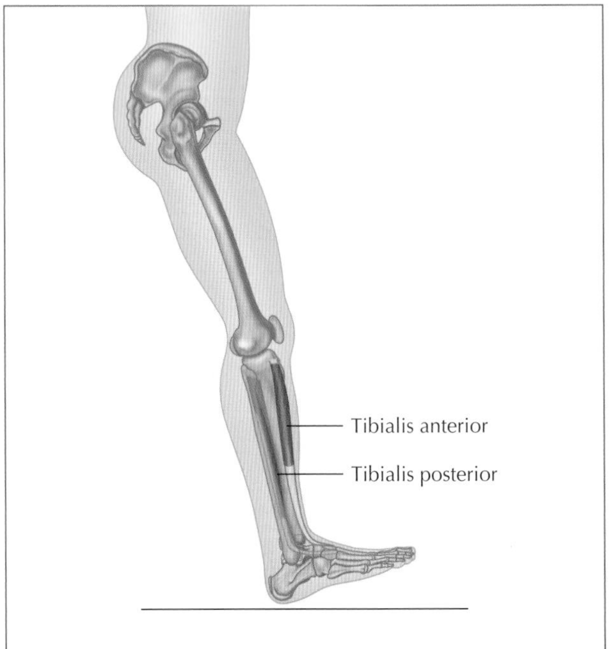

■ A myofascial link of the outer core

As a result of the ankle and foot being in a position of dorsiflexion and supination, the tibialis anterior is now part of a link system that we will call a *myofascial sling*. This sling, starting from the initial origin of the tibialis anterior, continues as the insertion of the peroneus longus (onto the first metatarsal and medial cuneiform, as in the case for the insertion of the tibialis anterior) to its muscular origin on the lateral side and head of the fibula. This bony landmark is also where the biceps femoris muscle inserts.

The sling now continues as the biceps femoris muscle toward its origin on the ischial tuberosity, where the muscle attaches to the tuberosity via the sacrotuberous ligament; often the biceps femoris directly attaches to this ligament rather than to the ischial tuberosity. Vleeming et al. (1989a) found that in 50% of subjects, part of the sacrotuberous ligament was continuous with the tendon of the long head of the biceps femoris.

The sling then carries on as the sacrotuberous ligament, which attaches to the inferior aspect of the sacrum and connects to the contralateral (opposite side) multifidi and to the erector spinae, which continue to the base of the occipital bone. This myofascial sling is known as the *posterior longitudinal sling (PLS)* (figure 4.3).

Even before you initiate the contact to the ground through heel-strike, dorsiflexion of the ankle causes a coactivation of the biceps femoris and peroneus longus just prior to heel-strike. This co-contraction therefore

Tibialis anterior
Tibialis posterior

Figure 4.2: *The position of the leg just before heel-strike*

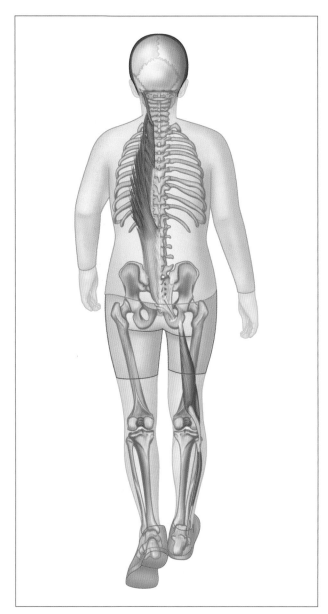

Figure 4.3: *A person walking, with the posterior (deep) longitudinal sling muscles highlighted*

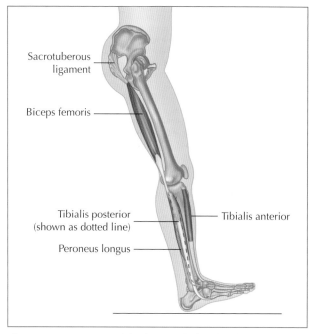

Figure 4.4a: *Position of the leg just before heel-strike, with the biceps femoris and sacrotuberous ligament tensioned*

You may also notice that the right ilium (figure 4.4b) undergoes posterior rotation during the swing phase, which will assist the force closure of the SIJ because of the increased tension in the sacrotuberous ligament.

You can also see from figure 4.4c, that there is now tension developing within the right sacrotuberous ligament because of the contraction of the biceps femoris as well as the posterior rotation of the right innominate; at the same time, the left innominate is rotating anteriorly and the sacrum has rotated on the left oblique axis (L-on-L). This specific motion of the hip-lumbopelvic complex occurs all at the same time as the right heel-strike.

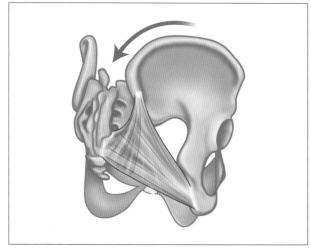

Figure 4.4b: *Right ilium in posterior rotation – sacrotuberous ligament tensioned*

serves to 'wind up' the thoracolumbar fascia mechanism as a means of stabilizing the lower extremity; this results in the storage of the necessary kinetic energy that will subsequently be released during the propulsive phase of the gait cycle.

The posterior longitudinal sling as described is being fascially tensioned; the increased tension is focused on the sacrotuberous ligament via the attachment of the biceps femoris, (figure 4.4a). This connection will assist the *force closure* (you can read more about this in a later chapter) mechanism process of the SIJ; in simple terms, this creates a self-locking and stable pelvis for the initiation of the weight-bearing gait cycle.

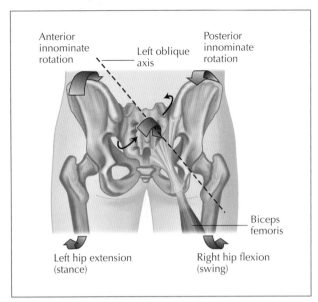

Figure 4.4c: *Right ilium in posterior rotation – left ilium in anterior rotation and sacrum rotated on the L-on-L axis*

Not only is the force closure being activated from the posterior longitudinal sling from the foot up towards the pelvis on the contact phase, it is also being activated from the head down to the pelvis from the rotatory motion of the thoracic spine as well as the natural swing of the arms, as this will aid propulsion during the walking cycle.

For the next phase towards mid-stance, your right leg moves from heel-strike to toe-off (stance phase), and your body weight begins to move over your right leg, causing your pelvis to shift laterally to the right. As the movement continues toward toe-off, your right pelvic innominate bone (innominate bone is the conjoined three bones of the ilium, pubis and ischium) begins to rotate anteriorly while your left innominate bone begins to rotate posteriorly.

As you proceed through the mid-stance phase of gait, this is where the hamstrings should reduce their tension because of the natural anterior rotation of the pelvis and the slackening of the sacrotuberous ligament so stability at this point is achieved and maintained through force closure. This is the point during the mid-stance phase where the Gmax on the right side should take the role of the continued movement of lower limb extension, as well as working in concert with the contralateral latissimus dorsi (left side). The active contraction of these two muscles increases the tension in the thoracolumbar fascia (posterior oblique sling), thus providing the necessary force closure stability to the right SIJ during the mid-stance phase of gait.

The Gmax simultaneously contracts with the contralateral latissimus dorsi – it is this muscle that will extend the arm through what is known as *counter-rotation*, to assist in propulsion. The thoracolumbar fascia, which is a sheet of connective tissue, is located between the Gmax and the contralateral latissimus dorsi; this fascial structure is forced to increase its tension because of the contractions of the Gmax and latissimus dorsi. This increased tension will assist in stabilizing the SIJ of the stance leg through the force closure mechanism.

In figure 4.5 you can see that just before heel-strike, the Gmax will reach maximum stretch as the latissimus dorsi is being stretched by the forward swing of the opposite arm. Heel-strike signifies a transition to the propulsive phase of gait, at which time the Gmax contraction is superimposed on that of the hamstrings.

The synergistic contraction of the Gmax and the contralateral latissimus dorsi creates a state of tension within the thoracolumbar fascia, which will be released in a surge of energy that will assist the muscles of locomotion. This stored energy within the thoracolumbar fascia helps to reduce the overall energy expenditure of

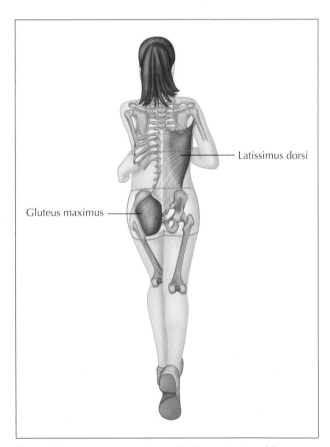

Figure 4.5: *A person running, with the posterior oblique sling muscles highlighted*

the gait cycle. Janda (1992, 1996) mentions that poor Gmax strength and activation is postulated to decrease the efficiency of gait.

As we progress from the mid-stance phase to heel-lift and propulsion, the foot begins to re-supinate and passes through a neutral position when the propulsive phase begins; the foot continues in supination through toe-off. As a result of the foot supinating during the mid-stance propulsive period, the foot is converted from a 'mobile adaptor' (which is what it is during the contact period) to a 'rigid lever' as the mid-tarsal joint locks into a supinated position. With the foot functioning as a rigid lever (as a result of the locked mid-tarsal joint) during the time immediately preceding toe-off, the weight of the body is propelled more efficiently.

■ Pelvis motion

During mid-stance phase of the walking cycle the right innominate bone starts to rotate anteriorly from an initial posteriorly rotated position, the tension of the right sacrotuberous ligament is reduced, and the sacrum will be forced to move (passively) into a right torsion on the right oblique axis (R-on-R). In other words, the sacrum rotates to the right and side bends to the left, because the left sacral base moves into an anterior nutation position (this is also known as *type I spinal mechanics*, as the rotation and side bending are coupled to opposite sides. The motion is illustrated in figure 4.6a.

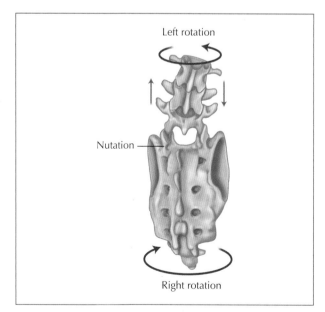

Figure 4.6a: *Sacral rotation and lumbar counter-rotation*

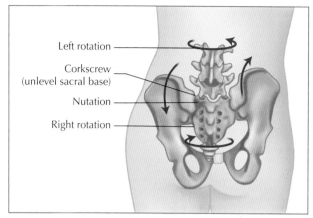

Figure 4.6b: *Sacral rotation and lumbar counter-rotation superimposed on the pelvic girdle*

We also need to mention and consider that, as the left side of the sacrum moves forward into nutation, the right side of the sacral base will move backward into counter-nutation *(R-on-R)*; this is mainly because of the slackening of the right sacrotuberous ligament and the continual anterior rotational movement of the right innominate bone during mid-stance.

Owing to the kinematics of the sacrum, the lumbar spine rotates left (opposite to the sacrum) and side bends to the right (type I mechanics) (figure 4.6b). The thoracic spine rotates right (same as the sacrum) and side bends to the left, and the cervical spine rotates right and side bends to the right. The cervical spine coupling is opposite to that of the other vertebrae, since its specific spinal motion is classified as *type II spinal mechanics* (type II means that rotation and side bending are coupled to the same side).

As the left leg moves from weight bearing to toe-off, the left innominate, the sacrum, and the lumbar and thoracic vertebrae undergo sacral torsion, rotation, and side bending in a similar manner to that described above, but with movements in the opposite directions.

■ Anterior oblique sling

The anterior oblique also works in conjunction with the stance leg adductors, ipsilateral internal oblique, and contralateral external oblique muscles (figure 4.7). These integrated muscle contractions help stabilize the body on top of the stance leg and assist in rotating the pelvis forward for optimum propulsion in preparation for the ensuing heel-strike.

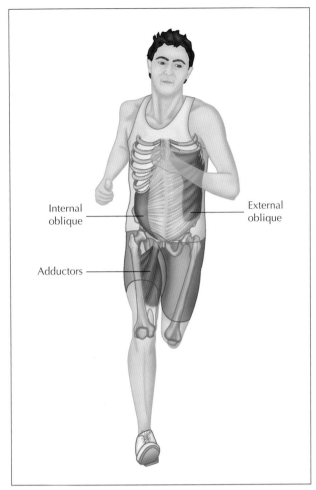

Figure 4.7: *A person running, with anterior oblique sling muscles highlighted*

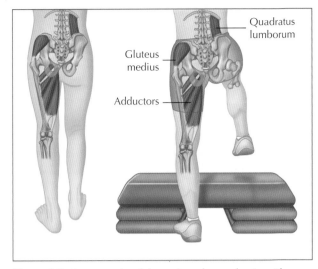

Figure 4.8: *An example of the swing phase of gait, with lateral sling muscles highlighted on the single-stance leg*

The abdominal oblique muscles, as well as the adductor muscle group, serve to provide stability and mobility during the gait cycle.

When looking at the EMG recordings of the oblique abdominals during gait and superimposing them on the cycle of adductor activity in gait, Basmajian and De Luca (1979) found that both sets of muscles (obliques and adductors) contribute to stability at the initiation of the stance phase of the gait cycle, as well as to the rotation of the pelvis and the action of pulling the leg through during the swing phase of gait. (This was also demonstrated by Inman et al. (1981).) As the speed of walking increases to running and sprinting speeds, the activation of the anterior oblique system becomes more prominent as well as a necessity.

The swing phase of gait utilizes the lateral sling system, as we have now entered the single-leg stance position. This sling connects the gluteus medius (Gmed) and the gluteus minimus (Gmin) of the stance leg, and the ipsilateral

(same side) adductors, with the contralateral (opposite) quadratus lumborum (QL) (figure 4.8). Contraction of the left Gmed and adductors stabilizes the pelvis, and activation of the contralateral QL will assist in elevation of the pelvis; this will allow enough lift of the pelvis to permit the leg to go through the swing phase of gait. The lateral sling plays a critical role, as it assists in stabilizing the spine and hip joints in the frontal plane and is a necessary contributor to the overall stability of the pelvis and trunk, and subsequently this has a knock on effect on the mechanics of the upper limb.

Not only does the lateral sling system provide stability that protects the working spinal and hip joints, but it is also a necessary contributor to the overall stability of the pelvis, trunk and of course the shoulder complex. Should the trunk and pelvis become unstable, the diminished stability will compromise one's ability to generate the forces necessary for moving the swing leg quickly, as required in many day to day working and sporting environments. Attempts to move the swing leg, or to generate force with the stance leg during gait and other functional activities, can easily disrupt the functionality of the SI joints as well as the lumbar spine and this results in dysfunction throughout the entire kinetic chain.

■ Gracovetsky's spinal engine theory

Serge Gracovetsky (1988) elaborated on a particular idea of spinal motion, which he discussed in his book *The Spinal Engine*. He considered the spine to be the 'primary engine' in the role for human locomotion and proposed that the legs were not responsible for gait, but were merely 'instruments of expression' and extensions of the spinal engine. He argued that the spine was not a rigid lever during the gait cycle and that its ability to produce axial compression and torsion was a fundamental driving force during locomotion.

In his discussions Gracovetsky says that during heel-strike, kinetic energy is not displaced into the earth as in the pedestrian model, but efficiently transmitted up through the myofascial system, causing the spine to resonate in the gravitational field. He did not view the spine as a compressive loading system, whereby the intervertebral discs act as shock absorbers; he regarded the outer annulus disc fibers and their accompanying facet joints as dynamic antigravity torsional springs that store and unload tensional forces to lift and propel the body in space. He also considered that the natural process of interlocking of the facet joints and intervertebral discs transmitted virtually all of the available counter-rotational pelvic torque that is needed to aid the inner and outer core muscles for locomotion.

Gracovetsky said:

> *'The spine is an engine driving the pelvis. Human anatomy is a consequence of function. The knee cannot be tested in isolation, as it is part of the overall function and purpose of the musculoskeletal system. The leg transfers the heel-strike energy to the spine. It is a mechanical filter. The knee is a critical part of that filter and improper energy transfer will affect spinal motion. Functional assessment of the spine ought to be part of the assessment of knee surgery.'*

Let us think back to the earlier concept of spinal and pelvis motion and it is this lumbar lateral flexion/rotation coupling that serves as the Gracovetsky spinal engine 'drivetrain.' For example, left lateral lumbar flexion will drive right rotation of the lumbar spine, and subsequently left rotation to the thoracic spine, and it continues through the whole of the shoulder complex.

What I would like to do now is return to the gait cycle and look at this concept in a slightly different way. Some authors have considered that the biceps femoris muscle of the hamstring group, along with its connection to the posterior longitudinal sling, effectively starts the spinal engine. The biceps femoris has been likened to the *pull cord* of the spinal engine in view of its action of inducing a 'force closure' mechanism in the SIJ. This closure of the SIJ will naturally lead to a subsequent transmission of force up into the osteo-articular-ligamentous tissues of the lumbosacral spine; this force will eventually continue

into the muscles of the lumbar and thoracic erector spinae.

EMG studies have demonstrated that the biceps femoris muscle is particularly active at the end of the swing phase of gait, through the early loading of the stance phase. During the transition from swing to stance, the heel contact phase of the gait cycle effectively closes the kinetic chain, and the biceps femoris can now perform its work in a manner that is commonly called a *closed kinetic chain*. Within the closed chain, the biceps femoris acts on its more proximal attachment within the chain, namely the pelvis. The biceps femoris attaches directly to the ischial tuberosity and also to the sacrotuberous ligament, sacrum, iliac crests, and up through the multifidi and lumbar erector spinae.

At heel contact the ipsilateral (same side) hip and contralateral (opposite side) shoulder is in a position of flexion, which effectively preloads the posterior oblique sling (see figure 4.5), specifically the ipsilateral Gmax and contralateral latissimus dorsi. This allows extra-spinal propulsion in a 'sling-like' manner, with the superficial lamina of the thoracolumbar fascia serving as an intermediary between these kinetically linked muscles.

The force transmitted through the osteo-articular-ligamentous structures induces 'form closure' of the spinal facet joints and rotation in the lumbar spine; coupled with a lateral flexion moment, the spinal engine *initiates and selects the gears* to drive the pelvis into a forward rotation. The induced lumbar rotation effectively stores elastic energy in the spinal ligaments and the annulus fibroses of the intervertebral discs, and it is this return of energy that drives gait.

In order to return the energy, the spine must be stabilized from above: this is accomplished via contralateral arm swing and trunk rotation produced by the contralateral Gmax and latissimus dorsi involvement. The coupling patterns of the spine have evolved to facilitate the return of this force. The counter-rotation is considered to be recruited directly from the spine and not from the legs.

Maitland (2001) mentions that the way our axial skeletal system alternately undulates in side bending and rotation as we walk is very interesting and extremely important to our overall well-being. It is a movement that is reminiscent of the undulating action of a snake as it slithers through the grass. The big difference between a snake and a human, of course, is that our snakelike spine has ended up having two legs on which to walk.

■ Clarification

Some of the information in this chapter may not seem to be immediately relevant to the subject of the shoulder. What I can say in my defense, however, is that often one might need to look at the bigger, overall picture with certain patients, especially if these patients have ongoing chronic neck, shoulder and arm pain – the underlying causative factor might well be connected to the walking cycle and to how the 'engine' of the spine is considered the primary drivetrain for us to be able to put one foot in front of the other. If this engine breaks down then we will naturally suffer the consequences somewhere in our body. You have only to watch someone trying to walk relatively normally when they have an issue such as plantar fasciitis, a meniscal tear in the knee, a degenerative hip joint, or even just a sling placed across one shoulder to protect a sprain of the AC joint or a shoulder dislocation. You will see how the body's compensatory mechanisms kick in to change our gait pattern, especially when we have an underlying joint or muscular pain of origin.

5

Differential diagnosis of shoulder pathology

When I teach the shoulder joint masterclass at my clinic within the University of Oxford, it is to students from all the corners of the earth, a fact that makes me feel truly honored. Nevertheless, when, during the course of the class, I discuss differential diagnosis of shoulder pain and upper limb pain, I have often found it disappointing how little knowledge many physical therapists have regarding other bodily structures and vital organs (viscera or viscus) that can be the underlying causative factor for the patient's presenting symptoms (or at least contribute to it). Medically trained personnel, whose initial training is generally longer, may have greater knowledge but hopefully this chapter will be of interest to all readers and serve as a reminder of the specific pathologies that can cause shoulder or upper limb pain. It is very important that pain from a musculoskeletal origin can be differentiated from a visceral pathology because they can easily mimic each other in terms of how they present, as we will read shortly.

An article I wrote many years ago discussed five individual patients that presented to my clinic with shoulder pain. What was of particular interest was that they all had something in common. Each was asked to place their arm by their side and to perform a movement of shoulder abduction as far as they could comfortably reach and to try to raise their arm over their head to the normal range of motion (typically classified as 180 degrees).

All were aware that something was 'not quite right' during the movement: three of them had actual pain on motion during abduction of their arm. The first patient was a 75-year-old male who had fallen off a ladder onto his right shoulder and when he presented to the clinic he was not able to even initiate abduction actively, even though I could take his arm to 180 degrees passively without any pain. The second patient was a 34-year-old female painter and decorator and she presented with pain only between 60 and 110 degrees of abduction (after a weekend of painting ceilings) – this is typically called a painful arc. The third patient was a 24-year-old rugby player. He had sustained an injury to the top of his shoulder when he was tackled in a game and he had pain towards the end of the range of motion for abduction. The fourth patient was a 55-year-old female. She had started to notice her shoulder was getting stiffer since doing a fitness class 6 weeks ago and now had limited movement of the shoulder joint and could not even lift the arm to 60 degrees without feeling restriction and subsequent pain. The fifth person was a 45-year-old male. He did not have the ability to abduct his shoulder past 20 degrees (but could initiate) and this had happened after doing some push-ups in the morning when he woke up. The patient could lift his arm to 20 degrees but could go no further without some pain and weakness and it appeared that the deltoid muscle was not working. At the time I considered this was due to a potential muscle weakness of some sort or possibly caused by a neurological problem.

My personal belief about treatment of the shoulder complex tends to chime with a methodology that was taught to me many years ago, when I was student of manual therapy. It is known as the K.I.S.S. principle (Keep it simple stupid!), or the *keep it simple* principle. I always say to my therapy students that if a patient presents with what they believe to be an 'actual shoulder' or upper limb problem and they are having an issue in terms of pain or restriction during abduction or even flexion of their shoulder to 180 degrees, it is probably a localized shoulder complex issue or pathology that would need addressing through hands-on physical therapy, whether that is considered to be the right or wrong approach. This approach currently seems to work well for me with my own patients and athletes.

Regarding the five case studies above (see also figure 5.1), the first patient had what I believed to be a full thickness tear (rupture) of the supraspinatus, the second an impingement syndrome of the subacromial bursa and/or a supraspinatus tendinopathy. The third patient, who presented with pain at the end range for abduction, sustained an acromioclavicular joint (AC joint) sprain, the fourth I diagnosed with a chronic frozen shoulder (adhesive capsulitis) and the last I considered to have an axillary nerve palsy due to the inability to activate the deltoid muscle during abduction (axillary nerve, which originates from the cervical nerve root level of C5 and specifically innervates the deltoid and teres minor muscles).

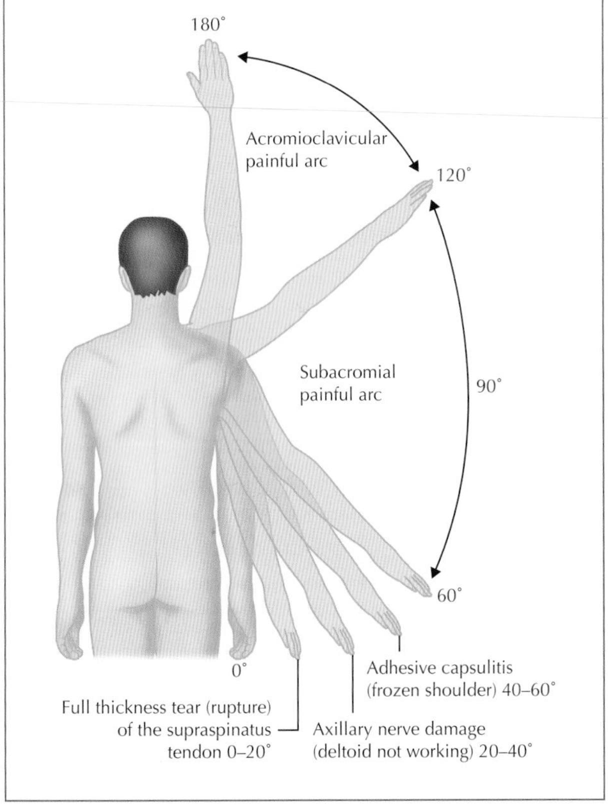

Figure 5.1: *Abduction of 0–180 degrees and the five specific conditions*

Regarding the last case study, many therapists with a good knowledge base might say it could be a C5 nerve root problem that is potentially causing the weakness with shoulder abduction, and that is perfectly correct because the person had weakness abducting their arm.

However, the C5 myotome also innervates the motion of elbow flexion and in this case the patient tested strong for contraction of the biceps muscle. Also, there was no weakness to other C5 innervated muscles like the supraspinatus or infraspinatus. In this case, therefore, it cannot be a C5 nerve root issue.

I used to be a vehicle electrician when I was in the military and I consider the axillary nerve to be similar to a sidelight or indicator on your car: if the bulb has blown or the wire has been cut (open circuit) then the light will cease to function. For the axillary nerve, if the little wire (nerve) that supplies the deltoid and teres minor has been damaged, this can subsequently cause the nerve to switch off (the muscle now becomes inhibited and/or the light bulb goes off or dims). As a result the muscles in question will test weak and will start to atrophy (waste) very quickly. However, everything else in the body (or car) will work as normal, and initially you might not notice a problem. It will not be long, though, before you are aware of the underlying issue.

So the next time someone walks into your clinic with shoulder pain, if you bear in mind what I have said regarding the motion of abduction, I am sure it will help you come to a diagnosis or a hypothesis of localized pathology or not.

To recap, if a patient is standing and is asked to abduct their arm to 180 degrees and the person is aware of something during this motion (e.g., pain, restriction, weakness) then there is a good likelihood that this patient has some dysfunction present that requires further investigation. However, if the patient in question is able to fully abduct as well as to flex their shoulder to 180 degrees, without mentioning anything, and the movement is fluid and pain free, then one needs to consider the following: does this patient actually have an underlying pathology with the shoulder complex? Remember what was discussed earlier concerning the scapulohumeral rhythm and the structures involved to allow this motion to happen? Simply lifting the arm above the head requires the precise interaction of the GH, ST, AC and SC joints, as well as the integration of all of the soft tissues and nerve innervations.

There are a multitude of reasons why patients or athletes present with shoulder pain and below I would like to discuss some of those conditions.

CASE STUDY

A lady in her mid 40s presented to the clinic, with pain generally located to the top of her right shoulder and upper trapezius muscle. This has been present for many months with no obvious cause. During the day the lady was not aware of her pain, but at night, while she was sleeping, the right shoulder was noticeably worse to the point she would wake up, take some medication and eventually fall back to sleep. The lady also mentioned something was not quite right with her middle to lower thoracic spine but she said her shoulder pain was the priority. On examination, I asked the lady to abduct her shoulder as far as she felt comfortable, and to my surprise she could easily reach a full range of motion to 180 degrees. It was the same when she was asked to flex the shoulder and also managed to reach the full 180 degrees of motion with no issues. Because the lady could abduct and flex the shoulder to full range, I considered that there *could not* be any underlying musculoskeletal issue present directly related with the region of shoulder complex.

This next sentence or two might sound a bit strange as I asked the patient the following: 'When you go to the toilet for a number two (defecation), have you noticed that your stool has a tendency to float on the surface, rather than sinking to the bottom of the bowl?' Unsurprisingly, the lady looked a little startled but responded by saying 'funny you should ask that question but yes, my stool does seem to float when I go to the toilet.'

Before I continue with the case study, ask yourself why I asked this particular question – what do you think was going through my thought processes? Before I actually answer this question, I want to mention something that was taught to me when I was studying osteopathy. One particular lecture that I found of great interest and remembered was on 'differential diagnosis of musculoskeletal pain in physical therapy.' The tutor had talked about a female patient that presented to him with right-sided shoulder pain who surprisingly had full range of motion (ROM) without any pain in all the tested movements. The tutor proceeded to discuss something known as the four 'F's – female, fair, fat and forty. You can probably guess that it relates to an overweight lady with fair coloring who is in early middle age. The patient in the case study certainly fitted this picture. Basically, the tutor had said if a patient comes to your clinic with right-sided shoulder pain and fits the criteria of the four Fs then one needs to consider that the *gall bladder* might be the underlying causative factor for their presenting symptoms of pain located to the right shoulder. Common pathologies that occur with the gall bladder are inflammation of the gall bladder (cholecystitis) and gallstones (cholelithiasis).

I am hoping at this point that I have whet your appetite enough for you to want to gain more underpinning knowledge of the subject matter and hopefully you are now trying to work out in your head the following: so how does the organ of the gall bladder cause right-sided shoulder pain? As far as I understand it there are two possible processes at work: one process is related to embryology and it is considered that when you are a foetus growing in your mothers womb, the gall bladder initially originates from the area near to the right shoulder and as you develop, the gall bladder naturally descends to its resting position underneath the lower rib cage located on the right side of the body. This means that if you have an inflamed gall bladder, or even gallstones, in some way the gall bladder remembers its original position from when it was forming inside of you as a foetus and subsequently pain is now present in the right shoulder.

The second process, which I am more inclined to believe, is the proximity of a nerve called the phrenic nerve and its relationship to the gall bladder. The phrenic nerve innervates the central component of the respiratory muscle of the diaphragm (it is a musculotendinous structure and not a viscus). This nerve originates from C3, C4 and C5 and there is a simple mnemonic that states *C3, 4, 5 keep the diaphragm alive*. This relates to spinal cord trauma, in that if you damage the spinal cord below the level of C5 then you should be able to breathe for yourself unassisted; however, if you damage the spinal cord above this level then you might need to have artificial respiration. However, the peripheral part of the diaphragm is innervated by the lower six intercostal nerves and subsequently, does not refer pain to the shoulder complex.

Let us now look at the scenario of an inflamed gall bladder. Because of its close proximity to the diaphragm and the phrenic nerve (figure 5.2a) there is a stimulus that excites the neurological system and subsequently a signal is relayed back to the origins of the nerve that is located to the area of the cervical spine from levels C3–5. If you look at a map of the neurological dermatomes, you will notice that C3–5 actually covers the area of the upper limb and in particular, the area of the shoulder region (figure 5.2b). Pain that is referred from the diaphragm is typically felt near the superior angle of the scapula, along the suprascapular fossa and even along the upper trapezius muscle, and it can be exacerbated when the patient coughs, sneezes, or deep breathes. What I am saying is this: if you have a pathological issue with your gall bladder then the chances of having right shoulder pain is increased because the pain signals are transmitted back to the cervical spine and the sensory input is then transported to the peripheral nerve and subsequent dermatomes.

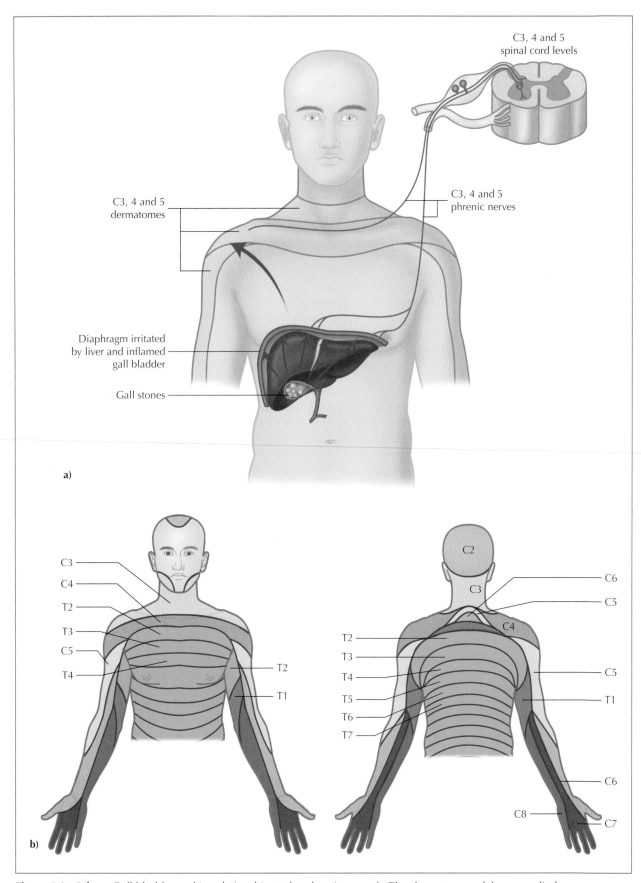

Figure 5.2a & b: *a. Gall bladder and its relationship to the phrenic nerve b. The dermatomes of the upper limb*

One could look at this as a *referred pattern of pain*. Let me give you an example: someone is having a myocardial infarction (heart attack). The person will naturally feel intense pain in the area of the central chest; however, most patients describe feeling other areas of pain or sensations and these can be felt in the mid thoracic spine, left arm and hand, and even towards the left side of face and jaw. What I want to do now is give an analogy for this process. Imagine you are travelling to London by train on a Monday morning at rush hour, arriving at, say, Paddington station. Hundreds of people will get off the train at the same time. The conductor directs them through the normal gates (relate this to chest pain). Nevertheless, because so many people are getting off the train, a queue forms and now the conductor diverts some people to alternative gates (left side of face and jaw), and if they also become busy, to another gate, which might be a few extra minutes walk away (arm and hand). I hope that this analogy makes some sense to you. To put it simply, if the gall bladder is inflamed then this organ can refer to the right shoulder via the phrenic nerve as well as to the area of the mid-lower thoracic spine. This is due to the sympathetic nerve celiac ganglia innervation of the gall bladder and because of the proximity of the gall bladder to the abdomen the patient could perceive pain to the right lower costal margin, which is located to the upper right quadrant of the abdomen.

Conclusion

Regarding the lady from the above case study, I mentioned to her that I thought it was the gall bladder that was responsible for her pain to her right shoulder as well as discomfort in the mid-lower thoracic spine. I discussed with her the function of the gall bladder in terms of breaking down fatty foods, etc., that and if this organ does not function correctly then the stool has a tendency to float. I also discussed through anatomical books and diagrams how the gall bladder caused pain to her right shoulder via the phrenic nerve. There is also a small area under the lower right costal margin (rib) that when palpated (especially with the patient breathing in), may cause a rebound tenderness (figure 5.3). This is known as Murphy's sign and is a positive finding for an inflamed gall bladder, especially if the same procedure is performed on the left side of the abdomen with no perceived pain from the patient.

I wrote a letter to my patient's GP, explaining my findings and she had a meeting with a gastrointestinal consultant who confirmed it was pathology with the gall bladder and removed it a few weeks later. The patient in question had a follow-up appointment a few weeks after the surgery and I was pleased to see that her shoulder and thoracic pain had disappeared.

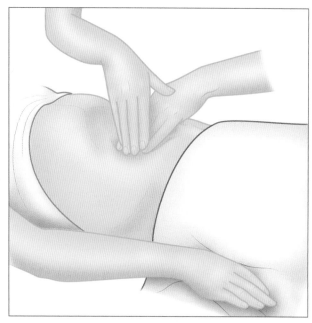

Figure 5.3: *Palpation for rebound tenderness of gall bladder pathology – Murphy's sign*

This type of condition is what is described as a *visceral-somatic* dysfunction because the organ (viscera) is the underlying causative factor for pain to present itself to the somatic/soma region (body), in this case pain the right shoulder.

Regarding pathology of the gall bladder, patients can also present with upper right abdominal pain, as well as nausea and vomiting, after eating fatty meals. They might also present with jaundice, low-grade fever and weight loss, especially if there is a cancer present.

■ Liver

The liver (hepatic) can suffer pathologies such as cirrhosis, tumors, and hepatitis. This organ has an association with the gall bladder and common bile duct (biliary) and these organs commonly present with musculoskeletal presentations to the area of the right shoulder, right upper trapezius (due to the liver's contact with the central portion of the diaphragm), thoracic spine, and interscapular regions of the upper body, as well as pain in the right upper quadrant of the abdomen (figure 5.4). The liver is the most common site for secondary cancer metastasis (especially in men older than 50 years of age) as a result of other primary cancer sites such as the stomach, lung, and pancreas, as well as breast cancers in women.

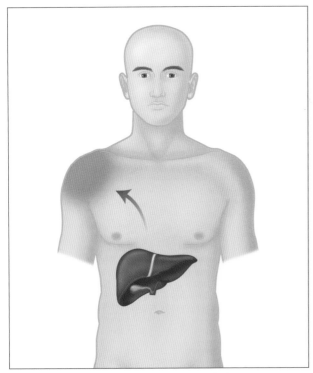

Figure 5.4: *Pain sites from the liver, gall bladder and common bile duct*

The sympathetic nerve fibers from the hepatic and biliary systems are connected through the splanchnic and celiac plexuses and have their origins from the thoracic spine, potentially giving interscapular pain and possibly intercostal pain. The splanchnic nerves synapse with the phrenic nerve, hence producing pain to the area of the right shoulder.

From a physical therapy perspective, the practitioner might be the first person who initially sees this patient, who presents with what they think is a simple musculoskeletal problem. It is of paramount importance that a detailed case history is taken, making close observations of the patient's physical appearance and well-being and looking for any obvious skin changes. The physical therapist will need to diversify and ask appropriate non-musculoskeletal questions that relate to the urinary and gastrointestinal systems. For example, one of the functions of the liver or biliary system is to convert bile from bilirubin, which gives the stool its natural brown color. If, due to some pathology, these systems lose the ability to excrete bilirubin, then the color of the urine can change and it becomes dark, almost like the color of coke or tea. This also has the effect of changing the stool from its normal brown appearance to a light color.

■ Spleen

CASE STUDY

I was reading a case study of a young male who was playing rugby one Sunday afternoon when he was tackled and hit the ground hard, landing on the left side of his body and feeling pretty winded. The physiotherapist gave him some assistance and said it would be best if he came off the pitch because they felt he needed to rest. After the game the player complained of left shoulder pain and the therapist said he might have damaged his rotator cuff and gave him some strengthening exercises. After a restful night the player woke up in the morning with severe pain to his left shoulder but still managed to go to work. While he was sitting at his desk he collapsed and was rushed to the emergency department, where a diagnosis of a ruptured spleen was made.

Think back to the proximity of the phrenic nerve to the aforementioned organs, as explained earlier; in this particular case the spleen is located on the left side of the body, at a similar level to the gall bladder and liver on the right side. A damaged or ruptured spleen can also refer pain but this time to the left shoulder (figure 5.5) rather than the right, as in the earlier case study: however, the C3–5 dermatomes are still involved because of the

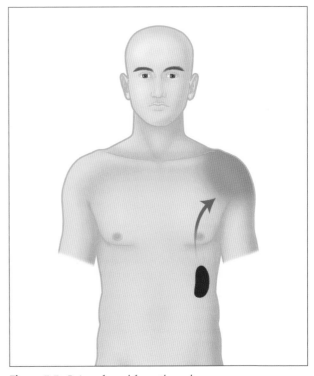

Figure 5.5: *Pain referred from the spleen*

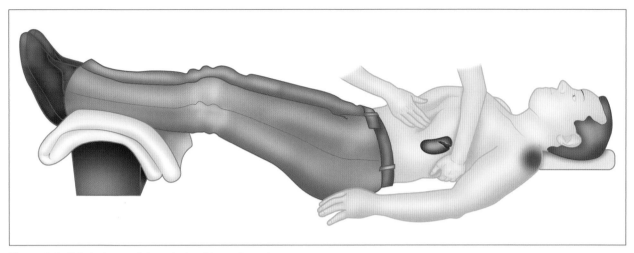

Figure 5.6: *Kehr's sign and the relationship to the spleen*

relationship to the phrenic nerve with the subsequent referral pattern to the region of the left shoulder. There are many problems that present to therapists, especially in a sporting context. It is very easy to come to a diagnosis of a rotator cuff tear when a player complains of shoulder pain. However, if the physiotherapist had assessed the player fully, then they would have probably seen a full range of motion into abduction and flexion of the shoulder complex, without any pain, and that in itself should have been a red flag for a medical referral. The history in this case would be beneficial and might have suggested a medical referral, because the patient had history of trauma with sudden onset of symptoms, especially with left shoulder pain. There is a sign called Kehr's sign and that is pain that typically presents itself to the tip of the shoulder. The most common cause of this pain in the left shoulder is a ruptured spleen (figure 5.6).

■ Lung carcinoma (Pancoast tumor)

A US radiologist called Henry Pancoast described a type of lung cancer that is called a *Pancoast tumor* and is defined primarily by its location at the extreme apex (very top) of the right *or* left lung (figure 5.7). The reason I am writing about lung carcinoma and the shoulder is because of the relationship to the lower roots of the brachial plexus and subclavian artery. When the tumor is progressing it can affect the nerves and blood vessels and potentially mimic a thoracic outlet syndrome (TOS). Thus the patient can present with pain to the areas of the shoulder, axilla, scapula, arm, and hand as well as atrophy/ weakness of the hand and arm muscles. Because of the location of these tumors within the apex, they are less likely to cause typical symptoms seen with general lung

cancer, such as shortness of breath, persistent cough, and coughing up blood.

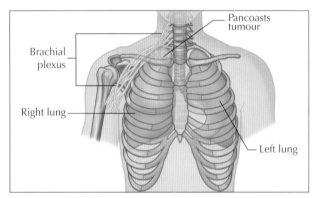

Figure 5.7: *Pancoast tumor*

Typically, later stages of a Pancoast tumor cause a *Horner's* syndrome, due to compression of the sympathetic ganglion (figure 5.8). The symptoms in severe cases include the following: drooping of the eyelid (ptosis), constriction of the pupil (miosis), and lack of sweating to one side of the face (anhidrosis).

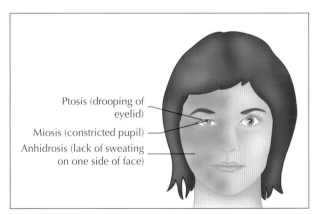

Figure 5.8: *Horner's syndrome*

Other symptoms of a Pancoast tumor are unexplained weight loss, loss of appetite, fatigue, sleep disturbance, chest tightness, and arm or hand weakness.

CASE STUDY

A 68-year-old woman was referred by her local doctor to a physiotherapy clinic for treatment of chronic shoulder pain. The patient had a 12-week ongoing history of constant, severe pain in the right shoulder. This pain also radiated beneath her scapula, into the right axilla (armpit) and around the right side of the chest wall. She mentioned an awareness of shortness of breath and complained of increased pain and chest tightness, especially on deep breathing.

The pain was exacerbated by walking a short distance, sitting, and even turning over in bed. On further questioning she also reported reduced appetite as well as sleep disturbance due to the discomfort and that she was a long-term heavy smoker.

On examination, this patient had a 'normal' shoulder in terms of range of motion but there were some cervical and thoracic spine movements that were restricted and painful; this was considered to be caused by age-related degenerative changes. There was no arm pain or paresthesia; however, the patient mentioned her right hand had symptoms of grip weakness, loss of dexterity (probably because of the compression from the tumor to the lower brachial plexus of C8/T1 – ulnar nerve) and a feeling of her arm 'not belonging to her.' On neurological testing there was no deficit in reflex testing nor was there any obvious weakness of the muscles for the corresponding myotomes for C5/6/7 within the upper limbs.

The patient had private health insurance and requested an MRI scan rather than a standard X-ray as soon as possible because she was naturally worried about her symptoms. The medical diagnosis was that of a large Pancoast tumor. Unfortunately, because of the size of the tumor it was considered inoperable so palliative care was given before the lady passed away a few months later. The patient did not present with Horner's syndrome in this instance because the tumor had not progressed far enough to compress the paravertebral sympathetic nerves.

■ Stomach and duodenal

Both the stomach and small intestine (duodenum) can be a source of pain to the right shoulder and in particular to the superior angle of scapula as well as to the area of the suprascapular region and the upper trapezius muscle. It is commonly considered that *Helicobacter pylori* (*H. pylori*) infection is the main cause of the majority of abdominal conditions that are specifically related to gastric or duodenal ulcers. Approximately 10% of ulcers are caused through chronic use of nonsteroidal anti-inflammatory drugs (NSAIDs) such as ibuprofen, naproxen and aspirin, which are often taken long term for arthritic types of medical conditions.

The physical therapist has to be continually aware of other presenting signs and symptoms because pain located to the midline of the epigastrium or upper abdomen as well as pain to the right shoulder could possibly be referred from the gall bladder and liver as well as from the stomach or small intestine. One has to be intuitive through correct questioning during the initial history taking, because there are almost certainly other signs and symptoms present that are associated with the above organs. For example, does the pain change during specific times, such as when eating meals? Have you noticed the stool is particularly dark (this darkness within the stool is called a melena, and can relate to a bleed that is located within the upper section of the alimentary canal, stomach or small intestine)?

CASE STUDY

A man in his mid twenties came to my clinic presenting with pain to his mid to lower thoracic spine and also mentioned an awareness of something that was not quite right in his right shoulder but he couldn't say quite what exactly. These symptoms had been present for many months and did not seem to be going away. When I assessed the patient and focused initially on the area of the thoracic spine, I found that he had particular spinal restrictions and tenderness to the area of T4–9. I also noticed that the skin overlying that area of the spine had trophic changes (dry, scaly, pimply skin) and would become hyperemic (reddening of the skin) quite quickly on light palpation. The muscles overlying the thoracic spine felt very firm to the touch and I considered them to be hypertonic (increased state of contraction). During the medical screening, I asked him about particular things that would exacerbate his symptoms and he replied by smiling and saying 'beer and curries' seemed to make his symptoms feel worse. I asked him how often he ate these and he said he had a few beers every evening and frequently enjoyed a spicy curry. I told this gentleman to see his general practitioner, because I felt an ulcer was responsible for his presenting symptoms (figure 5.9). I also mentioned that physical therapy in this instance would probably not be of any value. The patient telephoned me a few weeks later and confirmed my diagnosis of an ulcer, the cause of being *H. pylori* infection. He is now on medication for the infection and I am pleased to say that he has also reduced his regular intake of alcohol and curries. I am hoping that in time he makes a full recovery.

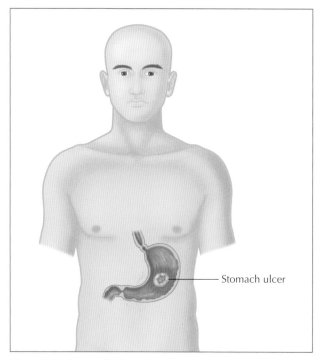

Figure 5.9: *Stomach ulcer*

Regarding the trophic changes to his thoracic spine, this was related to the sympathetic nerves from the stomach and small intestine being overstimulated, a condition called sympathetictonia (increased tone of the sympathetic nervous system); this condition alters the tone of the overlying muscles, as well as affecting the function of the sebaceous glands and hair follicles. In my medical notes, I remember writing down that he presented with a visceral-somatic (viscera (organ) responsible for causing pain to the soma (body)) dysfunction and the underlying cause was more than likely to be a peptic ulcer.

CASE STUDY

I had the privilege of knowing my very good friend Mark (renamed here to hide his true identity) for over ten years. Mark was a physical therapist who lived in Wales. When he approached his sixties he decided to do an online test for colon cancer, and unfortunately, the test was positive for carcinoma. Over the next few months he had the

majority of his colon removed, with continual treatments of chemotherapy and radiotherapy. I saw Mark a year or so after his diagnosis and he was a changed man. He must have lost over 4 stone (25 kg) in weight. The months passed and everything seemed to be going well. However, when Mark attended a course with me in Oxford in the November, he mentioned a swelling above his left clavicle (supraclavicular fossa) and complained of left shoulder discomfort. The GP had put him on medication and he could not venture into the sunlight because of the prescribed medication: the doctors had found something within his left lung, but didn't actually say what they found and further tests were needed.

I thought to myself that this would probably be the last time I would see my good friend and not surprisingly this became a reality: in late December he passed away. The diagnosis was stomach carcinoma and this was probably related to the initial primary colon cancer that caused secondary cancers that had metastasized to his stomach and lung. The left swelling that was present within the left supraclavicular fossa was probably due to metastasizing enlargements of the lymph nodes from the stomach cancer. It is a known fact that the left supraclavicular fossa can be one of the first signs of stomach cancer and malignancies of the stomach can actually be asymptomatic, and reach an advanced stage before giving any symptoms. This particular left-sided lymph node related to the above is called *Virchow's node* (named in 1848 after the German pathologist Rudolf Virchow) and has the scary alternative name of the 'devils' lymph node, for obvious reasons.

The thoracic duct (left side) in relation to the lymphatic system is like a reservoir (unlike the right side) and it is responsible for draining the lymphatic fluid for the majority of the body before it enters subclavian veins of the venous system. If there are metastases present then the thoracic duct can be blocked and this blockage causes a regurgitation of the lymphatic fluid into the surrounding lymph nodes (Virchow) (figure 5.10).

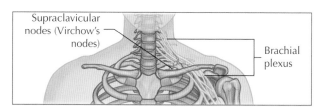

Figure 5.10: *Virchow's lymph nodes*

Pancreas

Generally speaking, the pancreas, especially in the case of carcinoma rather than pancreatitis (inflammation)), can be nonspecific and rather vague in terms of the presenting signs and symptoms. It has been clinically proven that lower back pain may be the only symptom that the patients present with. I can guarantee that if a patient walks into the clinic and presents with lower back pain the majority of physical therapists and medical practitioners will *not* suspect pancreatic carcinoma and will consider other musculoskeletal causes of back pain. However, some of the following signs and symptoms might also be present; if so, that should arouse suspicion:

- upper abdominal pain (epigastric) that radiates to the back
- unexplained weight loss and loss of appetite
- light colored stools
- dark urine
- constipation
- nausea and vomiting
- lower back pain
- left shoulder pain
- jaundice.

Patients with pathology of their pancreas tend to find relief by bending forward and bringing their knees to their chest and the symptoms are sometimes exacerbated by drinking alcohol, eating food and even walking or lying flat (supine) with legs straight.

CASE STUDY

Recently, one of the therapists whom I had had the privilege of teaching emailed me to say that she had a patient who presented with left shoulder pain as well as abdominal pains and increased weight loss over a short period of time. The GP said it was indigestion and sent her home; however, my therapist was concerned it was more than just indigestion and sent her back the next day. After further investigations, the patient was diagnosed with pancreatic cancer and unfortunately passed away quite soon after she was given the full diagnosis. The therapist in question messaged me the following week and said she had another patient. He was a male in his fifties who played badminton four times a week and cycled a lot and he came to her clinic with presenting symptoms mainly to his left groin that were relieved by *curling* up. He also mentioned left shoulder and some abdominal symptoms. He too was referred to the GP and unfortunately was also

diagnosed with pancreatic cancer and passed away a few weeks later.

Over the last few years I have lectured to many thousands of therapists from all corners of the earth. In these courses I have rarely talked about the pancreas causing shoulder and groin pain. This is mainly because I have so much information to cover in one day that it is difficult to include every single thing that therapists might see in their practice – the course would end up taking five days rather than one. However, from now on, I can guarantee that when teaching my shoulder and hip joint master class I will always talk about the pancreas, and I am truly pleased to look back at the email I received from my previous student and to see that she remembered my mentioning the shoulder pain/cancer link during the workshop she had taken (figure 5.11). I am very pleased to say that at least some of the knowledge I pass on can be of value, so thank you Kathryn Kemp for being on top of your game.

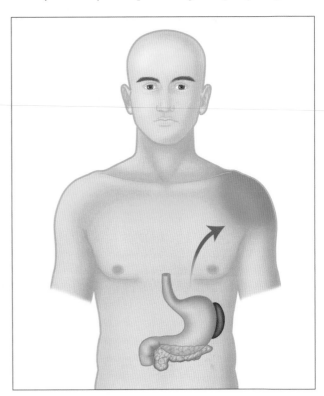

Figure 5.11: *Typical areas of pain associated with the pancreas*

Kidney

I have personally seen thousands of patients and I do not think I can recall any one of these having shoulder pain that was directly related to pathology of a kidney. Then again, maybe in my earlier years of training I might have missed this underlying causative factor of symptoms to the shoulder.

The kidney will potentially only cause ipsilateral (same side) shoulder pain if it contacts and causes increased pressure to the diaphragm and we know the relationship to the phrenic nerve (already discussed previously). It is not in the scope of this text to go through all the specific medical conditions that relate to the renal and urologic system; however, some of the signs and symptoms might be of concern to the physical therapist. Renal pain is commonly felt in the posterior subcostal and costovertebral region (figure 5.12). The pain can also be felt around the flank into the lower abdominal quadrant and even radiating into the testicular/genitalia area. As you can see from figure 5.12, lower back and possible ipsilateral shoulder pain might also be present.

Hopefully, after reading about the above specific medical conditions, my overall goal would be to make you more aware of some of the pathologies that can give rise to patients with so-called musculoskeletal presentations and in particular, pain that presents itself to the region of the shoulder complex. The underlying pathologies that I have discussed might be classified as *red flag conditions* and will require further investigation. Remember that many patients will come and see the physical therapist first with any painful symptoms rather than their primary care physician. We have a duty of care to the overall well-being of all of the patients that walk through our clinic door and we need to know *when to treat* and more importantly, *when not to treat and to refer to the medical profession*. That statement of when to refer has to be of the utmost priority because it can simply be a life or death situation, I hope you remember that when the time comes!

There are many other pathologies that I have not mentioned that can refer pain to the shoulder. However, my focus here is to try and make you aware of how the viscera actually refer pain to other structures within the musculoskeletal framework and especially to the region of the shoulder complex. With the correct questioning during the initial consultation and the appropriate orthopedic testing protocols, we can hopefully eliminate the musculoskeletal tissues as a source of a patient's presenting symptoms, especially if the practitioner cannot reproduce their symptoms during the physical therapy examination. It is time then to consider that the symptoms the patients are presenting with might actually be referred from pathology of the viscera rather than being musculoskeletal in origin.

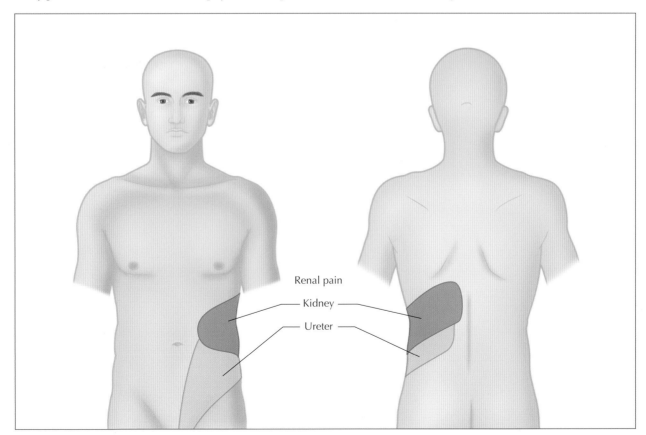

Figure 5.12: *Typical areas associated with renal and urologic pain*

6

The relationship of the cervical spine and nerves to the shoulder complex

It goes without saying that the cervical spine (CSP) has a direct relationship to all the unique components that make up the shoulder complex. There are at this moment probably thousands of people throughout the world that consider their presenting shoulder or upper limb pain to be actually coming from the shoulder joint or the associated structures. For the majority, however, it may be the cervical spine that is the underlying causative factor, not only of their presenting shoulder pain but also other symptoms they might have in the arm and hand.

My own thought process is that the cervical and shoulder are like a marriage or a conjoined partnership: simply speaking, if one breaks down or becomes dysfunctional (or maybe pathological as this is a medical relationship), then the other component will not be able to cope and has to compensate in one way or another. I always teach the following concepts: if one has a problem with the shoulder complex, then eventually this becomes a problem with/ the cervical spine and vice versa; that is, a problem with the cervical spine eventually becomes a problem with the shoulder complex. This latter concept probably makes more sense to me.

I have an interesting story to share with you. During the course of a soft tissue class I asked whether anyone attending had shoulder pain, since that was going to be the next topic we covered. Within a micro-second of myself saying those words, a gentlemen shot his hand up (waving his arm vigorously in the air to me from the back of the class), saying, "yes, I have a BIG problem with my shoulder" (while keeping his arm in the air!). I responded that I doubted that the pain was in the arm that was currently still in the air, especially given the speed he lifted it. No, said the man, it was the arm that was in the air that had the pain. There lies a problem, because to him it was a BIG problem with his shoulder; however, I would classify it as a LITTLE problem with his shoulder, especially after the assessment and treatment, as it was not actually his shoulder that was the causative problem of his pain. You can probably guess that his was a referred pain that he felt within the shoulder complex but that was radiating from his cervical spine.

CASE STUDY

A local personal trainer friend of mine who runs a cross-fit gymnasium referred one of his clients to me because he had difficulty performing one of the exercises in the routine. The exercise in question was to simply lie on your back on a bench and then to extend the elbows using two dumbbells (shown in figure 6.1). You can see that the left arm cannot extend as far as the right one and this was due to weakness. This exercise is designed to strengthen the triceps muscle group.

However, what I found interesting was the client in question did not mention that he had any form of pain or even any restriction in the neck, shoulder and arms; he simply had a weakness in performing that particular

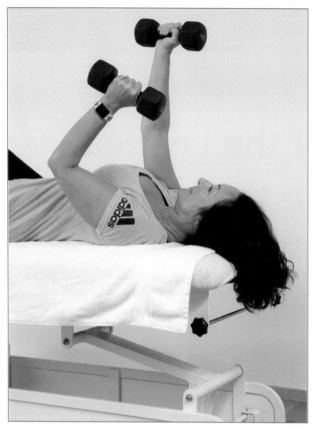

Figure 6.1: *Elbow extension exercise using the triceps – left side limited due to weakness*

maneuver. The personal trainer took a video of him performing the motion so that I could have a better understanding of the underlying problem. (I actually show this video to students on the neurological and cervical spine courses and ask them what they think is the problem.)

Some of you will be reading this and know straight away what the problem was; however, the majority will probably struggle, especially because he presented with no pain or restriction.

Later in this chapter I will be discussing power testing of the upper limb. This is what is called myotome testing. I remember watching a Canadian chiropractor who travelled over to treat a few of the Oxford University rowers that were previous Olympians from Canada. Initially, he would test the power (myotomes) of the upper and lower limb and when he felt he found a specific neurological weakness he would proceed to adjust/manipulate the specific level of the spine. After the treatment the chiropractor would then retest the power (myotome) of the motion and hopefully the power would be seen to test as normal (grade 5).

I have been trying to use similar concepts ever since, so when I tested the above client and focused on the power of elbow extension, I found the left side was very weak in comparison to the right side. If you look at the table of myotomes later in this chapter, you will notice that the C7 myotome could have been the level that was the underlying problem. The C7 nerve root passes between the level of C6 and C7 so it could also have been disc pathology. However, because there was no altered sensation or pain, then I considered he had a rotated vertebra (subluxation in some chiropractor terms) that was tensioning the exiting C7 nerve that subsequently gave him weakness on extending the left elbow.

An analogy I sometimes use is of a *dimmer switch*: if one turns the switch in one direction the light becomes dimmer – there is *less* current or power going to the light bulb; if we turn it the other way the bulb gets brighter. If the wire (nerve) is being turned or compressed for some reason (vertebral rotation) then the power (current) along the C7 nerve pathway is reduced, and subsequently the bulb becomes dimmer, or in this case the movement or power of elbow extension will test or show weakness.

My treatment consisted mainly of a specific cervical spinal mobilization and then a manipulation technique to the left side of C6/7, and an audible cavitation was heard. I then retested his power of left elbow extension and was very happy to say to the patient that the power had come back to normal. The personal trainer messaged me a few days later to say training had commenced and there was no weakness present.

The reason I discuss the above case study is to try and make you aware of an alternative way of assessing the upper limb through myotome testing of the neurological system. I know many therapists that consider pain located to the shoulder complex, arm and hands to *only* be coming from the cervical spine. That means all the treatments they perform are biased towards the cervical spine and the exiting nerve pathways rather than treating the painful areas the patients are presenting with.

■ Anatomy of the cervical spine

The human cervical spine has seven vertebrae (C1–7) and eight cervical nerves (C1–8), and the upper cervical complex is composed of the atlas (C1) and the axis (C2). In functional terms the vertebral column of the cervical spine should also include the occipital condyles, which transfer the weight of the head to the uppermost cervical vertebra (C1). This is a highly specialized vertebra aptly named after the Titan Atlas in classical mythology, whose role it was to support the whole of the world on his shoulders. The second cervical vertebra is known as the axis and this too is a specialized structure, since its function is mainly to assist in rotation of the head. The lower cervical spine, comprising the remaining five cervical vertebrae (C3 to C7), has structural features that are more typical of other spinal levels (figure 6.2).

General anatomy of a vertebra
Vertebral body
Spinous process
Transverse process
Facet joint
Intervertebral foramen
Spinal canal
Lamina
Pedicle
Intervertebral disc:
  nucleus pulposus
  annulus fibrosus

Intervertebral discs (figure 6.3)

Between adjacent vertebrae there is a structure known as an intervertebral disc; in total we have 23 of these soft tissue structures in the human vertebral column. A disc is made up of three components: a tough outer shell, called the annulus fibrosus; an inner gel-like substance in the center, called the nucleus pulposus; and an attachment to the vertebral bodies, called the vertebral end plate. As we get older, the center of the disc starts to lose water content, a process that will naturally make the disc less elastic and less effective as a cushion or shock absorber.

Nerve roots exit the spinal canal through small passageways between the vertebrae and the discs: such a passageway is known as an intervertebral foramen. Pain and other symptoms can develop when a damaged disc pushes into the spinal canal or nerve roots – a condition commonly referred to as a herniated disc.

Disc herniation
Herniated discs are often referred to as bulging discs, prolapsed discs, or even slipped discs. These terms are derived from the nature of the action of the gel-like content of the nucleus pulposus being forced out of the center of the disc. Just to clarify, the disc itself does not

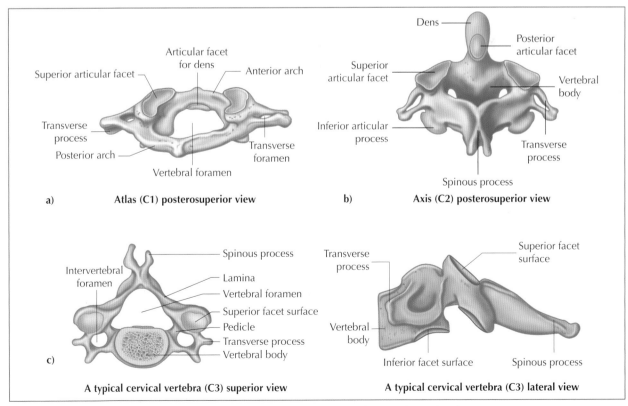

Figure 6.2a–c: *a: Anatomy of the atlas (C1); b: the axis (C2); c: a typical cervical vertebra from C3–7*

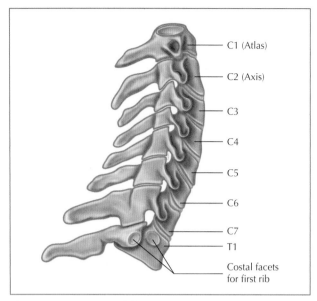

Figure 6.3: *Anatomy of the cervical spine and the intervertebral discs*

slip; however, the nucleus pulposus tissue that is located in the center of the disc can be placed under so much pressure that it can cause the annulus fibrosus to herniate or even rupture, as shown in figure 6.4. The severity of the disc herniation may cause the bulging tissue to press against one or more of the spinal nerves, which can cause local and referred pain, numbness, or weakness to the cervical spine as well as to the upper limb, arm and hand. Approximately 85–95% of a cervical spine disc herniation's will occur at the cervical segments C4–5, C5–6 or C6–7; the nerve compression caused by the contact with the disc contents will possibly result in perceived pain along either the C5, C6 or C7 nerve root pathway, as shown in figure 6.4.

Facet joints

Located within the cervical spine are the facet joints (anatomically known as the zygapophyseal joints); these structures can be responsible for provoking a lot of pain, especially to the shoulder region. The facet joints lie posterior and lateral to the vertebral body, and their role is to assist the spine in performing movements such as flexion, extension, side bending, and rotation. Depending on their location and orientation, these joints will allow certain types of motion but restrict others: for example, rotation is freely permitted (cervical spine) but has less range in lateral flexion.

Each individual vertebra has two facet joints: the superior articular facet, which faces upward and works similarly to

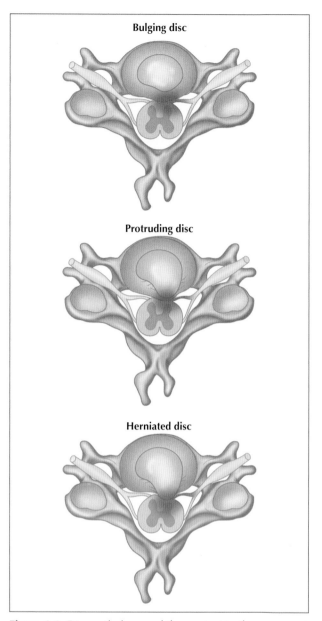

Figure 6.4: *Disc pathology and the contact to the nerve root*

a hinge, and the inferior articular facet located below it. The C4 inferior facet joint, for example, articulates with the C5 superior facet joint.

Like all other synovial joints in the body, each facet joint is surrounded by a capsule of connective tissue and produces synovial fluid to nourish and lubricate the joint. The surfaces of the joint are coated with cartilage, which helps each joint to move (articulate) smoothly. The facet joint is highly innervated with pain receptors, making it susceptible to producing neck, shoulder and arm pain.

Facet joint syndrome/disease
Facet joints have a tendency to slide over each other, so they are naturally in constant motion with the spine;

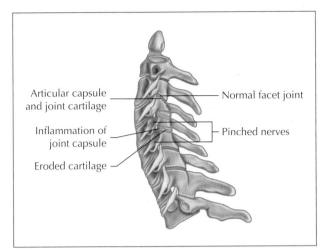

Figure 6.5: *Facet joint syndrome and cervical spondylosis*

like all types of weight-bearing joint, they can simply wear out and start to degenerate over time. When facet joints become irritated (the cartilage can even tear), this will cause the bone of the joint underneath the facet joint to start producing osteophytes, leading to facet joint hypertrophy, which is the precursor of facet joint syndrome/disease (figure 6.5) and eventually leads to a condition called spondylosis and is basically osteoarthritis (OA) of the spine. This type of syndrome or disease process is very common in many older patients presenting with ongoing chronic neck and shoulder pain.

Motion of the cervical spine

The cervical spine is capable of motion through all three axes/planes of movement allowing flexion/extension in the sagittal plane, side bending in the frontal plane and rotation in the transverse plane of motion. Circumduction is also possible as a gross movement, due to the summation of the other movements, even though this is not recommended. These movements are represented throughout the cervical spine; however, this is due to the specific shape of the facet joints, which assist in guiding the movements for the specific spinal cervical segments, and provide different emphasis of motion at different levels.

Motion of the atlas (C1) and axis (C2)

It is considered that 50% of the rotation (either left or right) of the cervical spine is mainly due to the atlas of C1 rotating on the axis of C2 due to this being a pivotal joint (figure 6.6). If we consider a normal range of motion

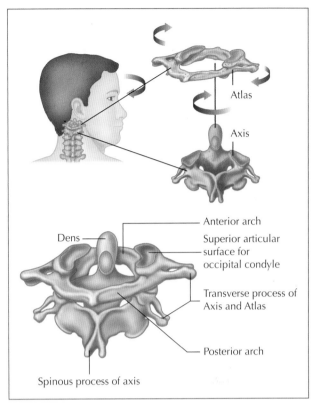

Figure 6.6: *C1 motion on C2*

for cervical rotation is approximately 80 degrees then 40 degrees of that movement will occur between the levels of C1 and C2.

■ Neurological anatomy

There are eight cervical nerves that exit the cervical spine. C1–4 will exit through the cervical plexus (figure 6.7) and C5–T1 will exit through the brachial plexus. However, there are only seven cervical vertebrae. The first (C1) through the seventh (C7) cervical nerves exit above the level of the cervical vertebra with the corresponding number (e.g., C1 nerve exits above the level of C1 vertebra), while the eighth cervical nerve exits below the seventh cervical vertebra and above the first thoracic vertebra (C8 nerve exits between the levels of C7/T1). The first thoracic nerve (T1 nerve root) then exits below the first thoracic vertebra (the T1 nerve root now exits between the levels of T1/T2). For example, if you have disc pathology between C5 and C6 then the exiting nerve root of C6 could be contacted by the disc pathology. However, in the lumbar spine and to the levels of L4 and L5 it will be the L4 exiting nerve root because it is the level below in the lumbar (and thoracic spine) as compared to the level above in the cervical spine.

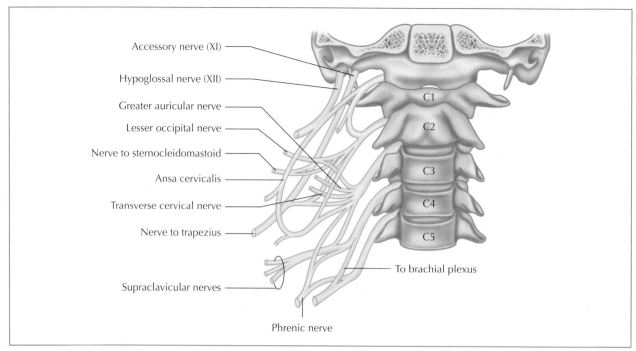

Accessory nerve (XI)

Hypoglossal nerve (XII)

Greater auricular nerve

Lesser occipital nerve

Nerve to sternocleidomastoid

Ansa cervicalis

Transverse cervical nerve

Nerve to trapezius

Supraclavicular nerves

Phrenic nerve

C1
C2
C3
C4
C5

To brachial plexus

Figure 6.7: *Anatomy of the cervical plexus and the levels of the exiting nerve roots*

Brachial plexus (figure 6.8)

The brachial plexus is composed of nerves emanating from the four lower cervical vertebrae and the first thoracic vertebra (C5–T1). The brachial plexus passes through the space that is formed between the scalenus anterior and scalenus medius muscle and is known as the interscalene triangle. The nerve roots of C5 and C6 join to form the *upper trunk.* The nerve roots of C8 and T1 join to form the *lower trunk.* C7 does not join with any other nerve root; it alone makes up the *middle trunk.* As the trunks pass beneath the clavicle, they then divide to form cords. The upper trunk and the lower trunk contribute to the middle trunk, to form the posterior cord. The middle trunk, in turn, sends a contribution with C5 and C6 to form the lateral cord. The remainder of C8 and T1 forms the medial cord.

The branches now continue and emanate from the cords; the lateral cord sends one branch to become the *musculocutaneous* nerve. The other branch of the lateral cord joins with a branch from the medial cord to form the *median* nerve. The second branch of the medial cord becomes the *ulnar* nerve and the posterior cord becomes the *axillary* and *radial* nerve.

It makes perfect sense in this chapter to cover the peripheral nerves that exit from the brachial plexus

(figure 6.9) and to focus a little bit more on their anatomy, sensory and motor function and then on how to assess them, without hopefully making it too complex to understand – neurological testing can be a hard to get your head around subject. (I have listened to expert explanations about neurology that make me start to lose the will to live!) However, I do not think it has to be that difficult if it is taught in a straightforward way. I will try my best to explain this fascinating subject simply.

In this section I want to discuss the five peripheral nerves that terminate from the brachial plexus, and these are the:

1. radial nerve
2. median nerve
3. ulnar nerve
4. musculocutaneous nerve
5. axillary nerve

1. Radial nerve

The posterior cord of the brachial plexus from the specific root levels of C5, 6, 7, 8 and T1 forms the radial nerve, continues behind the axillary region, follows the brachial artery in the arm and innervates the triceps muscle. The radial nerve continues and passes over the lateral epicondyle and through the cubital fossa and branches into the deep (posterior interosseous nerve) and superficial branch (figure 6.10).

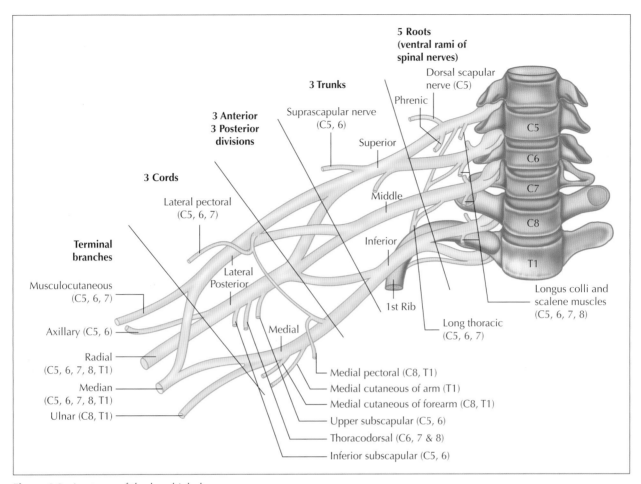

Figure 6.8: *Anatomy of the brachial plexus*

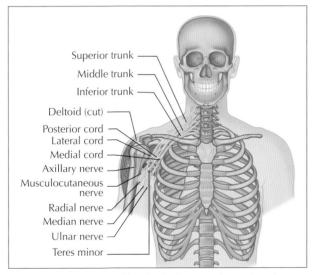

Figure 6.9: *Anatomy of brachial plexus and peripheral nerves*

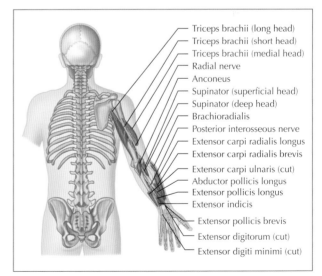

Figure 6.10: *Motor pathway of the radial nerve*

The radial nerve in terms of motor function initially supplies all three heads of the triceps muscles before it continues its journey into the forearm and hand, even though Rezzouk et al. (2004) found that the triceps long head muscle was innervated by the axillary nerve through 20 cadaver dissections and not one of them was supplied by the radial nerve.

Motor supply of the radial nerve
Triceps
Anconeus
Brachioradialis
Extensor carpi radialis longus

The deep branch of the radial nerve supplies the:

extensor carpi radialis brevis
supinator.

Posterior interosseous (deep branch continued) supplies the:

extensor digitorum
extensor digiti minimi
extensor carpi ulnaris
abductor pollicis longus

extensor pollicis brevis
extensor pollicis longus
extensor indicis.

The *sensory* component is supplied mainly from the posterior cutaneous nerve and supplies a strip of skin down the center of the back of the forearm and also the elbow joint. The superficial branch supplies the sensory innervation to the dorsal surface of the hand and the lateral three and half fingers as well as the web space between the thumb and index finger (figure 6.11).

Any form of trauma to the radial nerve may result in motor weakness of supination and/or extension of the wrist (wrist drop) and extension of the fingers with sensory loss to the posterior forearm, radial side of the forearm and the dorsal aspect of the 3½ digits (excluding the nail beds) and also the web space between the thumb and index finger.

Radial nerve strength test (figure 6.12)
Figure 6.12 shows the patient resisting the muscle of the thumb (extensor pollicis longus) to ascertain the motor contractibility of the radial nerve.

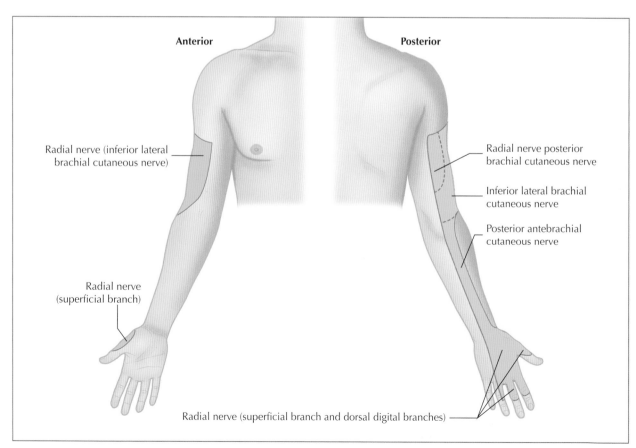

Figure 6.11: *Sensory functions of the radial nerve*

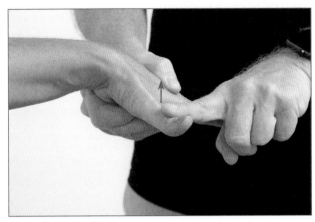

Figure 6.12: *Radial nerve strength tested through contracting extensor pollicis longus*

2. Median nerve

The median nerve (C5–T1) originates from the lateral (C5, 6) and medial (C8, T1) cords of the brachial plexus as well as having a branch from the middle trunk of C7 (continues into the lateral cord). The nerve continues through the axilla and lateral to the brachial artery and lies between the brachialis and biceps brachii muscles. The nerve will pass over the brachial artery so is situated medially as it continues its journey towards the cubital fossa; here it gives off an articular branch to the elbow joint.

The median nerve continues through the two heads of the pronator teres muscle and lies between the two muscles of the flexor superficialis profundus (FDP) and flexor digitorum superficialis (FDS), and now gives rise to two main branches in the forearm called the anterior interosseous nerve, which supplies the deep muscles in the forearm, and the palmar cutaneous nerve, which innervates the skin of the lateral palm. The median nerve then enters the hand through the carpal tunnel, where it terminates by dividing into two branches called the recurrent branch, which supplies the thenar muscles, and the palmar digital branch, which innervates the sensory supply to the palmar surface, the thumb, index finger and half the ring finger.

Motor supply of the median nerve

Superficial layer: pronator teres, flexor carpi radialis, palmaris longus
Intermediate layer: flexor digitorum superficialis
Deep layer: flexor digitorum profundus (lateral half), flexor pollicis longus, pronator quadratus

Hand muscles

The muscles listed below make up part of the thenar eminence and control movements of the thumb (pollux)

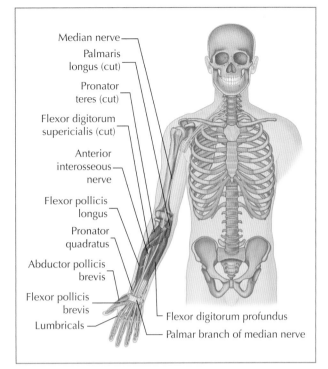

Figure 6.13: *Motor pathway of the median nerve*

and are called the LOAF muscles (figure 6.14), apart from the lateral two lumbricals, so can be known as the OAF muscles.

Lateral lumbricals (first and second)
Opponens pollicis
Abductor pollicis brevis
Flexor pollicis brevis

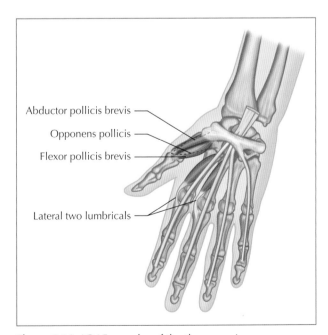

Figure 6.14: *LOAF muscles of the thenar eminence*

Sensory

The median nerve innervates the sensory supply for the palmar surface of the thenar eminence, the thumb, index, middle and half the ring finger as well as the associated nail beds (figure 6.15).

Median nerve strength test – pinch grip (figure 6.16)

Figure 6.16 shows the patient pinching their thumb and index finger. The therapist is trying to separate their thumb and finger and the patient is asked to resist this motion.

Trauma to the median nerve is normally within the carpal tunnel, hence the well known *carpal tunnel syndrome (CTS)*. It is commonly caused by swelling of the tendon sheath (tenosynovitis) due to repetitive motion of the fingers (typist) and also thickened ligaments. In extreme cases the thenar eminence muscles (LOAF) will atrophy (waste) due to the compression of the nerve. The median nerve can also be damaged at the elbow through a supracondylar fracture and this will cause paralysis of the flexors and pronators within the forearm with the appearance of permanent supination.

3. Ulnar nerve (figure 6.17)

The ulnar nerve (C8, T1) initially originates from the spinal roots of C8 and T1 and it forms the medial cords. The nerve continues its journey medially down the arm towards the elbow and continues posterior to the medial epicondyle of the humerus (the nerve is palpable at this area and is common site for injury). The nerve continues in the forearm and penetrates through the two heads of the flexor carpi ulnaris muscle and travels along the ulna bone and then at the wrist it continues through the tunnel of Guyon or Guyon's canal (located between the pisiform and hamate bones of the wrist) and terminates into the superficial and deep branches.

Motor

The ulnar nerve supplies the following muscles:

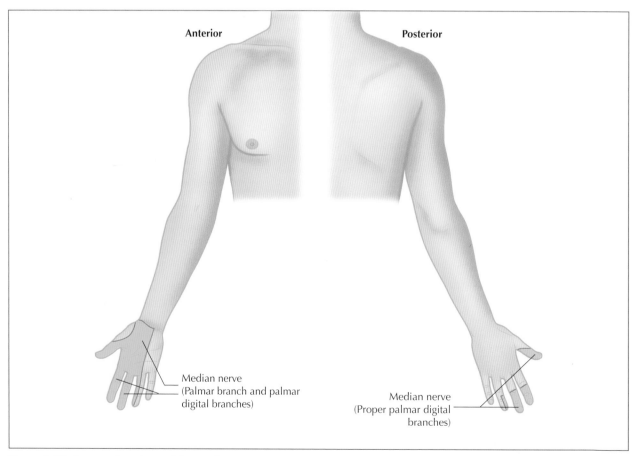

Anterior

Posterior

Median nerve
(Palmar branch and palmar digital branches)

Median nerve
(Proper palmar digital branches)

Figure 6.15: *Sensory functions of the median nerve*

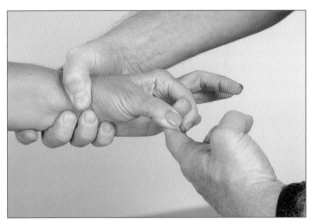

Figure 6.16: *Median nerve strength tested through a pinch grip test*

Forearm: flexor carpi ulnaris and flexor digitorum
    profundus (medial half)
Hand: the muscles below make up the hypothenar
    eminence and control the movements of: the little
    finger (digiti minimi)
abductor digiti minimi
opponens digiti minimi
flexor digiti minimi brevis.

The ulnar nerve also supplies the following muscles of the hand:

Medial two lumbricals
Adductor pollicis
Palmaris brevis
Interossei.

Sensory
The ulnar nerve innervates the medial side of the palm and the corresponding medial dorsal surface as well as the little finger and half the ring finger.

Ulnar nerve strength test (figure 6.18)
Figure 6.18 shows the patient resisting abduction of the little finger (abductor digiti minimi) to ascertain the motor contractibility of the ulnar nerve.

Damage to the ulnar nerve is common to the medial epicondyle of the elbow because of its susceptibility. The nerve can be compressed within the cubital tunnel and this is known as *cubital tunnel syndrome*. The nerve can also be stretched with the hand though the tunnel of Guyon, especially in cyclists because of the position

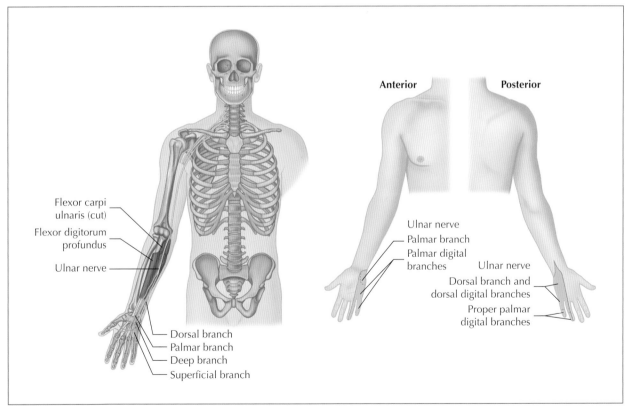

Figure 6.17: *Motor and sensory pathway of the ulnar nerve*

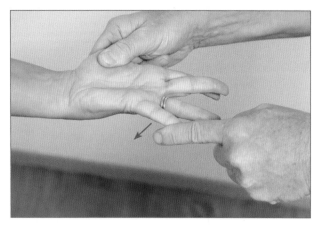

Figure 6.18: *Ulnar nerve strength tested through abducting the little finger*

of the hand in cycling is extended and ulnar deviated and stretches the nerve through the tunnel. In extreme cases the fingers are unable to abduct and adduct and movement of the little finger and ring fingers will be reduced; loss of sensation will be experienced to the area of the ulnar nerve innervation.

4. Musculocutaneous nerve

The spinal nerve root of C5 and C6 travels along the superior trunk with a connection from C7 of the

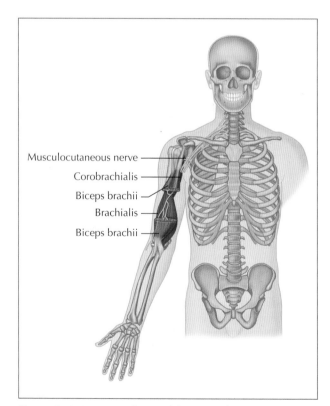

Figure 6.19: *Motor pathway of the musculocutaneous nerve*

middle trunk and continues to form the lateral cord and subsequently the musculocutaneous nerve. The nerve continues its journey down the arm and innervates the coracobrachialis and then the brachialis and biceps brachii. The nerve passes laterally to the tendon of the biceps before it enters the forearm to supply the necessary sensory innervation to the lateral forearm as the lateral cutaneous nerve.

Motor supply of the musculocutaneous nerve
Coracobrachialis
Brachialis
Biceps brachii.

Sensory supply is through the lateral cutaneous nerve and innervates the area of the skin to the lateral part of the forearm.

Damage to the musculocutaneous nerve is very rare because it is pretty well protected so there is no need to discuss any injuries to this nerve.

5. Axillary nerve (figure 6.20)

The spinal nerve roots of C5 and C6 travel along the superior trunk and connect to the posterior cord and continue to form the axillary nerve within the region of the axilla. The nerve is located posterior to the axillary artery and anterior to the subscapularis. It then divides into two branches called the posterior terminal branch, which supplies the teres minor muscle, and the anterior terminal branch, which supplies the deltoid muscle.

Motor supply of the axillary nerve
Deltoid
Teres minor.

Sensory supply of the axillary nerve is through the posterior terminal branch and continues as the upper lateral cutaneous nerves. It supplies the skin region inferior to the deltoid muscle and this is known as the "regimental badge area" because of the usual location of sergeant stripes or badge on the upper arm of a military uniform (figure 6.21).

Damage to the axillary nerve is normally through dislocation of the glenohumeral joint or a fracture to the surgical neck of the humerus with subsequent atrophy of the deltoid and teres minor muscles, to an extent that the acromion process and greater tubercle of the humerus can be seen and easily palpated. Shoulder abduction will be weak and difficult and sensory loss will be to the regimental badge area.

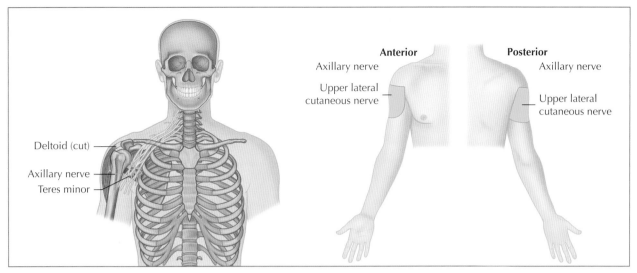

Figure 6.20: *Motor and sensory pathway of the axillary nerve*

■ Examination of the sensory system (dermatome)

A dermatome is a specific area of skin located on the body that is innervated by a single nerve root (figures 6.22 and 6.23).

Numbness, tingling, burning, and pain are abnormal feelings that may be felt in the shoulder and/or extremities. Sometimes these symptoms radiate from one area into another. Sciatica is a good example of pain that can radiate into the lower extremity.

Nerves originate from the spinal cord and divide into sensory and motor nerves. The sensory nerve gives sensation to specific areas of the skin and these are known as *dermatomes*. The dermatome patterns appear similar to a map on the body. The therapist may use a piece of cotton wool, pin or even a paperclip to test symmetrical feelings in the arms and legs. Abnormal responses by the patient when tested may be indicative of a specific nerve root problem.

Sensory tests

To truly assess the neurological sensory components of the dermatomes we can use some simple pieces of equipment such as cotton wool, a neurotip, or simply our fingers as we are able touch our patients gently and/or with pressure. I am not saying I include all the following tests but I use some of these in my assessment of the neurological system. The basic idea of these tests is to ascertain if the patient does actually have a neurological issue, as they might not be aware of contact to their skin through use of an external source.

Light touch
- Use the light touch of a finger, a piece of cotton wool or a piece of tissue paper.
- It is important to touch and not to stroke as a moving sensation.
- Ask the patient to close their eyes and tell you when they feel you touching them.
- Compare each limb in the same position.

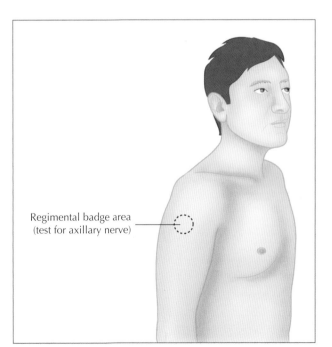

Figure 6.21: *Regimental badge area of the axillary nerve*

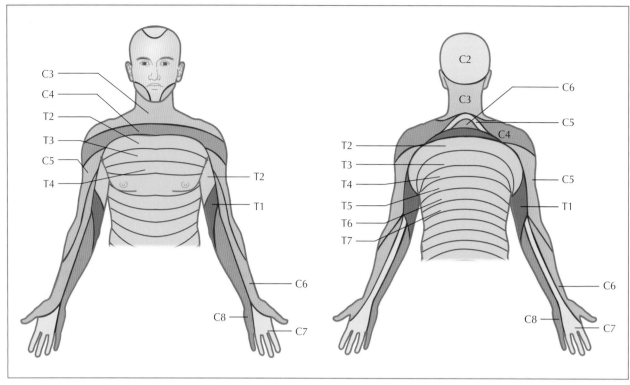

Figure 6.22: *Map of the dermatomes of the upper body: anterior view and posterior view*

- Keep the timing of each touch irregular to avoid anticipation by the patient, e.g. test C5 on the right arm then C7 on the left arm then C6 on the right arm, etc.
- Note any areas of reduced or increased sensation.

Sharp touch (pinprick)
- Test using a dedicated neurological testing pin.
- Use the sternal area of the chest to establish a baseline for sharpness before you begin.
- Follow the same progression as with light touch with the patient's eyes closed, comparing both sides of the upper limbs.
- Ask the patient to report the feeling of sharp or blunt

Temperature
- This is often overlooked but it can be important.
- An easy and practical approach is to touch the patient with the end of a patella hammer, as it will feel cold.

Dermatome location	Corresponding spinal level
Shoulders	C4, C5
Lateral forearm	C6
Thumb	C6
Middle finger	C7
Little finger	C8
Medial forearm	T1

- Compare the quality of temperature sensation on the specific dermatomes.

Vibration sense
- Use a tuning fork and ensure the tuning fork is vibrating.
- Place it on the sternum to start with so that the patient can feel the sensation.
- Then place it on one of the distal interphalangeal joints of one of the fingers.
- If no vibration is sensed, move backwards to the metacarpophalangeal joint, etc.

■ Examination of the motor system (myotome)

A myotome is a group of muscles that is innervated by a single nerve root.

Power testing

We ask the patient to contract the muscle group being tested to identify the corresponding myotome level and then the examiner will try to overpower that muscle group. Any weakness found during the testing might indicate a problem with that specific nerve root.

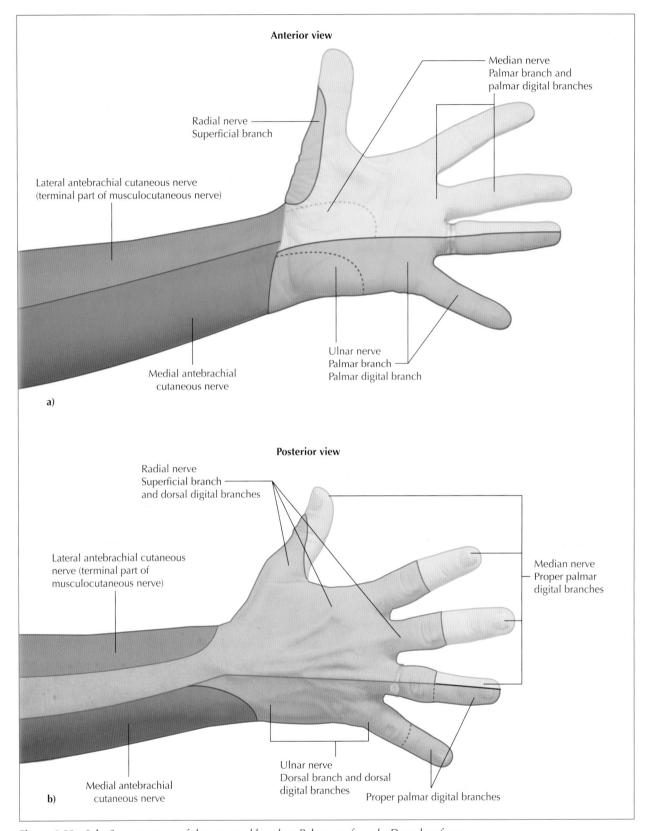

Anterior view

Radial nerve
Superficial branch

Median nerve
Palmar branch and
palmar digital branches

Lateral antebrachial cutaneous nerve
(terminal part of musculocutaneous nerve)

Medial antebrachial
cutaneous nerve

Ulnar nerve
Palmar branch
Palmar digital branch

a)

Posterior view

Radial nerve
Superficial branch
and dorsal digital branches

Lateral antebrachial cutaneous
nerve (terminal part of
musculocutaneous nerve)

Median nerve
Proper palmar
digital branches

Medial antebrachial
cutaneous nerve

Ulnar nerve
Dorsal branch and dorsal
digital branches

Proper palmar digital branches

b)

Figure 6.23a & b: *Sensory areas of the arm and hand. a: Palmar surface. b: Dorsal surface*

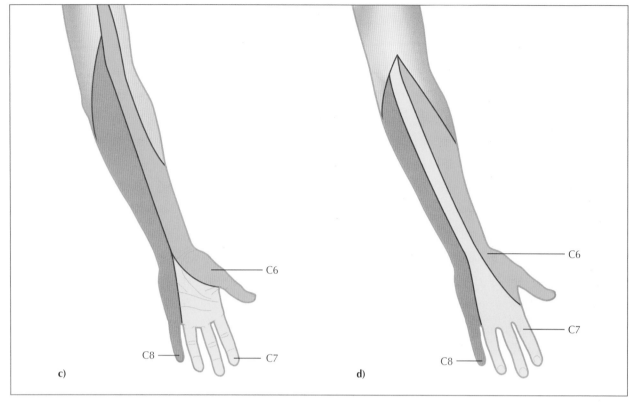

Figure 6.23c & d: *Dermatomes of the arm and hand. c: Palmar surface. d: Dorsal surface*

Myotome location	Spinal level
Cervical – flexion/extension	C1/2
Cervical – lateral flexion	C3
Shoulder elevation	C4
Shoulder abduction	C5
Elbow flexion	C5, C6
Wrist extension	C6
Elbow extension/wrist flexion/finger extension	C7
Finger flexion	C8
Abduction/adduction fingers	T1

Grading system for muscle power

0	No muscle contraction is visible
1	Muscle contraction is visible but there is no movement of the joint
2	Active joint movement is possible with gravity eliminated
3	Movement can overcome gravity but not resistance from the examiner
4	The muscle group can overcome gravity and move against some resistance from the examiner
5	Full and normal power against resistance

1. C1/2 myotome – cervical flexion and extension

Patient is sitting and the therapist applies a contact to the forehead and the patient is asked to flex the cervical spine against a resistance as shown in figure 6.24a. The therapist applies contact to the occipital and the patient is asked to resist cervical spine extension as shown by figure 6.24b.

2. C3 myotome – cervical lateral flexion

Patient is sitting and the therapist applies a contact to the lateral side of the forehead and the patient is asked to laterally flex the cervical spine against resistance, as shown in figure 6.25.

3. C4 myotome – shoulder elevation

Patient is sitting and the therapist applies a contact to the top of the shoulder. The patient is asked to elevate their shoulder girdle against resistance as shown by figure 6.26.

4. C5 myotome – shoulder abduction and elbow flexion

Patient is sitting and the patient is asked to abduct their shoulders (or one side at a time) to 90 degrees and the therapist applies a contact just above the elbow. The patient is asked to abduct their shoulders against the

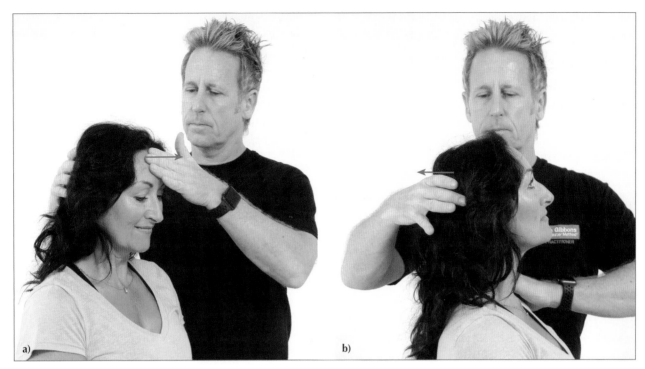

Figure 6.24a & b: *a: Resisted cervical flexion (C1/2). b: Resisted cervical extension (C1/2)*

resistance being applied by the therapist (figure 6.27a). The patient is now asked to flex their elbows to 90 degrees and the therapist applies contact to the lower part of the forearm. The patient is asked to flex their elbows against a resistance being applied by the therapist (figure 6.27b).

5. C6 myotome – elbow flexion and wrist extension

Elbow flexion has already been covered (figure 6.27), so this time the patient is asked to flex their elbows to 90 degrees. The therapist applies contact to the top of the wrist and the patient is asked to extend their

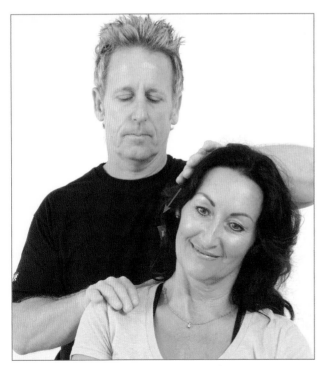

Figure 6.25: *Resisted cervical lateral flexion (C3)*

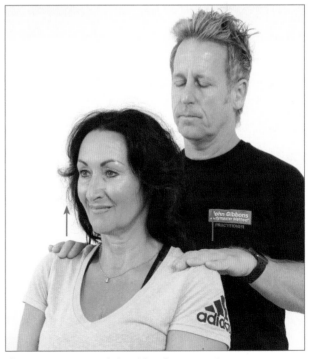

Figure 6.26: *Resisted shoulder elevation (C4)*

wrist against a resistance being applied by the therapist (figure 6.28).

6. C7 myotome – elbow extension, wrist flexion and finger extension

Patient is sitting and the patient is asked to flex their elbows to 90 degrees. The therapist applies a contact to the distal medial forearm and the patient is asked to extend their elbows against a resistance being applied by the

therapist (figure 6.29a). The patient is now asked to flex their wrist against a resistance (figure 6.29b). The last test for C7 is the patient is asked to extend their fingers against a resistance (figure 6.29c).

7. C8 myotome – finger flexion

Patient is sitting and the patient is asked to flex their fingers against a resistance (figure 6.30).

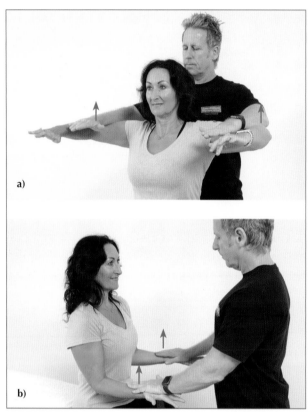

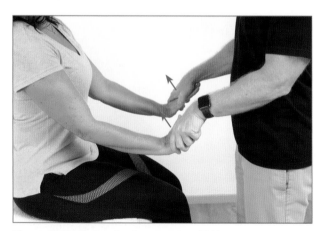

Figure 6.27a & b: *a: Resisted shoulder abduction (C5).* *b: Resisted elbow flexion (C5/6)*

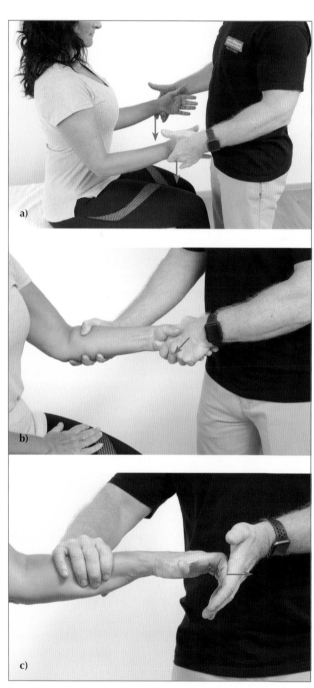

Figure 6.29a–c: *a: Resisted elbow extension. b: Resisted wrist flexion. c: Resisted finger extension (all C7)*

Figure 6.28: *Resisted wrist extension (C6)*

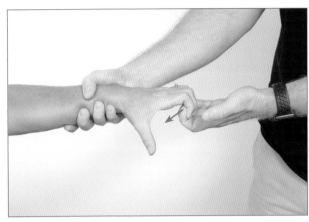

Figure 6.30: *Resisted finger flexion (C8)*

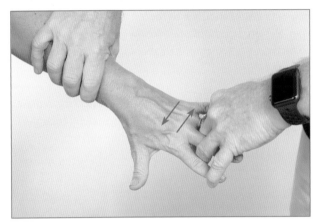

Figure 6.31: *Resisted finger abduction and adduction (T1)*

8. T1 myotome – adduction and abduction of the fingers

Patient is sitting and the therapist interlocks their fingers with the fingers of the patient and they are asked to abduct and adduct their fingers against a resistance (figure 6.31).

■ Deep tendon reflexes (DTRs)

Most people have experienced their general practitioner (GP) tapping their knees with a rubber hammer. The normal response is a knee jerk. This is an example of a reflex, which is an involuntary muscular response elicited by the patella or reflex hammer tapping the specific tendon.

When reflex responses are absent this could be a clue that the spinal cord, nerve root, peripheral nerve, or muscle has been damaged. When the reflex response is abnormal, it may be due to the disruption of the sensory (feeling) or motor (movement) nerves or both. To determine where the neural problem may exist, the therapist tests reflexes in various parts of the body.

Technique

- Ensure that the patient is comfortable and relaxed and that you can see the muscle being tested.
- Use a reflex/patella hammer to strike the tendon of the specific muscle and look for muscle contraction.
- Compare both sides.

Reflexes can be:

- hyperactive (3+++)
- normal (2++)
- sluggish (1+)
- absent (−)

C5 reflex testing – bicep

To test the biceps reflex (C5): with their arm relaxed, hold the patient's elbow between your thumb and remaining fingers, and ask the patient to resist elbow flexion so that you can feel the contraction of the biceps tendon. Place your thumb directly over the biceps tendon and you can elicit the reflex by tapping the hammer gently on your thumb (figure 6.32)

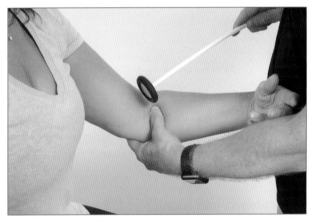

Figure 6.32: *C5 reflex testing*

C6 reflex testing – brachioradialis

The brachioradialis reflex (C6): ask the patient to relax their arm. Gently grasp the patient's wrist and ask them to elbow flex so that you can see the contraction of the brachioradialis muscle. Elicit the reflex by tapping gently over the brachioradialis tendon (or even the muscle belly as this also works) just above the wrist (figure 6.33).

C7 reflex testing – triceps

To test the triceps reflex (C7): hold the patient's (relaxed) arm across their lower chest/upper abdomen with one of your hands. Elicit the reflex by tapping over the triceps tendon just above and behind their elbow (figure 6.34).

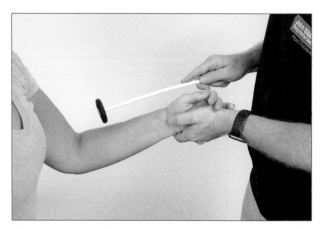

Figure 6.33: *C6 reflex testing*

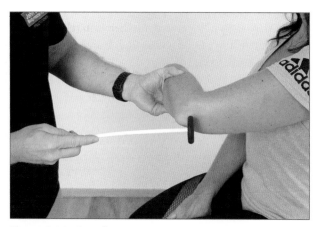

Figure 6.34: *C7 reflex testing*

If a reflex is difficult to elicit, try "reinforcement" – ask the patient to clench their teeth or interlock their fingers and try and pull their fingers apart, while you try to elicit the reflexes again.

Examples of interpretation of findings

Upper motor neurone (UMN) lesions usually produce hyper-reflexia (increased reflex), while lower motor neurone (LMN) lesions usually produce a hypo-reflexia (diminished or absent response).

Isolated loss of a reflex can point to a radiculopathy affecting that specific spinal segment, e.g., loss of biceps reflex if there is a C4–5 disc prolapse.

Quick reference table of specific reflexes

Area tested for reflex	Corresponding spinal level
Biceps	C5
Brachioradialis (forearm)	C6
Triceps (elbow)	C7

Assessment of the cervical spine

The physical therapist will need to ascertain if they consider the cervical spine to be involved in the symptoms for the patient's presenting shoulder pain. We could use the "keep it simple" process (KISS) by asking our patient to perform simple movements of rotation, flexion, extension and side bending to see if these motions of the cervical spine exacerbate the shoulder symptoms. If they do one can realistically say that the cervical spine needs further investigation.

Active range of motion (AROM)

The patient is asked to sit on a couch and they are instructed to rotate their neck as far as they comfortably can to the right and then to the left and to mention if they feel any symptoms, restriction or pain anywhere and to focus in particular to their shoulder, arm and hand (Figure 6.35).

The patient is then ask to slowly flex their neck by bringing the chin towards their chest and then to extend their neck by slowly looking up towards the ceiling and to mention if they feel any symptoms as before (figure 6.36).

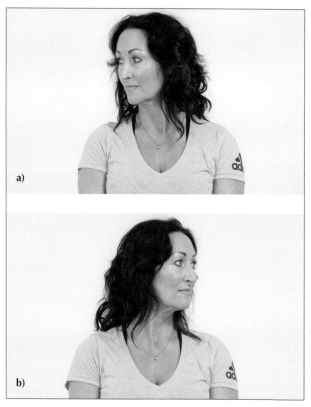

Figure 6.35a & b: *Patient rotates their neck to the right (a), and then to the left (b)*

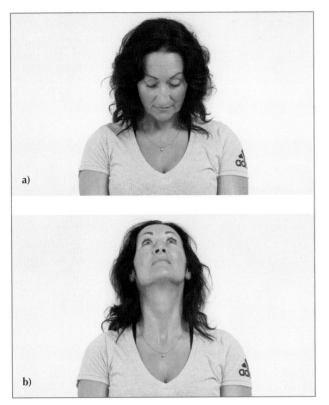

Figure 6.36a & b: *Patient flexes (a) and extends (b) their neck*

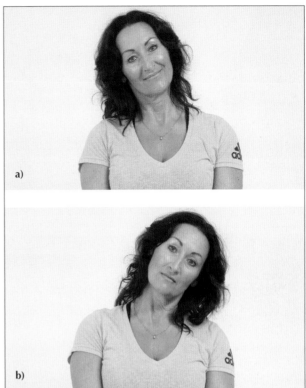

Figure 6.37a & b: *Patient side bends their neck to the right (a) and to the left (b)*

The patient is then asked to side bend (lateral flexion) their neck by bringing the right ear down towards their right shoulder and to repeat on the other side and to mention if they feel any symptoms as before (Figure 6.37).

Passive range of motion (PROM)

It is possible to perform all the above movements passively by the therapist in the sitting position; however, the movements are typically done with the patient in the supine position. Figure 6.38 shows a couple of examples of passive rotation and passive lateral flexion.

Please note: If the patient has any pain or restriction on the active movements but they are *pain free* when these movements are performed passively by the physical therapist then this normally indicates the soft tissues of the muscles and tendons are generally involved in the active motion. If on the other hand, active movements *and* passive movements cause increased symptoms to the patient, then one can assume that the cervical spinal joints are involved and will need further investigation.

Let me give you a couple of examples. A 20-year-old patient has strained one of their neck muscles, so when they move their neck to the left and to the right they will be aware of the pain. However, if I were to passively move their neck then probably the movement would be almost pain free. My second example is a 65-year-old patient with a confirmed degenerative cervical spondylosis (OA). When they move their neck to the left or to the right it will be very stiff, restrictive and possibly painful at certain ranges. If I was to passively move this patient's neck to the right and to the left, I will also feel the restrictive motion because of the underlying degenerative changes to the joints and the patient will more than likely be aware of some discomfort during the passive motions.

There are numerous other/special tests we can incorporate and some of these have already been covered earlier, such as the reflex and myotome testing, so we should already have a good idea if the cervical spine is involved with the patient's presenting upper limb symptoms. Below are some extra examples of the tests I might personally use in my clinic.

Special tests

In terms of cervical spine and special tests, I have already discussed and demonstrated what I would consider to be the best way of assessing the cervical spine and that is through the use of the C5–7 reflexes, as well as individual power testing of the specific spinal myotomes and sensory testing through the dermatomes. However, there are also

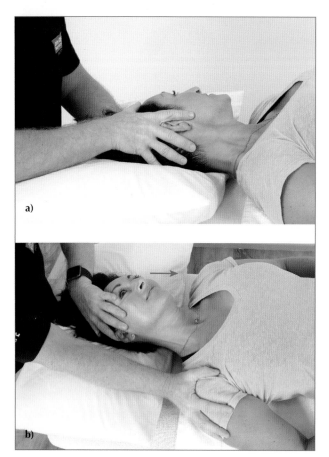

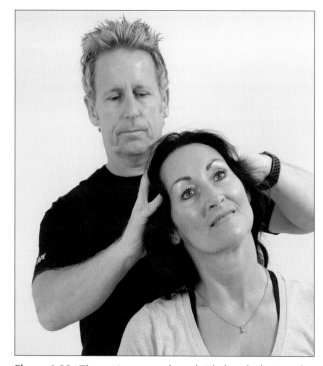

Figure 6.38a & b: *Passive ROM for the cervical spine. a: Rotation. b: Lateral flexion*

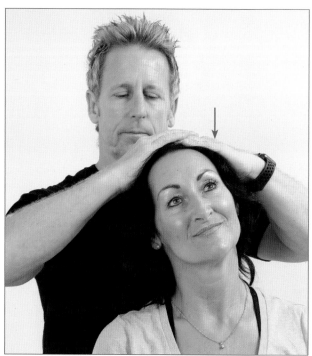

Figure 6.40: *The therapist applies a downward pressure on top of the patient's head*

some extra specific tests we can include to help with the overall diagnosis.

Spurling's compression test – cervical nerve root pain

This test for cervical nerve root pain was first described by Spurling and Scoville in 1944 and Anekstein et al. in 2012 described a few variations on the procedure. They suggested that a maneuver consisting of extension and lateral bending, which reproduced the patient's complaints in a tolerable fashion, be done first followed by addition of axial compression in the case of an inconclusive effect.

This test is performed with the patient in a sitting position and the therapist guides their head into extension and lateral flexion (figure 6.39). If there are no symptoms reproduced then the therapist gently applies a downward pressure to the top of the patient's head (figure 6.40). A positive sign is when the patient complains of pain that radiates into their shoulder or arm (dermatome).

Valsalva maneuver

This test was named after Antonio Maria Valsalva, a physician that specialized in the human ear. For example, the Valsalva maneuver is used in diving to equalize pressure within the middle ear for descent.

Figure 6.39: *The patient extends and side bends their neck to the right*

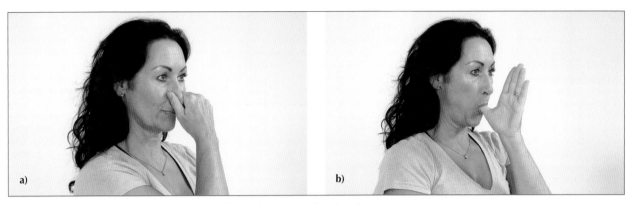

Figure 6.41a & b: *a: Valsalva maneuver. b: Alternative by sucking thumb*

With regards to the cervical spine and the nerves, the Valsalva motion can increase spinal pressure so any space-occupying lesion such as a disc prolapse with subsequent neural pain can be exacerbated through increasing pressure.

Figure 6 41a shows the patient performing the typical Valsalva maneuver by trying to equalize the pressure within the ears by blowing out through the pinched nostrils. Figure 6.41b is an alternative method, either sucking the thumb or blowing out on the thumb.

7

Differential diagnosis for pain located to the superior angle of the scapula

Pain that presents itself to the area of the superior scapula can be coming from a multitude of structures; pathologies that manifest from the viscera (as discussed in an earlier chapter), such as the gall bladder, pancreas and liver, and through certain pathological changes can contact and irritate the diaphragm with subsequent referral to the shoulder via the phrenic nerve. In this chapter I will mainly discuss the musculoskeletal causative factors that present to the superior angle of the scapula.

Imagine, one of your patient's comes in for a consultation and you ask them the most typical question in physical therapy: 'why have you come to see me today?' They respond by pointing to the top of the scapula and saying that it hurts 'here' (the area indicated by the circle of pain in figure 7.1).

As I mentioned in an earlier chapter, I came across an orthopedic surgeon who stated that the best diagnostic tool we have 'is the patient's finger.' Simply asking the patient to point to the area that hurts could be an accurate method of diagnosis for, say, a knee surgeon, who could reason that if, for example, the patient points to the inside of the knee then they might have a medial meniscus tear and might therefore benefit from surgery to correct the problem. In this context (and in all my books), however, I mention Dr Ida Rolf who invented the technique known as Rolfing, and who stated: 'Where the pain is, the

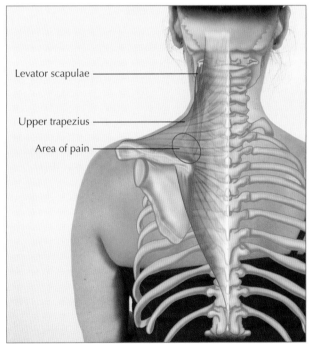

Figure 7.1: *Circle of potential pain that is located to the superior angle of the left scapula*

problem is not.' And as we have already seen in relation to other areas, when a patient points to the superior angle of the scapula and says this area of their body hurts we must always bear in mind that the underlying causative factor might not be under the patient's actual finger. This area is probably 'just the symptomology' and the actual cause of the pain is located far off, at some distance from the presenting symptoms.

Anatomically, first let us consider what structures are located directly within the drawn circle in figure 7.1. Before you start to list them (as I have below), think about how many patients and athletes have walked into your clinic with pain located to that area of the scapula. I know from my experience that it is a lot of people. If I was to offer a free 30-minute soft tissue treatment to my students on my courses or I offered the same free service to the general public, what part of their body do you think they would they want treating? Of course, I agree with what you are thinking: it would be the neck and shoulders for some and for others, the lower back, but the majority would choose a treatment to the neck and shoulder region.

Imagine the following scenario: you are an experienced physical therapist and a patient has presented with pain to the superior angle of the scapula. It is naturally very tempting (and, I agree, beneficial to the patient) for the physical therapist to start to perform soft tissue massage techniques to that area of the neck and shoulder – and let's be honest, it feels pretty fantastic. I also consider that it is natural to massage both sides of the upper trapezius muscles at the same time and I can guarantee that you have said the following words to your patients, 'those muscles feel pretty tight,' or that your patients have said these words to you, 'do those muscles feel tight?' I can guarantee your answer has been 'yes, those muscles are very tight.'

I am hoping that after reading that last paragraph, you have a smile on your face because what I have said is definitely true and you know it! Please do not get me wrong; there is absolutely nothing wrong with massaging the upper trapezius and, as I said above, it feels pretty good to have those muscles loosened up. However, I have heard lots of stories about inexperienced therapists that massage the area of the superior angle of the scapula and say to their patients, 'there are lots of "knots" in the muscles that need "working" out' and then proceed to be very aggressive with the treatment and subsequently cause a lot of discomfort to the patient. Think about this for one moment – those 'knots' they think they are feeling and working out are probably the actual tendon insertion point for the levator scapulae muscle. We know that we cannot actually get rid of that tendon structure

by massaging aggressively, so anyone tempted to do this should give up trying to get rid of those pseudo (false) knots and the patient will probably thank you for it.

For the patient in question in the above figure, the potential tissues that are located within the circle and those tissues mentioned below are possibly part of the overall picture that is/are responsible for the pain (symptoms) to the area of the superior scapula:

- levator scapulae
- upper trapezius
- scalenes
- supraspinatus
- rhomboids
- thoracic rib
- cervical rib (extra rib forming from the transverse process of C7).

Once the physical therapist has gone through a thorough subjective history and medical screening, he or she then proceeds to an objective assessment: this is where the therapist uses specialized orthopedic techniques and specific tests to thoroughly assess the musculoskeletal system and to hopefully come up with a potential diagnosis or hypothesis of at least what structures are involved with the patient's presenting symptoms.

One of the specific techniques employed by the therapist can be simple range of motion (ROM) tests that are initially performed by the patient; these are known as *active range of motion* (AROM) tests. This assessment is generally followed by a series of *passive range of motion* (PROM) tests; these tests are normally performed on the patient by the therapist, and are commonly used to check the integrity of the affected joint. Resisted testing comes next. This type of specific movement tests the power and involvement of the contractile tissues, i.e., muscles and tendons, as well as utilizing the specific myotomes of the nerve roots. For example, shoulder abduction will test the strength of the deltoid and supraspinatus muscles; however, it also tests the myotome for the C5 nerve root. So a weakness perceived during the testing might be because of a strain to the supraspinatus muscle; then again, the weakness could be a C4/5 disc pathology that is contacting the exiting C5 nerve root. The physical therapist also uses tactile palpatory awareness through the use of their fingertips to decide on the overall condition of the affected tissues, and will generally include specific special tests to complement the overall diagnosis.

■ Possible causative factors for the pain

The list below highlights some of the potential causes for the patient's presenting pain to the superior angle of the scapula.

1. Referral pain from cervical facet C4/5 or C5/6

The facet joints located within the middle levels of the cervical spine (C3–5) could be a constant source of pain in the shoulder area for many patients. Generally speaking, motion of the cervical in certain directions will probably exacerbate the shoulder pain. There is one test that I use in particular and I consider it works well for me to ascertain if the cervical spine is involved. I call it a 'facet load test' and it is described below.

Facet load test
This test is an adaption of the Spurling's test (see chapter 6). The patient adopts a seated position on the couch and is asked to sit upright and they are then asked to extend, rotate, and side bend their head towards the painful shoulder (figure 7.2a). If needed the therapist can also apply a little overpressure (figure 7.2b). If any movement exacerbates their symptoms then you know the cervical spine is involved with the patient's presenting shoulder pain.

2. Protective spasm/strain of upper trapezius or levator scapulae

These two muscles are probably treated the most in terms of massage therapy and it makes perfect sense to know if these muscles are involved in the patient's symptoms. I suggest a stretch of the tissue then to resist the muscle from this position to see if there is a strain present.

Upper trapezius stretch and resist
The patient adopts a sitting position and the therapist slowly side bends the patient's head away from the painful side (figure 7.3a). From this position the patient is asked to contract the upper trapezius against a resistance applied by the therapist (figure 7.3b).

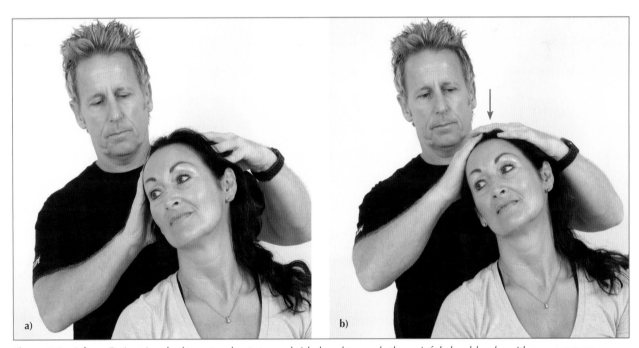

Figure 7.2a & b: *a: Patient is asked to extend, rotate, and side bend towards the painful shoulder; b: with overpressure applied from the therapist*

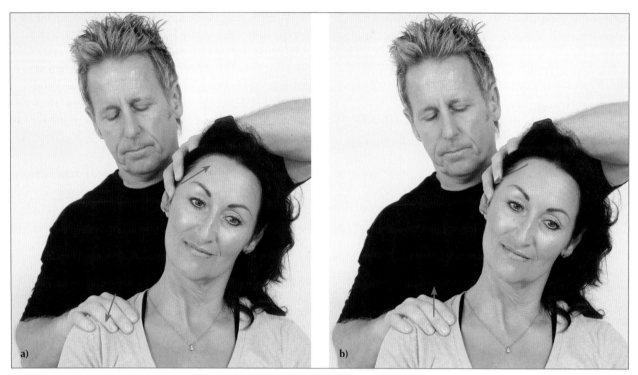

Figure 7.3a & b: *a: Upper trapezius stretch position; b: patient is asked to resist side bending of the cervical spine or shoulder elevation to activate the upper trapezius*

Levator scapulae stretch and resist

The patient adopts a sitting position and the therapist slowly flexes and rotates the patient's head away from the painful side (figure 7.4a). From this position the patient is asked to contract the levator scapulae against a resistance applied by the therapist by asking the patient to extend and rotate the cervical (figure 7.4b).

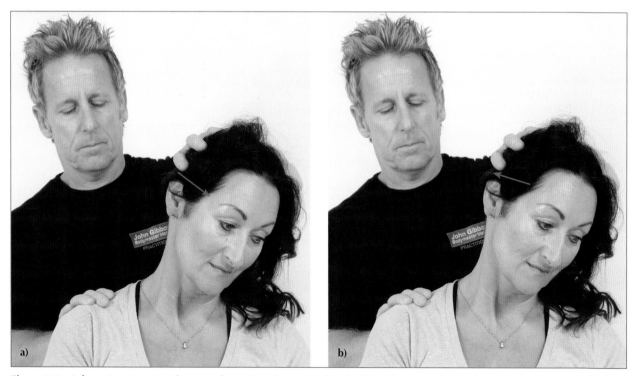

Figure 7.4a & b: *a: Levator scapulae stretch position; b: patient is asked to resist extension and rotation to the same side for the levator scapulae*

Dysfunction of the glenohumeral joint (GHJ)/ acromioclavicular joint (ACJ)/sternoclavicular joint (SCJ)

Obviously, this book is about the shoulder complex and the associated structures; from a biomechanics perspective, if the GH, AC, or SC joints are not functioning correctly then compensatory mechanisms will follow and this might cause the soft tissues to be overactive, with subsequent symptomology of pain perceived by the patients to the superior angle of scapula. There are numerous discussions throughout this text on assessing these areas so they will not be discussed here.

3. Intervertebral disc bulge of C4/5 or C5/6

When patients have pathology with the intervertebral disc then typically they tend to have more signs and symptoms rather than pain just to the superior scapula. For example, they might have shoulder and arm pain and this might be exacerbated when they cough and sneeze, rotate their neck to look for the seat belt in the car, etc. If, when they are discussing the symptoms, the patient happens to use words such as 'sharp,' 'shooting,' or 'stabbing' and if they have any form of altered sensations such as tingling or numbness then one must consider a neural structure is involved. I have discussed this type of pathology in a lot more detail in chapter 6 on the cervical spine.

4. Elevated or inspirated first rib

This is an interesting concept and there is lots of literature and many videos online that relate to the position of the first rib. The scalenes have an attachment to the first and second ribs so potentially if these muscles become shortened then they can either affect the attachment to the cervical spine (C2–7), or in this case cause the upper ribs to elevate. The lower aspect of the brachial plexus (C8/T1 of the ulnar nerve) and the subclavian artery and vein have to pass over the first rib and under the clavicle as they continue their journey down the arm (the vein is on its returning journey) and these three structures (i.e., brachial plexus and subclavian artery/vein) are collectively known as the neurovascular bundle of the thoracic outlet. If there is any form of compression to any of these structures then it is called a thoracic outlet syndrome (TOS) and there is no doubt they could be involved with the patient's symptomology because of the first rib that is fixed in a higher position than normal. The reason why the patient might have superior scapula pain is because of the unnatural position of the upper ribs and the subsequent altered biomechanics of the shoulder complex musculature during specific movements of abduction and flexion.

Test position for elevated rib

The patient adopts a sitting position and the therapist places their fingertips on the trapezius muscle and guides this muscle slightly posteriorly to access the first rib (figure 7.5a). The patient is asked to take a breath in and the first rib should be seen to rise and lower with the breathing motion (figure 7.5b).

5. Cervical rib (extra rib from the transverse process of C7)

This is a similar concept in one respect to the above pathology because if there is an extra rib present that is a continuation of the transverse process of the seventh

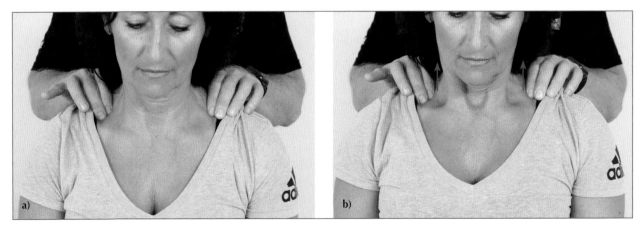

Figure 7.5a & b: *a: Palpation to ascertain position for the first rib; b: patient is asked to take a breath in and out and the position of the first rib is noted*

cervical vertebra, then this bony spur will eventually penetrate the already small space within the lower part of the exiting structures for the thoracic outlet and this could be why the patient has ongoing shoulder, arm and possibly hand pain with altered sensations, numbness and weakness. This condition is pretty rare but I have seen it present more often in females than males; however, it is not clear why this should be so.

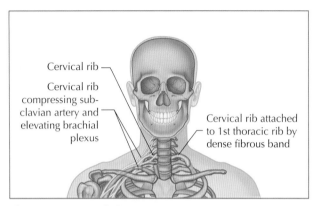

Figure 7.6: *Cervical rib present*

6. Relative shortness/tightness of the scalene muscles

The brachial plexus and the subclavian artery/vein (thoracic outlet) normally pass between the anterior and middle fibers of the scalene muscle groups. If for some reason this area becomes restricted or even fibrotic – there is a condition called *scalenus anticus syndrome* in which the anterior fibers have thickened and possibly become fibrosed – then the exiting neurovascular bundle is compromised. This might happen because the scalenes are working hard to stabilize the chest wall during repetitive motions. The scalenes, as you know from the text above, will lift the chest wall because they attach to the first and

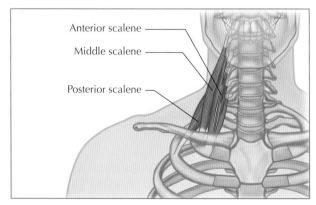

Figure 7.7: *A thickening on the anterior fibers of the scalenes (anticus syndrome)*

second ribs and are naturally involved in deep inhalation; however, if for some reason the diaphragm is not working as efficiently because the person is predominantly a chest breather due to asthma or other bronchial pathology, then the scalenes will be constantly working overtime. The scalenes can become shortened as a result of an adapted position of the upper chest wall (upper crossed syndrome), due, for example, to a daily posture sitting at an office desk for 8 hours of every day.

7. Positional

I have mentioned in an earlier chapter that symptomology of pain located to the shoulder complex can be linked to an *upper crossed syndrome* and this concept is related to a forward head posture, with subsequent rounded or protracted shoulders, potentially leading to shortened and tight pectorals and sternocleidomastoid, and possibly lengthened and weakened rhomboids, middle fibers of the trapezius, and serratus anterior.

8. Upper lobe of lung, referring to the trapezius

Visceral pain through disease has to be considered from time to time as the causative factor for the patient's pain, no matter where that might be located. This is especially important for this particular book, when patients present with shoulder pain that you consider is not musculoskeletal in nature. When I discussed visceral pain in an earlier chapter I mentioned a case study in which the patient had been a smoker of many years who presented to the clinic with shoulder and arm pain. The diagnosis was a lung carcinoma called a Pancoast tumor; it was located to the apical (top) part of the lung and had infiltrated the upper ribs and brachial plexus. Any type of disease process (not just cancer) that affects the respiratory system can be a source of pain to the shoulder region.

9. Diaphragm

Again, recapping a passage in an earlier chapter, the diaphragm is innervated by the phrenic nerve, which originates from the level of C3–5 from the cervical spine; the dermatome from C3–5 can cause a referred pattern of pain that can radiate to the area of the shoulder (a *dermatome* is an area of skin that is supplied from a single nerve root) and the pain sensation from the diaphragm muscle (if you remember) is generally felt to the superior angle of the scapula, suprascapular fossa and along the trapezius muscle. Remember that the respiratory muscle will only give shoulder pain if the central portion is affected as the lower intercostal nerves innervate the peripheral aspect of the diaphragm, so these nerves do not refer to the shoulder region. Typically, the patient will probably be more aware of their shoulder pain on deep inhalation, coughing, and sneezing.

As you can see, there are many possible causes of the patient's presenting pain. This list is not exhaustive and highlights just some of the many avenues to consider when confronted with a common complaint of 'shoulder/trapezius pain.'

Other possibilities of pain located to the superior angle

Some readers may have read another book that I wrote called *The Vital Glutes*, and may (or may not) be thinking 'hey, what about the glutes!' Some of the musculoskeletal pathology above was mentioned there, as was the possibility of shoulder pain being caused by the glutes. In relation to this possibility, I want to illustrate the statement from Dr Ida Rolf mentioned above with a case study taken from my own clinic at the University of Oxford. As I become more experienced, not only as a lecturer but also as a practicing sports osteopath, I am convinced that many issues patients and athletes present with are purely symptoms rather than actual causes. This was one of the main driving forces that inspired me to write a whole book on the gluteal muscles, on which a small part of this chapter is based.

To highlight the relevance of this chapter the information below is taken from a real case study patient who came to my clinic for a consultation.

CASE STUDY

The patient in question was a woman of 34 years who was a physical trainer for the Royal Air Force. She presented to the clinic with pain located to the superior aspect of her left scapula (figure 7.8). The pain would come on four miles into a run, forcing her to stop because it was so intense. The discomfort would then subside, but quickly return if she attempted to start running again. Running was the only activity that caused the pain. Her complaint

had been ongoing for eight months, had worsened over the past three, and was starting to affect her work. There was no previous history or related trauma to trigger the complaint.

She saw numerous soft tissue practitioners, who all focused their treatment on the upper limb soft tissues. The treatments she had received were all biased toward the application of soft tissue massage techniques to the affected area, namely the trapezius, levator scapulae, pectoralis major, sternocleidomastoid (SCM), scalenes, as they had told her she presented with an upper crossed syndrome. Because the pain was still present, she was advised to see an osteopath, who treated her cervical spine with manipulations to the area of the left C4/5 and also performed a muscle energy technique (MET) for what they said was an inspirated first rib. She then saw a chiropractor who also used manipulative techniques on the facet joints of her cervical spine – C4/5 and C5/6. Lastly, she visited a physiotherapist trained in acupuncture and exercise therapy and she used muscle energy techniques and trigger point releases to the soft tissues of trapezius and levator scapulae with specific dry needling techniques, but which were used in a localized area, which offered relief at the time but made no difference when she attempted to run more than four miles. She had not undergone any scans (e.g., MRI or X-ray).

Taking a holistic approach

I think it is a good idea just to pause for a moment and think about the above paragraph and how *all* of the therapists *only* focused on the presenting complaint. This is the surgeon's *diagnostic finger* resurfacing its ugly head again – the patient pointed to the pain and the therapists treated what the patient pointed at! The strategy of 'treating where it hurts' was not working for this patient, as I hope you agree.

Let us now assess the case study patient globally rather than focusing locally (to the pointed finger), remembering the most important fact – *the pain only comes on after running four miles.*

When I see a new patient for the first time, no matter what the presenting pain is, I normally assess the pelvis for position and movement, as I consider this area of the body in particular to be the foundation for everything that connects to it. I often find in clinic that when I correct a dysfunctional pelvis, my client's presenting symptoms tend to settle down. However, when I assessed this particular patient, I found her pelvis was level and moving correctly. I then went on to test the firing patterns of the gluteus maximus (referred to as the *Gmax* for the remainder of this text), which I often do with patients and athletes who participate in regular sporting activities. However, I only test the firing pattern sequence once I feel that the pelvis is in its correct position; the logic here is that you often get a positive result of the muscle misfiring (I call it gluteal amnesia, this means the glute muscles are taking a nap) when the pelvis is slightly out of position.

With the patient in question, I found a bilateral weakness/misfiring of the Gmax, but the firing on the right side seemed a bit slower than when I tested the left side (more details in the next chapter on how to test the firing of the Gmax). As I had not found any dysfunction in the pelvis, I pursued this line of approach a little further.

Before we continue I would like to pose a few questions for you to think about:

- How can a weakness of the Gmax on the right side cause pain to the region of the left shoulder?
- Is there a link between the Gmax and the opposite trapezius and levator scapulae, and if so, how is this possible?
- From a physical therapy perspective, what can be done to correct the issue?
- What has happened to cause it in the first place?

To answer these questions, we need to look at the functional anatomy of the Gmax, and the relationship of the Gmax to other anatomical structures.

Gmax function

The Gmax operates mainly as a powerful hip extensor and a lateral rotator, but it also plays a part in stabilizing the sacroiliac joint (SIJ) by helping it to 'force close' while going through the gait cycle.

Some of the Gmax muscular fibers attach to the sacrotuberous ligament, which runs from the sacrum to the ischial tuberosity. This ligament has been termed the *key ligament* in helping to stabilize the SIJ. To gain a better understanding of this action, we first need to consider two concepts, namely form closure and force closure, which are both associated with stability of the SIJ (explained in more detail in the next chapter).

Form closure is formed by the natural shape of the sacrum and the fact that it is wedged between the two ilia bones and this provides some stability; however, form closure of the SIJ is not perfect and movement is possible, which means stabilization during loading is required. This is achieved by increasing compression across the joint at the moment of loading; the surrounding ligaments, muscles, and fascia are responsible for this. The mechanism of compression of the SIJ by these additional forces is called *force closure*.

When the body is working efficiently, the forces between the innominate bones and the sacrum are adequately controlled, and loads can be transferred between the trunk, pelvis, and legs. So how do we link this to the patient's complaint? In one of my previous articles (Gibbons 2008), about training the Oxford rowing team, I wrote about the posterior oblique 'sling.' This structure directly links the right Gmax to the left latissimus dorsi via the thoracolumbar fascia (figure 7.8). The latissimus dorsi has its insertion on the inner part of the humerus, and one of the functions of this muscle is to keep the scapula against the thoracic cage and aid in depression of the scapula.

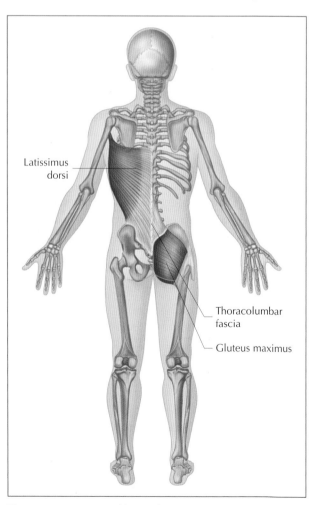

Figure 7.8: *Posterior oblique sling*

Piecing it all together

So what do we know? We know that the right side of the patient's Gmax is slightly slower in terms of its firing pattern and that this muscle plays a role in the force closure process of the SIJ. This tells us that if the Gmax cannot perform this function of stabilizing the SIJ, then something else will assist in stabilizing the joint. The left latissimus dorsi is the synergist that helps stabilize the right Gmax and, more importantly, the SIJ. As the patient participates in running, every time her right leg contacts the ground and goes through the gait cycle, the left latissimus dorsi is overcontracting. This causes the left scapula to depress, and the muscles that resist the downward depressive pull will be the upper trapezius and the levator scapulae. Subsequently, these muscles start to fatigue; for the patient in question, this occurs at approximately four miles, at which point she feels pain in her left superior scapula.

Treatment

You might think the easy way to treat the weakness found within the Gmax is to simply prescribe strength-based exercises. However, in practice this is not always the correct solution, as sometimes the short and tight antagonistic muscle is responsible for the apparent weakness. The muscle in this case is the iliopsoas, rectus femoris and adductors (hip flexors), and shortening of these hip flexors can result in a weakness inhibition of the Gmax. My answer to this complex puzzle of the presenting left shoulder pain was to promote lengthening using muscle energy techniques (METs) to the patient's right iliopsoas, rectus femoris, and adductor muscles to see if it promoted and *rebooted* the firing activation of the right Gmax, while at the same time introducing specific strength control exercises for the right Gmax.

Prognosis

I advised the patient to abstain from running and to get her partner to assist in lengthening the iliopsoas, rectus femoris, and adductors twice a day. Strength exercises were also advised twice daily until the follow-on treatment (these exercises are discussed in my vital glutes book). I reassessed her 10 days later and found normal firing activation for the right Gmax on the hip extension firing pattern test, and also found a reduction in the tightness of the associated iliopsoas, rectus femoris, and adductors. Because of these positive results, I advised her to run as far as she felt comfortable. I was not sure if my treatment was going to correct the problem, but she reported that she had no pain during or after a six-mile run. The patient is still pain free and continues to regularly use the Gmax strengthening exercises and the lengthening techniques that were prescribed for the tight and shortened hip flexor muscles.

■ Conclusion

This case study I personally feel will demonstrate (hopefully) that very often the underlying cause of a condition or problem may not be local to where the symptoms/pain presents, which means that all avenues need to be fully considered. I hope that the information from this chapter and in particular the case study has intrigued you enough to *'think, before you treat'* patients with superior scapula pain!

Remember, this book (and this goes for all my books to date) is what I call a *jigsaw puzzle journey* – if you stick with it, the picture will eventually become a lot clearer.

8

The relationship of the pelvis, the sacroiliac joint and the gluteals to the shoulder complex

The incidence of shoulder and cervical (neck) pain continues to increase, so what I would like to do in this chapter is to discuss the muscular as well as skeletal relationships that affect the core and lumbo-pelvic-sacral stability and how it relates to the function or even dysfunction of the shoulder complex. We will then have to decide how to incorporate this knowledge into an assessment, treatment, and rehabilitative plan, especially for patients and athletes who present with pain associated to the area of the upper limb and specifically to the region of the shoulder complex.

CASE STUDY

I have personally seen thousands of the athletes at the University of Oxford, where I am currently based. However, I would like to tell you about one in particular. Anil was a student at Oxford and was very competitive at cricket and a member of the university cricket team. He would always complain of pain to his right shoulder, especially after bowling. He told me that many physical therapists had looked at him over the last few years, with most of them recommending certain typical shoulder exercises, but they had produced no real change in his symptoms. He also produced an MRI scan that confirmed he had damaged the rotator cuff muscle group; in particular, there was a partial thickness tear to the supraspinatus muscle and some thickening/inflammation of the subacromial bursa.

On examination I did find him to have some pain and restriction through 70–110 degrees of shoulder abduction, so this painful arc confirmed the involvement of the rotator cuff. I told Anil that I would *not* be treating the right shoulder initially and that I was going to look at the function and stability of the left side of the pelvis and in particular the left gluteal muscles. He looked rather bemused and even annoyed that I was not going to treat the painful right shoulder; however, I mentioned an athlete that I had seen previously with left shoulder pain while running – the causative factor was inhibition or weakness/misfiring to the right gluteus maximus (Gmax) muscle and the left latissimus dorsi muscle was now compensating and contracting to take the role of the weak Gmax to provide a 'force closure' to the right sacroiliac joint during the running cycle.

When I assessed Anil I found him to be relatively unstable while standing on the left leg and he struggled to activate the left gluteus medius (Gmed) compared to standing on the right leg. When I tested the firing pattern of the left Gmax, I found this muscle to be slow compared to the right side. I tested the length of the antagonistic (opposite) muscles, i.e., psoas, rectus femoris, and the adductors, and found them to be relatively shortened on the left side. The treatment plan consisted of lengthening these tight muscular structures, while strengthening the weak Gmax and Gmed. Anil noticed a marked improvement almost immediately over the next few weeks and he is now at the point whereby the right shoulder does not cause him any more pain or restriction, especially after bowling.

If you think just for a minute about why Anil improved by doing what I suggested, imagine that when you plan to bowl a ball in cricket, you are naturally running pretty fast and when you are about to bowl you will have to contact the ground with the left leg, while at the same time, the right arm is about to throw the ball. If the left Gluteal muscles are weaker for some reason then the right latissimus dorsi muscle is going to stabilize the left sacroiliac joint through force closure (recall the earlier case study of left shoulder pain and right Gmax inhibition), the problem you have now is that the athlete will want to raise the right arm to throw the ball; however, the right latissimus muscle is also contracting to improve the sacroiliac joint stability on the left (opposite) side. As the right arm is abducting by the supraspinatus muscle, the simultaneously contracting right latissimus muscle will end up resisting the abduction (acting like a brake) because it needs to stabilize the left SIJ (because the glutes is not performing its natural function). I mention here David and Goliath (biblical warrior defeated by the young David in the Book of Samuel), David being the small supraspinatus and Goliath the large latissimus muscle. In this case, however, the larger muscle wins the battle and the smaller muscle loses, or in this case the supraspinatus muscle will end up suffering the consequences of losing the battle with ongoing tears and recurrent inflammation; so no matter what one does to stabilize the shoulder with exercises, the patient will never get better unless they take a complete rest from bowling.

This book is about the upper limb and shoulder complex; however, in this chapter I want to briefly focus on the pelvis, the SI joint and the gluteal muscles and to discuss if these associated areas can be related to the patients presenting with upper limb symptomology. Think of Dr Ida Rolf's precept that wherever you think the pain is coming from, it is not. Maybe, just maybe, for certain individuals, the area of the pelvis, SIJ and even the gluteal muscles might be part of the causative factor for their pain located to the region of the upper limb.

Sacroiliac stability: form and force closure

First, we will look at stability of the pelvis. Two main factors affect the stability of the pelvis (or to be more precise the sacroiliac joint): form closure and force closure. These two mechanisms collectively assist in a process known as the *self-locking mechanism*.

Form closure arises from the anatomical alignment of the bones of the innominate and the sacrum, where the sacrum forms a kind of keystone between the wings of the pelvis. The SIJ transfers large loads and its shape is adapted to this task. The articular surfaces are relatively flat, which helps to transfer compression forces and bending movements. However, a relatively flat joint is vulnerable to shear forces. The SIJ is protected from these forces in three ways. First, the sacrum is wedge (triangular) shaped and thus is stabilized between the innominate bones, similarly to a keystone in a Roman arch, and is kept in a state of 'suspension' by the ligaments acting upon it. Second, in contrast to other synovial joints, the articular cartilage is not smooth but rather irregular. Third, a frontal dissection through the SIJ reveals cartilage-covered bone extensions protruding into the joint – the so-called 'ridges' and 'grooves.' They seem rather irregular, but are in fact complementary to each other, and this unusual irregularity is very relevant as it serves to stabilize the SIJ when compression is applied.

According to Vleeming et al. (1990a), after puberty most individuals develop a crescent-shaped ridge running the entire length of the iliac surface with a corresponding depression on the sacral side; this complementary ridge and groove are now believed to lock the surfaces together and increase stability of the SIJ.

If the articular surfaces of the sacrum and the innominate bones fitted together with perfect form closure mobility would be practically impossible. However, form closure of the SIJ is not perfect and mobility – albeit small – is possible, and therefore stabilization during loading is required. This is achieved by increasing compression across the joint at the moment of loading; the anatomical structures responsible for this compression are the ligaments, muscles, and fasciae. The mechanism of compression of the SIJ by these additional forces is what is commonly called *force closure*. When the SIJ is compressed, friction of the joint increases and consequently reinforces form closure (figure 8.1). According to Willard et al. (2012), force closure reduces the joint's 'neutral zone,' thereby facilitating stabilization of the SIJ.

Force closure is accomplished as follows: the first method is by a forward type of motion by the sacrum that is called nutation; this is achieved either by anterior motion of the sacral base or by posterior rotation of the innominate bone (figure 8.2a). These two types of motion result in a tightening of the sacrotuberous, sacrospinous, and

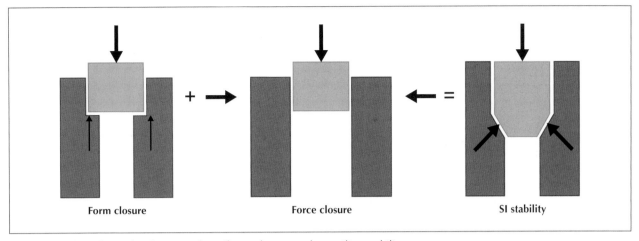

Figure 8.1: *The relationship between form/force closure and sacroiliac stability*

interosseous ligaments; this tightening assists in activating the force closure mechanism, thereby increasing the compression of the SIJ. Counternutation, on the other hand, which is a posterior type of motion performed by the sacrum or an anterior motion of the innominate bone (figure 8.2b), decreases the stability of the SIJ because of the reduced tension in the above-mentioned ligaments.

In the second method, force closure is assisted by the activation/contraction of the inner and outer core muscles (local and global muscle systems), as mentioned in the early chapters.

The terms *form closure* and *force closure* delineate the active and passive components of this self-locking mechanism and were first identified by Vleeming et al. (1990a, 1990b). Below is a quote from Vleeming et al. (1995) that I personally believe explains the above text.

'Shear in the sacroiliac joints is prevented by the combination of specific anatomical features (form closure) and the compression generated by muscles and ligaments that can be accommodated to the specific loading situation (force closure). If the sacrum would fit the pelvis with perfect form closure, no lateral forces would be needed. However, such a construction would make mobility practically impossible.'

■ Sacroiliac stability

Several ligaments, muscles, and fascial systems contribute to force closure of the pelvis: these are collectively referred to as the *osteo-articular-ligamentous system*. Recall that when the body is working efficiently, the shear forces between the innominate bones and the sacrum are adequately controlled, and loads can then be transferred between the trunk, pelvis, and legs (figure 8.3).

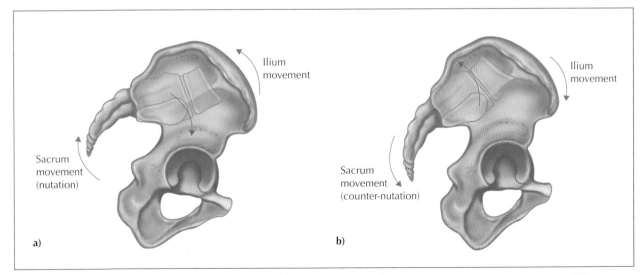

Figure 8.2a & b: *a: Nutation and posterior rotation of the innominate. b: Counternutation and anterior rotation of the innominate*

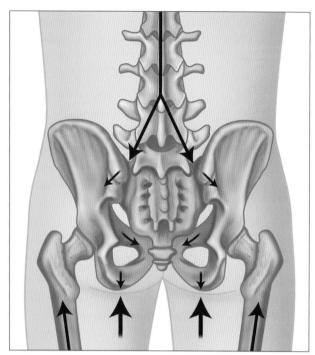

Figure 8.3: *Weight transfer forces through pelvis and sacroiliac joints*

Vleeming and Stoeckart (2007) mention that various muscles are involved in force closure of the SIJ, and that even muscles such as the rectus femoris, sartorius, iliacus, Gmax, and hamstrings have adequate lever arms to influence movement in the SIJ. The effect of these muscles is dependent on open or closed kinematic movements, and whether the pelvis is sufficiently braced.

As you will read shortly, there is one muscle in particular that plays a highly significant role in stabilizing the SIJs: this muscle is the gluteus maximus (Gmax), and we will also be discussing the gluteus medius (Gmed) as this muscle too has a relationship with the pelvis. Some of the Gmax fibers merge and attach onto the sacrotuberous ligament as well as onto a connective tissue structure known as the *thoracolumbar fascia*.

Vleeming et al. (1989a) demonstrated this fact on 12 cadaver dissections; they found that the Gmax muscle was directly attached to the sacrotuberous ligament in all cases.

The Gmax connects, via the thoracolumbar fascia, to the contralateral latissimus dorsi to form what is known as the *posterior oblique myofascial sling* (see also section entitled The outer core unit: the integrated myofascial sling system (global system). It has been shown that weakness, or possibly a misfiring sequence, of the Gmax will predispose the SIJ to injury by decreasing the function of this (posterior oblique) myofascial sling. A weakness or misfiring of the Gmax is

a potential cause of a compensatory overactivation of the contralateral latissimus dorsi, with potential for neck and shoulder pain; walking and running impose high loads on the SIJ, so this weight-bearing joint will need to be self-stabilizing in order to reduce the effect of the altered compensatory mechanism.

Research has shown that sacral nutation (a nodding type of movement of the sacrum between the innominate bones) is the best position for the pelvic girdle to be at its most stable. Nutation occurs when moving (for example) from a sitting position to standing, and full nutation occurs during forward or backward bending of the trunk. This motion of sacral nutation tightens the major ligaments (sacrotuberous, sacrospinous, and interosseous) of the posterior pelvis, and the resulting tension increases the compressive force across the SIJ. The increased tension provides the required stability that is needed by the SIJ during the gait cycle as well as when simply rising from a sitting to a standing position.

Vleeming et al. (1989b), showed how load application to the sacrotuberous ligament, either directly to the ligament or through its continuations with the long head of biceps femoris or the attachments of the Gmax, significantly diminishes forward rotation of the sacral base. They demonstrated that this increases the coefficient of friction, thus decreasing movement of the SIJ by force closure.

■ Force closure ligaments

The main ligamentous structures that influence force closure (figure 8.4) are: (1) the sacrotuberous ligament, which connects the sacrum to the ischium and has been termed the *key* or *lead* ligament; and (2) the long dorsal sacroiliac ligament, which connects the third and fourth sacral segments to the PSIS and is also known as the *posterior sacroiliac ligament*.

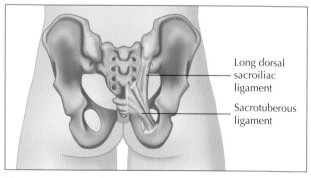

Long dorsal sacroiliac ligament

Sacrotuberous ligament

Figure 8.4: *Sacrotuberous ligament (key) and the long dorsal sacroiliac ligament*

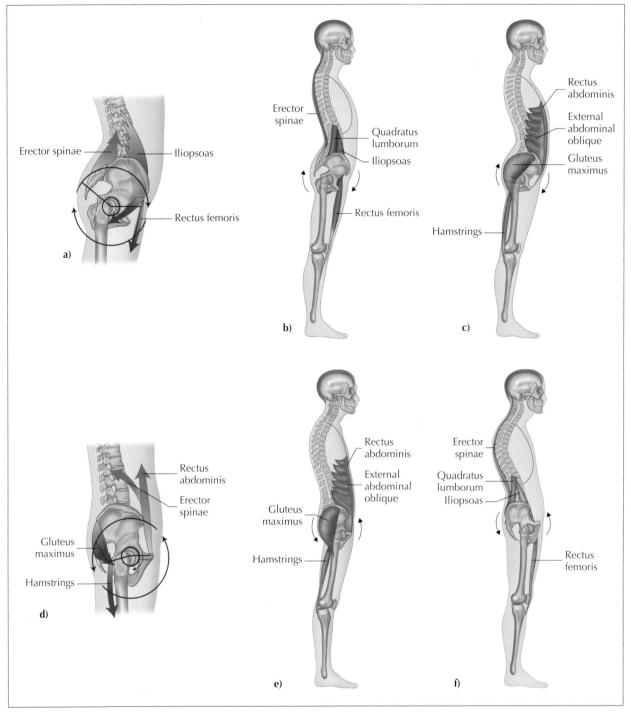

Figure 8.5a–f: *a: Sagittal plane (anterior) pelvis force couple; b: anterior tilt: muscles held in a shortened position; c: anterior tilt: muscles held in a lengthened position; d: sagittal plane (posterior) pelvis force couple; e: posterior tilt: muscles held in a shortened position; f: posterior tilt: muscles held in a lengthened position*

Ligaments can increase articular compression when they are tensed or lengthened by the movement of the bones to which they attach, or when they are tensed by the contraction of muscles that insert onto the bones.

Tension in the sacrotuberous ligament can be increased in one of three ways:

1. posterior rotation of the innominate bone relative to the sacrum

2. nutation of the sacrum relative to the innominate bone

3. muscular contraction of any one of the four muscles that have a direct attachment to the sacrotuberous ligament, namely the biceps femoris, piriformis, Gmax, and multifidus.

The main ligamentous tissue to restrain counternutation of the sacrum, or anterior rotation of the innominate, is the long dorsal sacroiliac ligament (posterior sacroiliac ligament). This is a less stable position (compared with the position of nutation) for the pelvis to resist horizontal and/or vertical loading, since the SIJ is under less compression and is not self-locked. The long dorsal ligament is commonly a source of pain and can be palpated just below (inferior to) the level of the PSIS.

By themselves, ligaments cannot maintain a stable pelvis: they rely on several muscle systems to assist them. There are two important groups of muscles that contribute to stability of the lower back and pelvis: collectively they are called the *inner unit* (core) and the *outer unit* (myofascial sling systems). The inner unit consists of the transversus abdominis (TVA), multifidus, diaphragm, and muscles of the pelvic floor – also collectively known as the *core*, or *local stabilizers*. The outer unit consists of several 'slings,' or systems of muscles (global stabilizers and mobilizers that are anatomically connected and functionally related).

■ Force couple

Definition: A *force couple* is a situation where two forces of equal magnitude, but acting in opposite directions, are applied to an object and pure rotation results, as mentioned by Abernethy et al. (2004).

Any altered positioning of the pelvis caused by potential muscle imbalances will subsequently affect the rest of the kinetic chain and this change to the biomechanics will subsequently alter the pelvic relationship to the upper limb. There are several force couples responsible for maintaining proper positioning and alignment of the pelvis. The force couples responsible for controlling the position of the pelvis in the sagittal and frontal planes are shown schematically in figures 8.5a–f and 8.6.

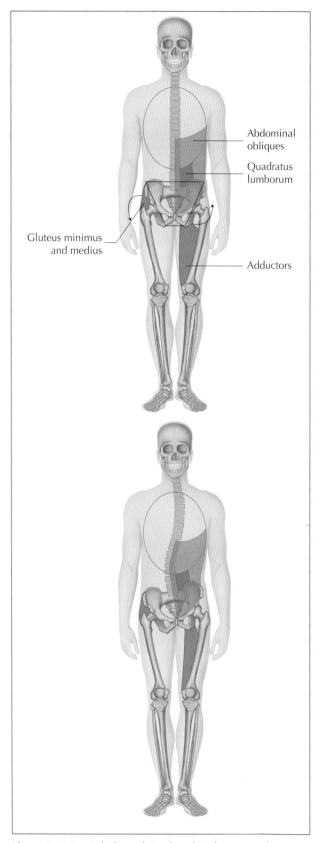

Figure 8.6: *Frontal plane (lateral) pelvic force couples*

■ Functional anatomy of the gluteus maximus (Gmax)

I want to focus on the gluteus maximus (Gmax) and how this muscle could be responsible for many of the complaints that patients and athletes present with, especially painful symptoms in the area of the upper limb. The Gmax, I feel, is relatively neglected by most physical therapists I come into contact with. Perhaps the reason for this neglect is that the Gmax does not normally itself present with pain, and hence this amazing and functional muscle is left on what I call the *neglect shelf*.

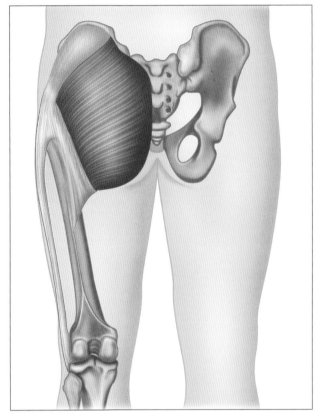

Figure 8.7: *Anatomy of the Gmax*

Origin: Outer surface of the ilium behind the posterior gluteal line and a portion of the bone superior and posterior to it. Adjacent posterior surface of the sacrum and coccyx. Sacrotuberous ligament. Aponeurosis of the erector spinae.

Insertion: *Deep fibers of distal portion*: gluteal tuberosity of the femur.
Remaining fibers: iliotibial tract of the fasciae latae.

Action: Through its insertion into the iliotibial tract, helps to stabilize the knee in extension.

Upper fibers: laterally rotate and abduction of hip joint.
Lower fibers: extend and laterally rotate hip joint (forceful extension as in running or standing up from sitting). Extend trunk.

Nerve: Inferior gluteal nerve (L5, S1, S2).

Function of the Gmax

From a functional perspective, the Gmax performs several key roles in controlling the relationship between the femur, pelvis, trunk and the upper limb. This magical muscle is capable of abducting and laterally rotating the hip, which helps to control the alignment of the knee with the lower limb. For example, in stair climbing, the Gmax will laterally rotate and abduct the hip to keep the lower limb in optimal alignment, while at the same time the hip extends to carry the body upward onto the next step. When the Gmax is weak or misfiring, the knee can be seen to deviate medially and the pelvis can also be observed to tip laterally.

The Gmax also has a role in stabilizing the SIJs and has been described as one of the force closure muscles. Some of the Gmax fibers attach to the sacrotuberous ligament and the thoracolumbar fascia, which is a very strong, non-contractile connective tissue that is tensioned by the activation of muscles connecting to it. One of the connections to this fascia is the latissimus dorsi. The Gmax forms a partnership with the contralateral latissimus dorsi via the thoracolumbar fascia; this partnership connection is known as the *posterior oblique sling* (see figure 8.8). This sling increases the compression force to the SIJ during the weight-bearing single-leg stance in the gait cycle.

Misfiring or weakness in the Gmax reduces the effectiveness of the posterior oblique sling, which will predispose the SIJs to subsequent injury. The body will then try to compensate for this weakness by increasing tension via the thoracolumbar fascia by in turn increasing the activation of the contralateral latissimus dorsi. As with any compensatory mechanism, 'structure affects function' and 'function affects structure.' This means that other areas of the body are affected: for example – and the focus of this book – the shoulder mechanics are altered since the latissimus dorsi has attachments on the humerus and scapula. If the latissimus

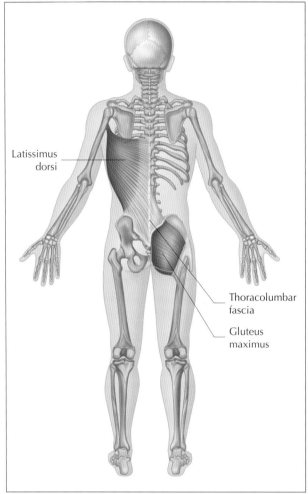

Latissimus dorsi

Thoracolumbar fascia

Gluteus maximus

Figure 8.8: *Posterior oblique sling and the connection with the latissimus dorsi*

dorsi is particularly active because of the compensation, this can be observed as one shoulder appearing lower than the other during a step-up or a lunge type of motion

The Gmax plays a significant role in the gait cycle, working in conjunction with the hamstrings. Just before heel-strike, the hamstrings will activate, which will increase the tension to the SIJs via the attachment on the sacrotuberous ligament. This connection assists in the locking mechanism of the SIJs for the weight-bearing cycle. From heel-strike to mid-stance of the gait cycle, the Gmax increases its activation and the hamstrings decrease theirs. The Gmax significantly increases the stabilization of the SIJs during early and mid-stance phases through the attachments of the posterior oblique sling.

Weakness or misfiring in the Gmax will cause the hamstrings to remain active during the gait cycle in order to maintain stability of the SIJs and the position of the

pelvis. The resultant overactivation of the hamstrings will subject them to continual and abnormal strain.

Generally speaking, the Gmax follows a trait of becoming weakened if the antagonistic muscles have become short and tight. The main muscles that have shortened can cause a neurological inhibition to the Gmax, and theses are the iliopsoas, rectus femoris, and adductors, as they all are classified as *hip flexors*, which are the antagonistic muscles to the hip extension action of the Gmax.

The assessment and treatment of the iliopsoas and other associated shortened antagonistic muscles will not be discussed here and the reader is directed to *The Vital Glutes* (Gibbons 2014). However, if you have a good understanding of the muscles mentioned above and you were to normalize the tight and shortened antagonistic muscles by the use of lengthening techniques then this will promote a normal neutral position of the pelvis and lumbar spine, and in turn hopefully have the effect of 'switching' the weakened Gmax back on and subsequently reducing the pain to the area of the shoulder complex.

■ Assessment of the Gmax

In this section I will discuss the hip extension firing pattern test, which is used for determining the correct firing order of the hip extensors (including the Gmax muscle). The aim of the test is to ascertain the actual firing sequence of a group of muscles to ensure that all are firing correctly, just like the cylinders of an engine. A misfiring pattern will commonly be found in athletes and patients.

Hip extension firing pattern test (figure 8.9)

The normal muscle activation sequence is:

Gluteus maximus
Hamstrings
Contralateral lumbar extensors
Ipsilateral lumbar extensors
Contralateral thoracolumbar extensors
Ipsilateral thoracolumbar extensors.

The hip extension firing pattern test is unique in its application. Think of yourself as a car with six cylinders in your engine: basically that is what your body is – an engine. The engine has a certain way of firing and so does your body. For example, the engine in a car will not fire its individual cylinders in the numerical order 1–2–3–4–5–6; it will fire in a pre-defined optimum sequence, say 1–3–5–6–4–2. If we have our car serviced and the mechanic mistakes two of the leads and puts them back incorrectly, the engine will still work but not very efficiently; moreover, it will eventually break down. Our bodies are no different: in our case, if we are particularly active but have a misfiring dysfunction, our bodies will also break down, ultimately causing us pain.

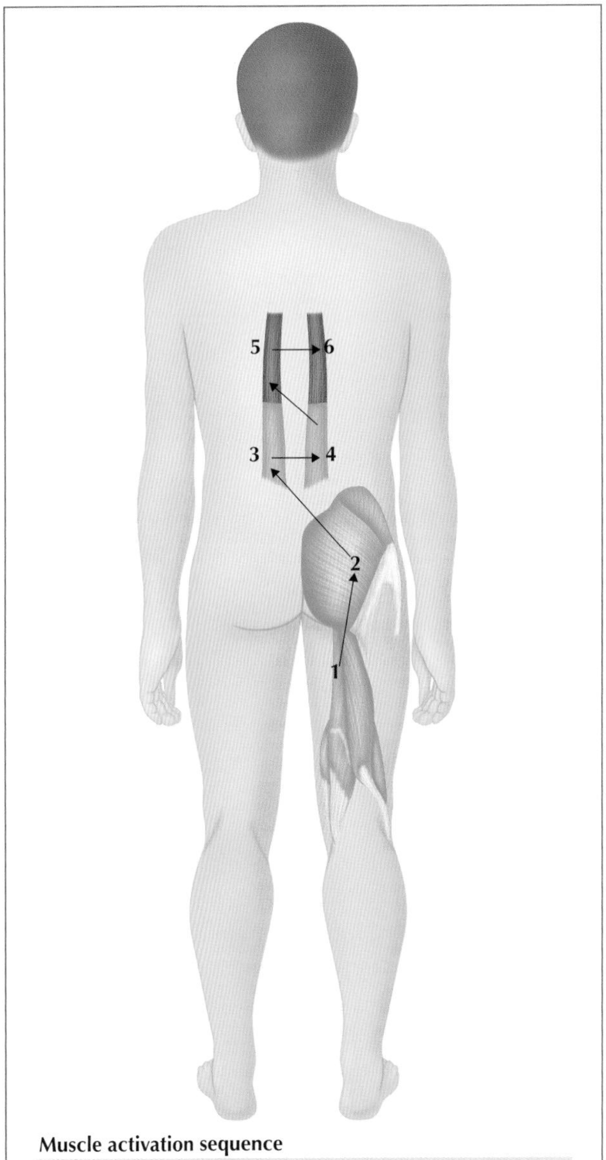

Sequence 1

The therapist places their fingertips lightly on the patient's left hamstrings and left Gmax (figure 8.10a&b), and the patient is asked to lift their left leg 2 in (5 cm) off the couch (figure 8.10c). The therapist tries to identify which muscle fires first and notes the result of this first sequence in table 8.1.

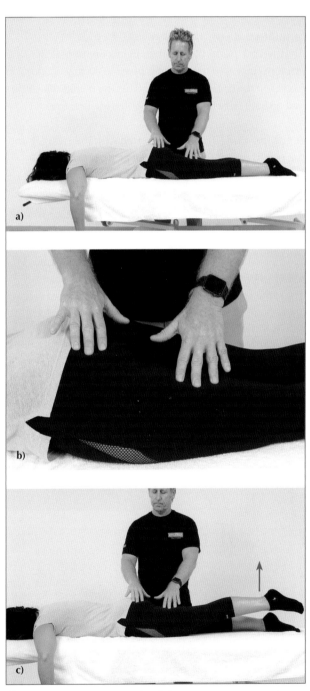

Figure 8.10a–c: *Hip extension firing pattern sequence 1. a: The therapist lightly palpates the patient's left hamstrings and Gmax; b: close-up view of the therapist's hand position; c: the patient lifts their left leg off the couch*

Muscle activation sequence

1. Hamstrings
2. Gluteus maximus
3. Contralateral lumber extensors
4. Ipsilateral lumber extensors
5. Contralateral thoracolumbar extensors
6. Ipsilateral thoracolumbar extensors

Either group may normally activate first

Figure 8.9: *Correct firing pattern in hip joint extension*

Table 8.1: Hip extension firing pattern – left side

	1st	2nd	3rd	4th
Gluteus maximus	○	○	○	○
Hamstrings	○	○	○	○
Contralateral erector spinae	○	○	○	○
Ipsilateral erector spinae	○	○	○	○

Table 8.2: Hip extension firing pattern – right side

	1st	2nd	3rd	4th
Gluteus maximus	○	○	○	○
Hamstrings	○	○	○	○
Contralateral erector spinae	○	○	○	○
Ipsilateral erector spinae	○	○	○	○

Sequence 2

The therapist places their thumbs lightly on the patient's erector spinae, and the patient is asked to lift their left leg 2 in (5 cm) off the couch (figure 8.11a&b). The therapist identifies and notes in table 8.1 which erector muscle fires first.

Sequences 1 and 2 are then repeated with the right leg and the results recorded in table 8.2. Having done this, the therapist can determine whether or not the muscles are firing correctly. The firing pattern should be: (1) gluteus maximus; (2) hamstrings; (3) contralateral erector spinae; and, lastly, (4) ipsilateral erector spinae.

If, when palpating in sequence 1, the gluteus maximus is found to fire first you can safely say that this is correct. The same applies in sequence 2: if the contralateral erector spinae contracts first this is also the correct sequence.

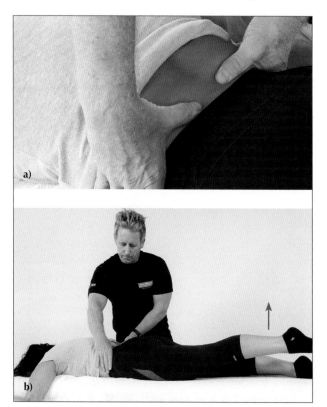

Figure 8.11a&b: *Hip extension-firing pattern sequence 2. a: The therapist lightly palpates the patient's erector spinae; b: the patient lifts their left leg off the couch*

However, if you feel that the hamstrings are number 1 in the sequence, or that the ipsilateral erector spinae is number 1 and the gluteus maximus is not felt to contract, you can deduce that this is a misfiring pattern. If the misfiring dysfunction is not corrected our body (the engine) will start to break down and a compensatory pattern of dysfunction will be created.

I have found that in a lot of patients, the hamstrings and the ipsilateral erector spinae are typically first to contract and the Gmax is number four in the sequence. In these cases the erector spinae and the hamstrings will become the dominant muscles in assisting the hip in an extension movement. This can cause excessive anterior tilting of the pelvis with a resultant hyperlordosis, which can lead to inflammation of the lower lumbar facet joints.

An example of a misfiring sequence is shown in figure 8.12 and demonstrates a typical dysfunctional pattern that I see on a regular basis. You will notice that the first muscle to contract is the right hamstrings (1), then the ipsilateral erector (2), then the contralateral erector (3), and finally the Gmax (4). I did not add in the thoracolumbar erector muscles because the 1–4 is dysfunctional and as mentioned earlier once 1–4 is corrected I find that 5 and 6 regain a normal firing sequence.

To correct the misfiring sequence, and before one is tempted to strengthen, we need to first look at the length of the antagonistic muscles as mentioned in the previous paragraph and by using METs in particular we normalize these shortened and tight tissues. So the simple process when it comes to correcting a misfiring Gmax is to 'lengthen before you strengthen.'

Note that the firing patterns of muscles 5 and 6 have not been discussed in this chapter, because we need to make sure that the correct firing order of muscles 1–4 is established. I also find, as stated above, that when the muscle 1–4 firing sequence has been corrected, the firing pattern of muscles 5 and 6 is generally self-correcting and tends to follow the normal firing pattern sequence.

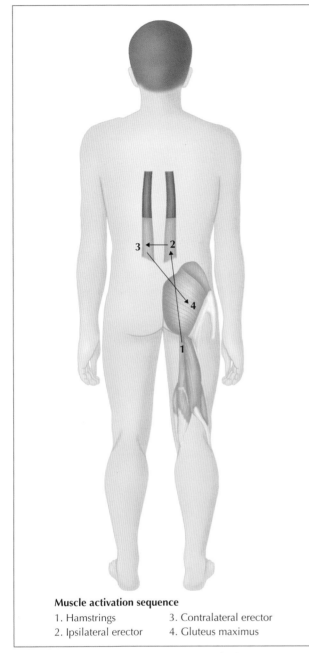

Muscle activation sequence

1. Hamstrings   3. Contralateral erector
2. Ipsilateral erector 4. Gluteus maximus

Figure 8.12: *Dysfunctional firing pattern for hip extension*

■ Functional anatomy of the gluteus medius (Gmed)

Origin: Outer surface of the ilium, inferior to the iliac crest, between the posterior gluteal line and the anterior gluteal line.

Insertion: Oblique ridge on the lateral surface of the greater trochanter of the femur.

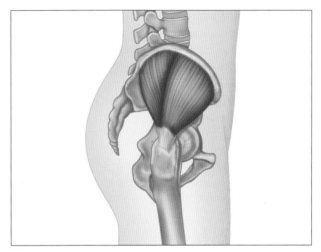

Figure 8.13: *Anatomy of the Gmed*

Action: *Upper fibers*: laterally rotate and abduction of the hip joint.
Anterior fibers: medially rotate and flexion of the hip joint.
Posterior fibers: laterally rotate and extend the hip joint.

Nerve: Superior gluteal nerve (L4, L5, S1).

Function of the Gmed

The Gmed is predominantly used in the gait cycle, especially during the initial contact with the ground and the stance phase of the cycle. Simplistically speaking, the Gmed is responsible for maintaining the position of the pelvis as we walk from point A to point B.

The Gmed should be assessed in every running injury to the upper and lower body that a patient may present with. Many athletes present to my clinic with overuse running types of injury to the lower limb and trunk, and the majority of them present with poor Gmed function. I have come to the conclusion that the strength and control of this muscle is probably the most important overall component in achieving a biomechanically efficient running pattern. This is not so surprising when you consider that during running you are always either completely in the air or dynamically balanced on one leg. All physical therapist practitioners should be able to assess and restore the Gmed function.

Let us take a closer look at the anatomy of the Gmed: the muscle attaches to the entire length of the iliac crest, to the external ilium between the posterior and anterior gluteal lines, to the gluteal fascia, to the posterior border of the TFL, and to the overlying ITB. The Gmed is divided into three distinct portions – anterior, middle, and posterior – which collectively form a broad conjoined tendon that wraps around, and inserts onto, the greater trochanter of the femur. The more vertical anterior and middle portions of the Gmed appear to be in a better position for abducting the hip than is the more horizontal posterior portion.

There has been much debate over whether the Gmed is primarily activated during medial rotation or during lateral rotation. In 2003, a study by Ireland et al. demonstrated that hip abduction and lateral rotation were significantly weaker in female subjects with patellofemoral pain than in matched controls. This weakness of lateral rotation was attributed to Gmed dysfunction. In contrast, Earl (2005) observed the highest activation of the Gmed in tasks that involved a combination of abduction and medial rotation.

As mentioned above, the Gmed has a posterior fiber in its structure as well as an anterior component; it is the posterior fibers that we as therapists are concerned with. The Gmed posterior fibers work in conjunction with the Gmax, and these muscles control the position of the hip into an external rotation, which helps to align the trunk, pelvis, hip, knee, and lower limb as the gait cycle is initiated.

As an example, consider a patient who is asked to walk while the therapist observes the process. When the patient puts their weight on their *left* leg at the initial contact phase of the cycle, the Gmed is responsible in part for the stability mechanism acting on the lower limb; this will also assist in the overall alignment of the lower limb. The patient continues with the gait cycle and now enters the stance phase. The Gmed in this phase is responsible for abducting the *right* hip, which is then seen to start to lift slightly higher than the *left* side. This process is very important, as it allows the *right* leg to swing during the swing phase of gait.

If there is any weakness in the *left* Gmed, the body will respond in two ways during the gait cycle: either the pelvis will tip down on the contralateral side to the stance leg (*right* in this case), giving the appearance of a Trendelenburg pattern of gait (figure 8.14a); or a compensatory Trendelenburg pattern will be adopted,

in which the patient will be observed to shift their whole trunk excessively to the weaker hip (figure 8.14b).

When we stand on one leg, we activate the lateral sling, which consists of the Gmed, Gmin, adductors on the ipsilateral side, and the QL on the contralateral side (figure 8.15a&b). As explained earlier, if we present with weakness, this is probably a result of overactivation in other muscles owing to the compensation process. Patients who present with weakness in their Gmed (posterior fibers) tend to have overactivity of the contralateral (opposite) quadratus lumborum (QL) adductors and ITB via the connection from the TFL; the piriformis can also have an overactive role if the Gmed posterior fibers are shown to be weak.

The Gmed is key to dynamic pelvic stability. In my experience, runners with poor dynamic pelvic stability will shorten their stride length and adopt a more shuffling pattern to reduce the ground reaction force at contact and thereby decrease the amount of muscle control required to maintain pelvic posture.

Gmed weakness will have implications all the way down and of course all the way up the kinetic chain. From heel contact to the mid-stance phase, a weakness of the Gmed allows the potential for the following:

- Trendelenburg or compensatory Trendelenburg pattern of gait
- lumbar spine to increase lateral flexion and coupled rotation so potentially causes pathology as well as pelvic and sacral torsions
- iliopsoas can compensate due to decreased pelvic stability and the hip, lumbar and thoracic spine mechanics are now altered
- hypertonicity in the contralateral (opposite side) quadratus lumborum and the relationship to its attachment onto the diaphragm so breathing mechanics can be affected
- alters the biomechanics of the shoulder complex and cervical spine due to the connection of the myofascial slings
- hypertonicity in the ipsilateral (same side) piriformis and TFL muscles and the IT band
- medial drifting of the knee into a valgus position, causing a patella mal-tracking syndrome
- internal rotation of the lower limb (tibia), relative to the position of the foot
- excessive pronation of the subtalar joint (STJ).

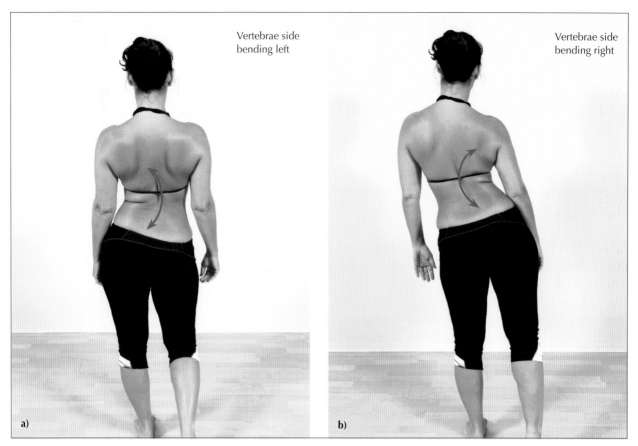

Vertebrae side bending left

Vertebrae side bending right

Figure 8.14a & b: *a: Trendelenburg gait; b: compensatory Trendelenburg gait*

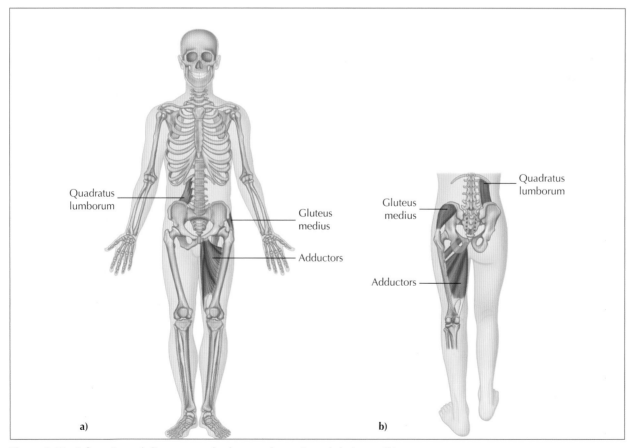

Figure 8.15a & b: *a: Lateral sling system; b: the muscles activated during walking*

■ Assessment of the Gmed

Whenever I look at patients who present with upper or lower limb issues as well as spinal pain, part of my assessment process includes checking the strength of the gluteal muscles and in particular the Gmed. In this section I will discuss the hip abduction firing pattern test, which is used for determining the correct firing order of the hip abductors.

Hip abduction firing pattern test

To check the firing sequence on the left side, the patient adopts a side-lying posture with both legs together and their left leg on top. In this sequence, three muscles will be tested: Gmed, TFL, and QL. The therapist palpates the QL muscle by placing their right hand lightly on the muscle. Next, to palpate the Gmed and TFL, the therapist places their finger on the TFL and their thumb on the Gmed (figure 8.16).

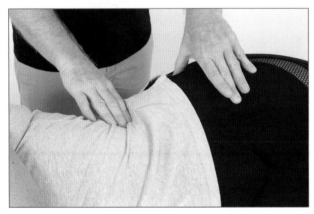

Figure 8.16: *Palpation of the QL, Gmed, and TFL*

The patient is asked to lift their left leg into abduction, a few inches from their right leg, while the therapist notes the firing sequence (figure 8.17). It is important to check for any compensatory or cheating recruitment. The idea of this test is that the patient must be able to abduct their hip without (1) hitching the left side of their pelvis (hip hitching would mean they were activating the quadratus lumborum), (2) falling into an anterior pelvic tilt, or (3) allowing their pelvis to tip backward.

The correct firing sequence should be gluteus medius, followed by TFL, and finally QL at around 25 degrees of pelvis elevation. If the QL or the TFL fires first, this indicates a misfiring sequence, resulting in adaptive shortness.

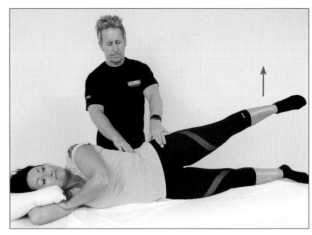

Figure 8.17: *As the patient abducts their left hip, the therapist notes the firing sequence*

Once we have ascertained the firing sequence for hip abduction, we have to decide on the next step. Most patients feel that they need to strengthen the weak Gmed muscle by going to the gym, especially if they have been told it is weak, and they do lots of side-lying abduction exercises. The difficulty in strengthening the apparent weak Gmed muscle is that this particular exercise will not, I repeat *not*, strengthen the Gmed, especially if the TFL and QL are the dominant abductors. The piriformis will also get involved, as it is a weak abductor, which can cause a pelvic/sacroiliac dysfunction, further complicating the underlying issue.

So the answer is to initially postpone the strengthening of the Gmed and focus on the shortened/tight tissues of the adductors, TFL, and QL. In theory, by lengthening the tight tissues, the lengthened and weakened tissue will become shorter and automatically regain its strength. If, after a period of time (two weeks has been recommended), the Gmed has not regained its strength, specific and functional strength exercises for this muscle can be added.

Gluteus medius anterior fibers strength test

To test the left Gmed, the patient adopts a side-lying posture, with their left leg uppermost. The therapist palpates the patient's Gmed with their right hand, and the patient is asked to raise their left leg into abduction, a few inches away from the right leg, and hold this position isometrically to start with. Placing their left hand near the patient's knee, the therapist applies a downward pressure to the leg. The patient is asked to resist the pressure (figure 8.18); if they are able to do so, the Gmed is classified as *normal*.

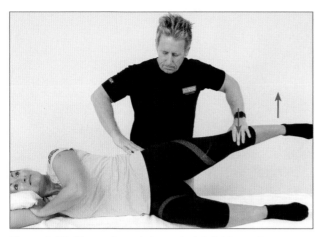

Figure 8.18: *The patient abducts their left hip against resistance from the therapist*

Gluteus medius posterior fibers strength test

In testing the left side, to put more emphasis on the posterior fibers of the Gmed, the therapist controls the patient's left hip into slight extension and external rotation (figure 8.19). The therapist applies a downward pressure as before and if the patient is able to resist this force, the Gmed posterior fibers are classified as *normal*. If you want to assess muscular endurance as opposed to strength, ask the patient to hold the abducted leg and maintain the position for at least 30 seconds.

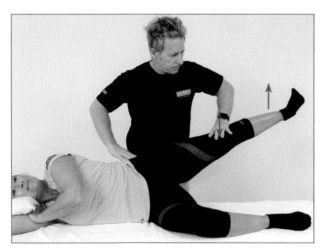

Figure 8.19: *External rotation and slight extension of the hip, which emphasizes the posterior fibers of the Gmed. The therapist applies a downward pressure to the patient's abducted hip*

■ Conclusion

This chapter aims to make the reader aware that pain presenting itself to the upper limb, neck and shoulder complex just might be as a result of the function and stability of the pelvis, the SIJ, and the relationship to the gluteal muscles. It does not focus on the treatments that might follow your findings, though I have given a few suggestions. This is because there is not enough space here for this potentially extensive topic and the author has written many other texts that discuss and treat these fascinating areas of the pelvis and gluteal muscles. Anyone interested in following up this subject should look at the appendix for suggestions on further reading.

It goes without saying that when (because they will) patients and athletes walk in to your consulting room, you do not know exactly what they will be presenting with – everyone has their own unique story to tell. As we are all different in one way or another, to me it makes perfect sense to ascertain the function of the Gluteal muscles (Gmax and Gmed) in everybody, no matter where the pain presents, because these gluteal muscles (out of all the muscles we have, and there are over 600) are the ones that are truly unique, and I personally believe they are generally not considered sufficiently and are often neglected. So please, next time you see someone with pain, spend some time and take these muscles off the *neglect shelf* and you might be quietly surprised by the results!

9

Muscle energy techniques (METs) and their link to the shoulder complex

Many years ago, when I was studying osteopathy, we only had a few short lectures on muscle energy techniques in the five-year degree program. At the time I felt the tutor in question did not really understand the simple fundamental components of METs and these techniques were taught with so little real passion my fellow students were almost put off using them. Fortunately for some of my class members I was already teaching METs on sports therapy courses so I spent a few more hours going through the concepts with them. I was (and still am) disappointed that METs were almost brushed to one side during my degree – hand on heart, I would have used an MET of some sort (or at least a modified version of the technique) on EVERY single patient I have EVER seen. METs are an osteopathic technique so every osteopath should be competent in using them. One of my goals (I have many!) is to teach the same concepts to all physical therapists throughout the world and I hope I am able to convey something of my own passion when I teach these wonderful techniques.

In later chapters you will read and learn about specific techniques that can be incorporated into a treatment plan to help correct shoulder complex dysfunctions and these techniques will also have a great effect on all aspects of the range of motion of the cervical spine. I consider the techniques I will be demonstrating in this chapter to be some of the best soft tissue techniques that one can use to correct any soft tissue or spinal joint anomalies. You might have already guessed what these are – *muscle energy techniques* (METs).

Since I discuss in this book how to treat specific dysfunctions associated with the shoulder complex as well as many of the dysfunctions that are also associated within the cervical spine. I need to explain the role of METs, so that you have a better understanding of when and why to employ this type of soft tissue treatment. Physical therapists have a toolbox of various techniques at their disposal to help release and relax muscles, which will then assist the patient's body to promote the healing mechanisms. METs, first described by Fred Mitchell in 1948, are one such tool, which if used correctly can have a major influence on a patient's well-being. (The reader is referred to Gibbons (2011) for a fuller account of METs.)

Definition: *Muscle energy techniques (METs) are a form of osteopathic manipulative diagnosis and treatment in which the patient's muscles are actively used on request, from a precisely controlled position, in a specific direction, and against a distantly applied counterforce.*

METs are unique in their application, in that the patient provides the initial effort and the practitioner just facilitates the process. The primary force comes from the contraction of the patient's soft tissues (muscles), which is then utilized to assist and correct the presenting musculoskeletal dysfunction. This treatment method is generally classified as a *direct* form of technique as opposed to *indirect*, since the use of muscular effort is from a controlled position, in a specific direction, and against a distant counterforce that is usually applied by the practitioner.

■ Some of the benefits of METs

When teaching the concept of METs to my students, one of the main benefits I emphasize is their use in normalizing joint range, rather than in improving flexibility. This might sound counterintuitive; what I am saying is if, for example, your patient cannot rotate their neck (cervical spine) to the right as far as they can to the left, they have a restriction of the cervical spine in right rotation. The normal rotational range of the cervical spine is 80 degrees, but let us say the patient can only rotate 60 degrees to the right. This is where METs come in. After an MET has been employed on the tight restrictive muscles, hopefully the cervical spine will then be capable of rotating to the full range of 80 degrees – the patient has made all the effort and you, the practitioner, have encouraged the cervical spine into further right rotation. You have now improved the joint range to 'normal.' This is not stretching in the strictest sense – even though the overall flexibility has been improved, it is only to the point of achieving what is considered to be a normal joint range.

Depending on the context and the type of MET employed, the objectives of this treatment can include:

- restoring normal tone in hypertonic muscles
- preparing muscles for subsequent stretching
- increasing joint mobility
- strengthening weak muscles.

Restoring normal tone in hypertonic muscles

Through the simple process of METs, we as physical therapists try to achieve a relaxation in the hypertonic shortened postural muscles. If we think of a joint as being limited in its ROM, then through the initial identification of the hypertonic structures, we can employ the techniques to help achieve normality in the tissues. Certain types of soft tissue (massage) therapy can also help us achieve this relaxation effect, and generally an MET is applied in conjunction with massage therapy. I feel that massage therapy with motion is one of the best tools a physical therapist can use to assist relaxing shortened tissues.

Preparing muscles for subsequent stretching

In certain circumstances, what sport your patient or athlete participates in will be determined by what range of motion (ROM) they have at their joints. Everybody can improve their flexibility, and METs can be used to help achieve this goal. Remember, the focus of METs is to try to improve the normal ROM of a joint, rather than developing the length of the muscle.

If you want to improve the patient's flexibility past the point of normal, a more aggressive MET approach might be necessary. This could be in the form of asking the patient to contract a bit harder than the standard 10–20% of the muscle's capability. For example, we can ask the patient to contract using, say, 40–70% of the muscle's capability. This increased contraction will help stimulate more neurological motor units to fire, in turn causing an increased stimulation of the Golgi tendon organ (GTO). This will then have the effect of relaxing more of the muscle, allowing it to be lengthened even further. Either way, once an MET has been incorporated into the treatment plan, a flexibility program can follow.

Increasing joint mobility

One of my favorite sayings when I teach muscle-testing and function courses is: 'A stiff joint can cause a tight muscle, and a tight muscle can cause a stiff joint.'

Does this not make perfect sense? When you use an MET correctly, it is one of the best ways to improve the mobility of the joint, even though you are initially relaxing the muscles. This is especially the case with the use of METs to correct any dysfunctions that you found within the shoulder complex, which is covered in a later chapter. The focus of the MET is to get the patient to contract the muscles; this subsequently causes a relaxation period that I call 'a window of opportunity,' allowing a greater ROM to be achieved within that specific joint.

Typically, chiropractors will perform only manipulations to improve the mobility of the vertebra; however, if one thinks about it logically, then soft tissue techniques like METs will greatly assist in the overall mobility, especially prior to manipulations because METs work on a contract–relax–lengthen theory and by utilizing this simple but superb concept, it will be a win–win situation not only for the patient but the therapist as well.

Strengthening weak muscles

METs can be used in the strengthening of weak or even flaccid muscles, as the patient is asked to contract the muscles prior to the lengthening process. The therapist should be able to modify the MET by asking the patient to contract the muscle that has been classified as *weak*, against a resistance applied by the therapist (isometric contraction), the timing of which can be varied. For example, the patient can be asked to resist the movement using approximately 20–30% of their maximum capability for 5–15 seconds. They are then asked to repeat the process five to eight times, resting for 10–15 seconds between repetitions. The patient's performance can be noted and improved over time.

■ Physiological effects of METs

There are two main effects of METs and these are explained on the basis of two distinct physiological processes:

- post-isometric relaxation (PIR)
- reciprocal inhibition (RI).

When we use METs, certain neurological influences occur. Before we discuss the main process of PIR/RI, we need to consider the two types of receptor involved in the stretch reflex:

- muscle spindles, which are sensitive to change, as well as speed of change, in length of muscle fibers
- GTOs, which detect prolonged change in tension.

Stretching the muscle causes an increase in the impulses transmitted from the muscle spindle to the posterior horn cell (PHC) of the spinal cord. In turn, the anterior horn cell (AHC) transmits an increase in motor impulses to the muscle fibers, creating a protective tension to resist the stretch. However, increased tension after a few seconds is sensed within the GTOs, which transmit impulses to the PHC. These impulses have an inhibitory effect on the increased motor stimulus at the AHC; this inhibitory effect causes a reduction in motor impulses and consequent relaxation. This implies that the prolonged stretch of the muscles will increase the stretching capability, because the protective relaxation of the GTOs overrides the protective contraction due to the muscle spindles. A fast stretch of the muscle spindles, however, will cause immediate muscle contraction, and

since it is not sustained, there will be no inhibitory action (figure 9.1). This is known as the *basic reflex arc*.

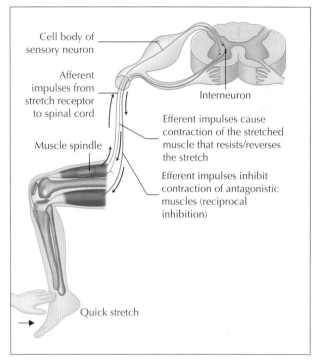

Figure 9.1: *The stretch reflex arc. A quick 'stretch by hand' to activate the muscle spindles*

Post-isometric relaxation (PIR)

PIR results from a neurological feedback through the spinal cord to the muscle itself when an isometric contraction is sustained, causing a reduction in tone of the muscle, which has been contracted (figure 9.2) This reduction in tone lasts for approximately 20–25 seconds, so you now have a perfect window of opportunity to improve the ROM as during this relaxation period the tissues can be more easily moved to a new resting length.

Reciprocal inhibition (RI)

When RI is employed, the reduction in tone relies on the physiological inhibiting effect of antagonists (opposite muscles) on the contraction of a muscle (figure 9.2). When the motor neurons of the contracting agonist muscle receive excitatory impulses from the afferent pathway, the motor neurons of the opposing antagonist muscle receive inhibitory impulses at the same time, which prevent it contracting. It follows that contraction or extended stretch of the agonist muscle must elicit relaxation or inhibit the antagonist; however, a fast stretch of the agonist will facilitate a contraction of the agonist (stretch reflex).

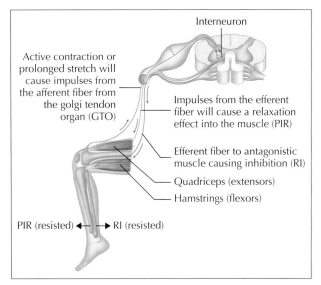

Figure 9.2: *Post-isometric relaxation (PIR) and reciprocal inhibition (RI)*

In most applications of METs, the point of bind, or just short of the point of bind, is the preferred position in which to perform an MET. Clearly, an MET is a fairly mild form of lengthening/stretching compared with other techniques, so one can assume its use is therefore more appropriate in the rehabilitation process. It should be borne in mind that most problems with muscle shortening will generally occur in postural/tonic muscles. Since these muscles are composed predominantly of slow-twitch fibers, a milder form of stretching is perhaps more appropriate.

■ MET procedure

- The patient's limb is taken to the point where resistance is felt, i.e. the point of bind. It can be more comfortable for the patient if you ease off to a point slightly short of the point of bind in the affected area that you are going to treat, especially if these tissues are in the chronic stage.
- The patient is asked to isometrically contract the muscle to be treated (PIR) or the antagonist (RI), using approximately 10–20% of the muscle's strength capability against a resistance that is applied by the therapist. The patient should be using the agonist if the method of approach is PIR; this will release the tight, shortened structures directly. (See the PIR example below.)
- If the RI method of MET is used, the patient is asked to contract the antagonist isometrically; this will induce a relaxation effect in the opposite muscle group

(agonist), which would still be classified as the *tight* and *shortened* structures. (See the RI example below.)
- The patient is asked to slowly introduce an isometric contraction, lasting between 10 and 12 seconds, avoiding any jerking of the treated area. This contraction, as explained above, is the time necessary to load the GTOs, which allows them to become active and to influence the intrafusal fibers from the muscle spindles. This has the effect of overriding the influence from the muscle spindles, which inhibits muscle tone. The therapist then has the opportunity to take the affected area to a new position with minimal effort.
- The contraction by the patient should cause no discomfort or strain. The patient is told to relax fully by taking a deep breath in, and as they breathe out, the therapist passively takes the specific joint that lengthens the hypertonic muscle to a new position, which therefore normalizes joint range.
- After an isometric contraction, which induces a PIR, there is a relaxation period of 15–30 seconds; this period can be the perfect time to stretch the tissues to their new resting length.
- Repeat this process until no further progress is made (normally three to four times) and hold the final resting position for approximately 25–30 seconds.
- A period of 25–30 seconds is considered to be enough time for the neurological system to lock onto this new resting position.
- This type of technique is excellent for relaxing and releasing tone in tight, shortened soft tissues.
- A refractory period (the brief period needed to restore the resting potential) of about 20 seconds occurs with RI; however, RI is thought to be less powerful than PIR. Therapists need to be able to use both approaches, because the use of the agonist may sometimes be inappropriate owing to pain or injury. Since the amount of force used with an MET is minimal, the risk of injury or tissue damage will be reduced.

■ MET method of application

'Point of bind' (or 'restriction barrier')

In this book the word 'bind' is mentioned many times. The *point of bind*, or *restriction barrier*, occurs when the palpating hand/fingers of the therapist first feels a soft tissue resistance. Through experience and continual practice, the therapist will be able to palpate a resistance of the soft tissues as the affected area is gently taken into the position of bind. This position of bind is *not* the position of stretch – it is the position just before the point of stretch. The therapist should be able to feel the difference and not wait for the patient to say when they feel a stretch has occurred.

Acute and chronic conditions

The soft tissue conditions that are treated using METs are generally classified as either *acute* or *chronic*, and this tends to relate to tissues that have had some form of strain or trauma. METs can be used for both acute and chronic conditions. *Acute* involves anything that is obviously acute in terms of symptoms, pain, or spasm, as well as anything that has emerged during the previous three to four weeks. Anything older and of a less obviously acute nature is regarded as *chronic* in determining which variation of MET is suitable.

If you feel the presenting condition is relatively acute (occurring within the last three weeks), the isometric contraction can be performed at the point of bind. After the patient has contracted the muscle isometrically for the duration of 10 seconds, the therapist then takes the affected area to the new point of bind.

In chronic conditions (persisting for more than three weeks), the isometric contraction starts from a position just before the point of bind. After the patient has contracted the muscle for 10 seconds, the therapist then goes through the point of bind and encourages the specific area into the new position.

PIR versus RI

How much pain the patient is presenting with is generally the deciding factor in determining which method to initially apply. The PIR method is usually the technique of choice for muscles that are classified as *short* and *tight*, as it is these muscles that are initially contracted in the process of releasing and relaxing.

On occasion, however, a patient may experience discomfort when the agonist, i.e. the shortened structure, is contracted; in this case it would seem more appropriate to contract the opposite muscle group (antagonist), as this would reduce

the patient's perception of pain, but still induce a relaxation in the painful tissues. Hence, the use of the RI method, using the antagonists, which are usually pain free, will generally be the first choice if there is increased sensitivity in the primary shortened tissues.

When the patient's initial pain has been reduced by the appropriate treatment, PIR techniques can be incorporated (as explained earlier, PIR uses an isometric contraction of the tight shortened structures, in contrast to the antagonists being used in the RI method). To some extent, the main factor in deciding the best approach is whether the sensitive tissue is in the acute stage or in the chronic stage.

After having used PIR and RI on a regular basis, I have found that the best results for lengthening the hypertonic structures are achieved with PIR (provided the patient has no pain during this technique). However, once I have performed the PIR method, if I feel more ROM is needed in the shortened tight tissue, I bring into play the antagonists using the RI method for approximately two more repetitions, as explained in the RI example below. This personal approach for my patients has had the desired effect of improving the overall ROM.

PIR example

To illustrate the PIR method of MET treatment, we are now going to apply the procedure to the adductor pollicis muscle (*pollicis* relates to the thumb, or pollex). You might consider it more appropriate to demonstrate how METs work by means of an example related to the shoulder complex; however, I wanted the therapist to be able to practice the technique on themselves first, so that they can better understand the MET concept. Once the technique has been understood and subsequently practiced using this simple example, the therapist will then be ready to tackle more complex METs with the aim of helping to restore function to the area of the shoulder and cervical spine.

Place your left (or right) hand onto a blank piece of paper and, with the hand open as much as possible, draw around the fingers and the thumb (figure 9.3).

Remove the paper and actively abduct the thumb as far as you can, until a point of bind is felt. Next, place the fingers of your right hand on top of the left thumb and, using an isometric contraction, adduct your thumb against the downward pressure of the fingers, so that an isometric

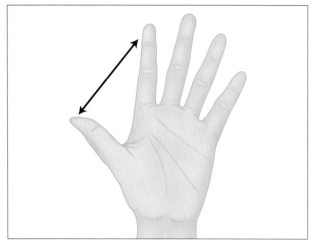

Figure 9.3: *The distance between the thumb and finger is measured*

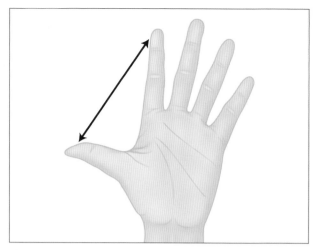

Figure 9.5: *The hand redrawn after the MET treatment using PIR and RI*

contraction is achieved (figure 9.4). After applying this pressure for 10 seconds, breathe in, and on the exhalation passively take the thumb into further abduction (but do not force the thumb). Repeat this sequence two more times and on the last repetition, maintain the final resting position for at least 20–25 seconds.

Now place your hand back on the piece of paper and draw around it again (figure 9.5); hopefully you will see that the thumb has abducted further than before.

RI example
To apply the RI method, follow the same procedure as for the PIR method, i.e. go to the point of bind by still abducting the thumb. From this position of bind, instead

of adducting the thumb (PIR) against a resistance, perform the opposite movement and abduct your thumb (using the abductor pollicis brevis/longus muscle) against a resistance (figure 9.6). After applying this pressure for 10 seconds, breathe in, and on the exhalation passively take the thumb into further abduction (again, do not force the thumb). Repeat this sequence one or two more times and on the last repetition, maintain the final resting position for at least 20–25 seconds.

As before, place your hand back on the piece of paper and draw around it again (figure 9.5); hopefully you will see that the thumb has abducted further than previously.

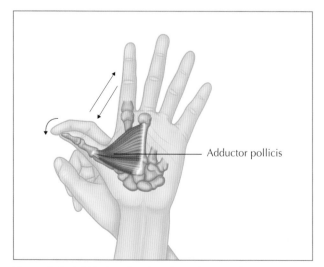

Figure 9.4: *Adducting the thumb against a resistance applied by the opposite hand (PIR method)*

Adductor pollicis

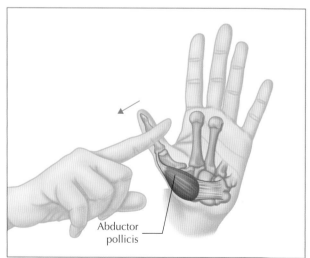

Abductor pollicis

Figure 9.6: *Abducting the thumb against a resistance applied by the opposite hand (RI method)*

■ Conclusion

I always say to my students during the MET course, that if the above example works as well as it does simply with using the thumb then we should be able to incorporate and utilize the same process and apply METs to any hypertonic tissue we find during the assessment and treatments of all of our patients. METs can be applied to anywhere in the body (not just to the shoulder complex) where you feel there is restrictive tissue and/or joint stiffness and, as with the thumb, after the treatment you should notice some positive changes.

10

Muscle length testing of the shoulder complex and cervical spine

The muscles listed below are the ones I consider to be specifically related to the shoulder complex and cervical spine.

1. Upper trapezius
2. Levator scapulae
3. Sternocleidomastoid
4. Scalenes
5. Coracoid muscles: pectoralis minor, biceps short head and coracobrachialis
6. Latissimus dorsi
7. Pectoralis major
8. Subscapularis
9. Infraspinatus.

Table 10.1 can be used as a guide to help you assess your patients and athletes. The table is also found at the end of the book in the Appendix and you are able to print these out free of any copyright to use in your own clinic.

In this chapter, I will demonstrate how to assess for each of these muscles, which have a natural tendency to shorten and subsequently become tight. After the testing procedure has been explained, I will demonstrate in the

Table 10.1: Postural assessment sheet – Upper body

Patient Name:			
Key: E = Equal in length			
L/R = Short on left or right side			
Muscles	**Date:**	**Date:**	**Date:**
Upper trapezius			
Levator scapulae			
Sternocleidomastoid			
Scalenes			
Coracoid muscles • Pectoralis minor • Biceps brachii short head • Coracobrachialis			
Latissimus dorsi			
Pectoralis major			
Subscapularis			
Infraspinatus			

Chapter 11 specific METs to encourage these short/tight muscles to lengthen to their natural resting length, so that we can assist and hopefully normalize the dysfunctional position.

■ Upper trapezius

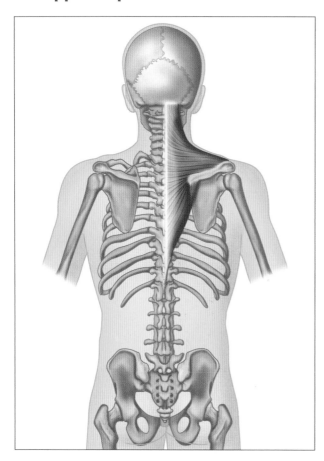

Origin: Base of skull (occipital bone). Spinous processes of seventh cervical vertebra (C7) and all thoracic vertebrae (T1–12).

Insertion: Lateral third of clavicle. Acromion process. Spine of scapula.

Action: *Upper fibers*: Pull the shoulder girdle up (elevation). Help prevent depression of the shoulder girdle when a weight is carried on the shoulder or in the hand. *Middle fibers*: Retract (adduct) scapula. *Lower fibers*: Depress scapula, particularly against resistance, as when using the hands to get up from a chair. *Upper and lower fibers together*: Upwardly rotate scapula, as in elevating the arm above the head.

Nerve: Accessory XI nerve. Ventral ramus of cervical nerves (C2, C3, C4).

Assessment of upper trapezius

The patient is in a sitting position for this test. The therapist passively side bends the patient's neck to the right while palpating the left trapezius with their left hand (figure 10.1). The therapist needs to be aware of the bind of the tissue, rather than the patient saying that they feel a stretch. The bind is where the 'slack' is taken out of the tissue before the position of stretch is achieved – it is very important to understand this process of bind as opposed to stretch.

If a range of motion of 45 degrees is achieved, a normal length of trapezius is noted. The test is repeated on the contralateral side for comparison.

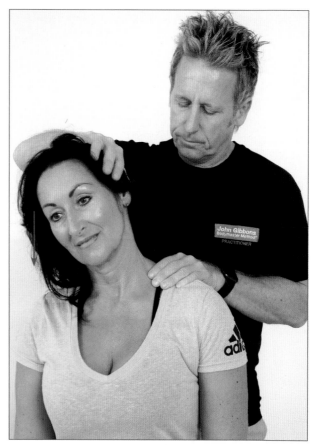

Figure 10.1: *The therapist slowly bends the patient's head to the right while stabilizing the patient's shoulder with their hand*

Alternative assessment of trapezius

Scapulohumeral rhythm test
The patient is asked to abduct the right shoulder and the movement is observed. The first 30 degrees of motion comes purely from the glenohumeral joint; after 30 degrees, the scapula starts to upwardly rotate. The ratio is generally 2:1 – that is, for every 2 degrees of motion from the glenohumeral joint, there is 1 degree of scapula rotation. For example, at 90 degrees of abduction, 60 degrees would have been performed by the glenohumeral joint and 30 degrees of scapula rotation.

A normal scapulohumeral rhythm is shown in figure 10.2a, while figure 10.2b indicates a 'reverse' scapulohumeral rhythm pattern of motion, as the 'upper trapezius' on the right is seen to be overactive and assisting the motion of shoulder abduction. This altered

rhythm can be seen very clearly with a condition called adhesive capsulitis or frozen shoulder.

This limited range of motion is due to restricted movement of the glenohumeral joint that can be caused by adhesive capsulitis (frozen shoulder); the scapula thoracic articulation will be the joint of compensation and will be seen to elevate and rotate excessively.

Scapulohumeral rhythm test with palpation

To confirm the activation or possibly the overactivation of the upper trapezius during the motion of shoulder abduction, the therapist can place their left hand over the patient's right trapezius while the patient performs the movement (figure 10.3). The therapist notes when they feel the upper trapezius contract. If the contraction is felt within the first 30 degrees of shoulder abduction, the upper trapezius will be classified as overactive.

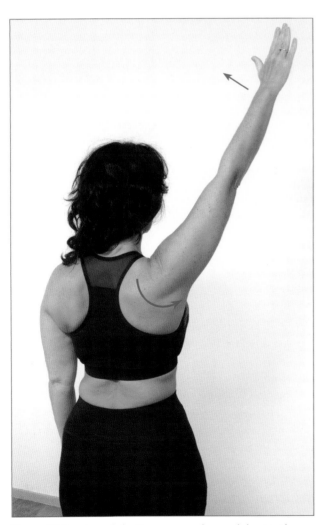

Figure 10.2a: *Arm abduction – normal scapulohumeral rhythm*

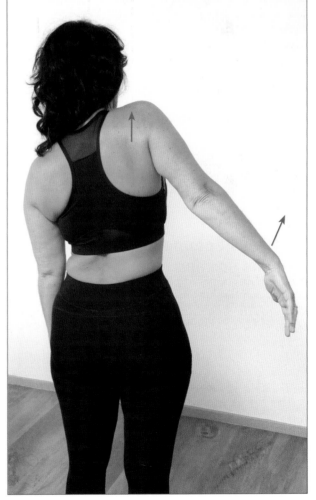

Figure 10.2b: *Arm abduction – reverse scapulohumeral rhythm*

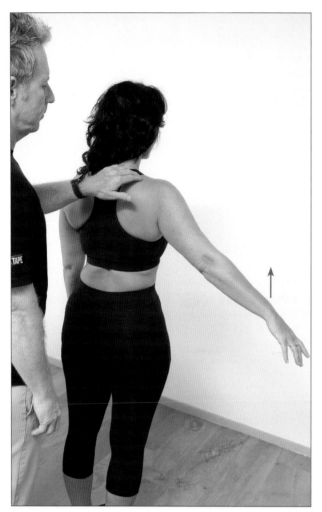

Figure 10.3: *The patient abducts their right arm as the therapist palpates the upper trapezius for overactivation*

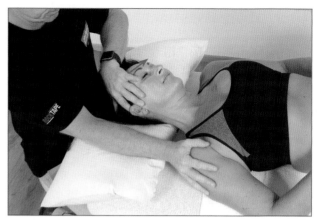

Figure 10.4: *Assessment of the upper trapezius from a supine position*

■ Levator scapulae

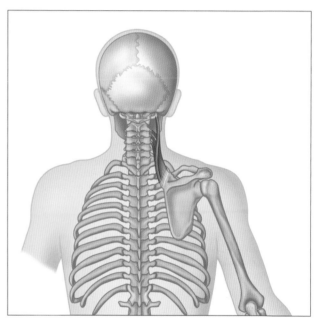

Assessment of upper trapezius from a supine position

The patient adopts a supine position with their knees bent, as this helps relax the lumbar spine (figure 10.4). Sitting at the cephalic end of the couch, the therapist places their left hand to cradle the patient's temporal bone and their right hand on top of the patient's right shoulder. Slowly, the therapist passively side bends the patient's head to the left while stabilizing the motion from the right shoulder. When the therapist feels the bind from the right upper trapezius, a measurement is taken. A value less than 45 degrees would be classified as short.

Origin: Transverse processes of the first three or four cervical vertebrae (C1–4).

Insertion: Upper medial (vertebral) border of the scapula (i.e., portion above the spine of the scapula).

Action: Elevates scapula and assists in lateral flexion of the cervical spine.

Nerve: Dorsal scapular nerve (C4, C5) and cervical nerves (C3, C4).

Assessment of levator scapulae

This test for the levator scapulae is very similar to the testing of the upper trapezius. Also, the muscles mentioned have a similar action, i.e., both can elevate the shoulder girdle and side bend the cervical spine. One difference between them is that the upper trapezius assists the upward rotation of the scapula, whereas the levator scapulae assists in downward rotation of the scapulae.

One method of testing the levator scapulae (left side) is from the seated position shown in figure 10.5. The therapist gently assists the motion of the head and controls the cervical spine into approximately 30 degrees of right rotation. Once the cervical spine is in the position of rotation, the therapist then encourages cervical flexion and will try to approximate the patient's chin onto

their chest. The therapist's left hand prevents the scapula from elevating. When the therapist feels a bind, the range of motion is noted. If the chin can approximate the chest with no resistance, the levator scapulae are classified as normal.

■ Sternocleidomastoid

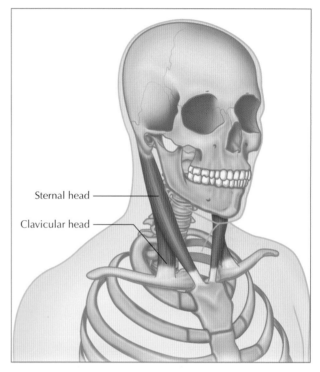

Origin: *Sternal head*: Anterior surface of upper sternum. *Clavicular head*: Medial third of clavicle.

Insertion: Mastoid process of temporal bone (bony prominence just behind the ear).

Action: *Contraction of both sides together*: Flexes neck (draws head forwards). Raises sternum, and consequently the ribs, during deep inhalation. *Contraction of one side*: Tilts the head towards the same side. Rotates head to face the opposite side (and also upwards as it does so).

Nerve: Accessory XI nerve, with sensory supply for proprioception from cervical nerves (C2, C3).

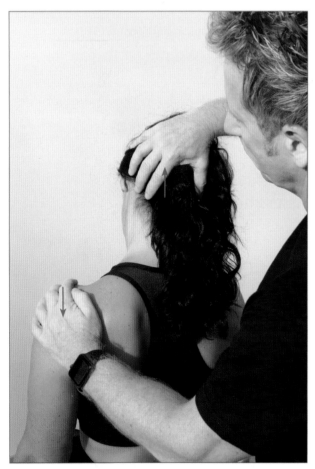

Figure 10.5: *Hand positions for assessment of left levator scapulae with the therapist stabilizing the shoulder*

Assessment of sternocleidomastoid

The patient is asked to adopt a supine position, knees bent and arms placed by their sides. They are then asked to perform a curl-up from the supine position. The therapist observes the position of the chin and the forehead as the patient performs the curl-up. Figure 10.6 indicates a normal sternocleidomastoid (SCM) as demonstrated by the forehead leading in a curl-up exercise. Here, the patient has the ability to hold the chin tucked while flexing the trunk.

If the chin pokes forwards while attempting a curl-up (i.e., the chin leads the movement), the SCM is classified as shortened (figure 10.7).

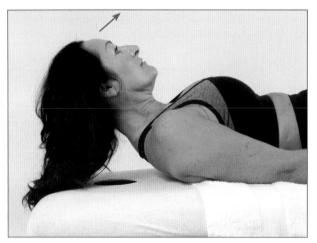

Figure 10.6: *The forehead is leading the movement – normal SCM*

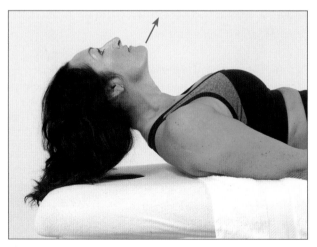

Figure 10.7: *The chin leads the movement – shortened SCM*

■ Scalenes

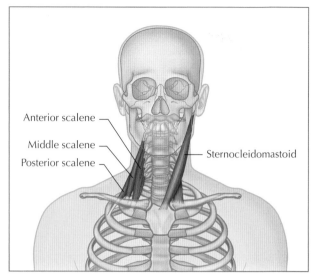

Anterior scalene
Middle scalene
Posterior scalene
Sternocleidomastoid

Origin: Transverse processes of cervical vertebrae.

Insertion: *Anterior and medius*: First rib. *Posterior*: Second rib.

Action: *Acting together*: Flex neck. Raise first rib during a strong inhalation. *Individually*: Laterally flex and rotate neck.

Nerve: Ventral rami of cervical nerves (C3–8).

Assessment of scalenes

To assess for relative shortness of the scalenes, one must be aware of the position of the cervical spine and its relationship to the vertebral arteries.

Vertebral artery test
Important note: The test that I am about to describe puts the cervical spine into an extended and rotated position. When you are performing the test, if you notice anything strange about the movements of your patient's eyes, or if the patient feels strange or even faint, then you must stop the test immediately, as the vertebral artery is being compromised. If the test demonstrates a positive result for compression of the vertebral artery, you must avoid taking the cervical spine into an extended and rotated position. A safer approach for the treatment of the cervical spine using METs will be from a more flexed position. If you are still unsure, seek the advice of a qualified medical practitioner.

Assessment of the right scalenes

The patient is asked to adopt a supine position, with their knees bent and their head off the end of the couch. The therapist controls the position of the head and gently takes the patient's cervical spine into an extended position (figure 10.8), followed by a side bend to the left and a rotation to the right (figure 10.9).

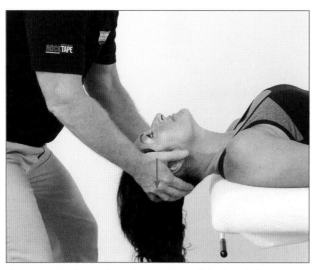

Figure 10.8: *Controlling the position of the head, the therapist gently takes the patient's cervical spine into an extended position*

Full rotation of approximately 80 degrees should be achieved. If there is a bind before the full rotation is achieved, the right scalenes are classified as tight.

Another way of looking at the specific tightness of the scalenes: The therapist supports the head and gently takes the cervical spine into extension (figure 10.8), side bend to the right, then rotation to the left (to test the left side); or into extension, a side bend to the left, then rotation to the right (to test the right side). A feeling of resistance prior to full rotation (80 degrees) indicates hypertonicity.

Observation test for the relative shortness of the scalene muscle group

The scalenes are accessory muscles for inspiration. To identify relative shortness, the therapist can observe the respiration cycle with the patient in a supine position (figure 10.10).

The patient is asked to breathe in and out normally while the therapist lightly palpates the sternum with their right hand and the area of the diaphragm with their left hand. On the inspiration phase, the therapist observes and feels for motion. If the upper chest is seen to move prior to the diaphragm on inspiration, this indicates possible dysfunction and overactivity of the scalenes.

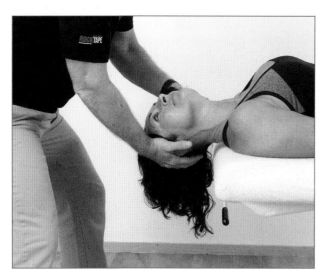

Figure 10.9: *From the extended position, the therapist gently takes the patient's cervical spine into a side bend to the left and a rotation to the right*

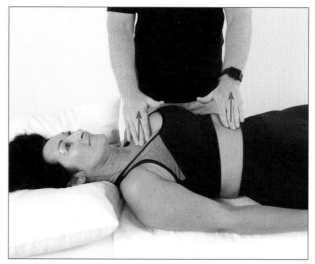

Figure 10.10: *The patient lies in a supine position while the therapist observes and palpates the sternum and diaphragm during the respiration cycle*

■ Latissimus dorsi

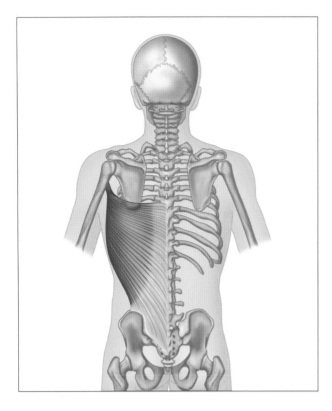

Origin: A broad sheet of tendon which is attached to the spinous processes of lower six thoracic vertebrae and all the lumbar and sacral vertebrae, (T7–S5). Posterior part of iliac crest. Lower three or four ribs. Inferior angle of the scapula.

Insertion: Twists to insert in the intertubercular sulcus (bicipital groove) of the humerus, just below the shoulder joint.

Action: Extends the flexed arm. Adducts and medially rotates the humerus (i.e., draws the arm back and inwards towards the body). One of the chief climbing muscles, since it pulls the shoulders downwards and backwards, and pulls the trunk up to the fixed arms (therefore also active in crawl swimming stroke). Assists in forced inspiration, by raising the lower ribs.

Nerve: Thoracodorsal nerve (C6, C7, C8), from the posterior cord of the brachial plexus.

Assessment of latissimus dorsi

Arm elevation test

To assess tightness of the latissimus dorsi, we can perform a maneuver known as the arm elevation test. The therapist supports the patient's arms and takes them over their head and in a fully flexed position, and then slowly lowers them towards the couch (figure 10.11a) and the therapist tries to sense if there is any bind and if the arm wants to adduct.

It can be seen in figure that the patient's right arm is held in a position of adduction (figure 10.11b), as compared to the left side. You will also notice that the patient's right elbow is flexed; this also indicates a tightness of their right latissimus dorsi.

Alternative assessment for latissimus dorsi

The therapist controls the patient's right arm into an abducted position, and senses for bind of the latissimus dorsi. To confirm any tightness, the arm is allowed to slightly adduct away from the midline.

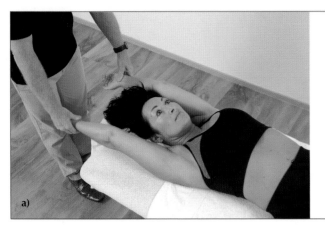
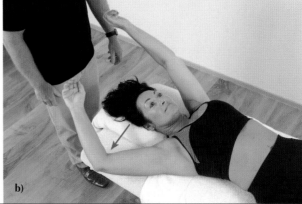

Figure 10.11a & b: *a: Arm elevation test. b: Tightness of the right latissimus dorsi is indicated*

From the adducted position of the arm, the therapist tries to straighten the elbow (figure 10.12). If the latissimus dorsi is tight, the arm will be seen to come back to the original position of adduction, confirming that the muscle is held in a shortened position.

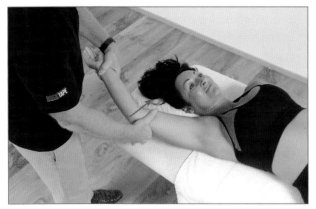

Figure 10.12: *The therapist applies pressure to straighten the elbow*

■ Pectoralis major

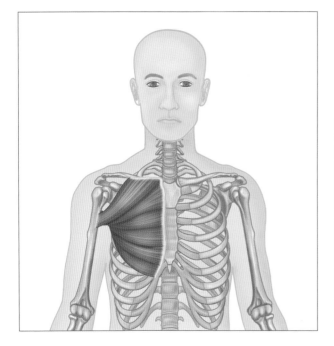

Origin: *Clavicular head*: Medial half or two-thirds of front of clavicle. *Sternocostal portion*: Sternum and adjacent upper six costal cartilages.

Insertion: Upper shaft of humerus.

Action: Adducts and medially rotates the humerus. *Clavicular portion*: Flexes and medially rotates the shoulder joint, and horizontally adducts the humerus towards the opposite shoulder. *Sternocostal portion*: Obliquely adducts the humerus towards the opposite hip. One of the main climbing muscles, pulling the body up to the fixed arm.

Nerve: *Nerve to upper fibers*: Lateral pectoral nerve (C5, C6, C7). *Nerve to lower fibers*: Lateral and medial pectoral nerves (C6, C7, C8, T1).

Assessment of pectoralis major

Arm elevation test

This test is similar to the one that was described for the assessment of the latissimus dorsi, the major difference being the position of the patient's arms. The therapist supports the patient's arms in a fully flexed position, and then slowly lowers them towards the couch. If the arms are unable to contact the couch when lowered, one can assume a shortness condition of the pectoralis major.

Figure 10.13a demonstrates the test and indicates that the right and left sides appear to be tight since neither arm is touching the couch. If you look closely, you will see the patient's left arm is held higher off the couch than the right side, which indicates that the left side is the tighter structure. However, you should also note that the right side is tight as well.

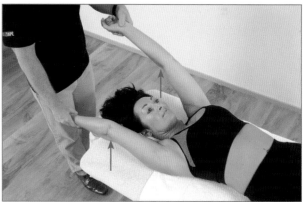

Figure 10.13a: *The left arm is seen to be higher, compared to the right side*

If there is a limited range of motion then the therapist is able to palpate the sternal fibers of the pectoralis major (figure 10.13b) to feel for a 'bind' just to clarify that it is the muscle restricting the motion and not a restriction from the shoulder joint.

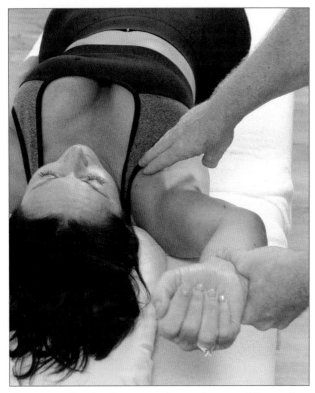

Figure 10.13b: *The therapist palpates the sternal fibers of the pectoralis major to make sure of the bind*

■ Pectoralis minor and coracoid muscles (biceps brachii, coracobrachialis)

Pectoralis minor

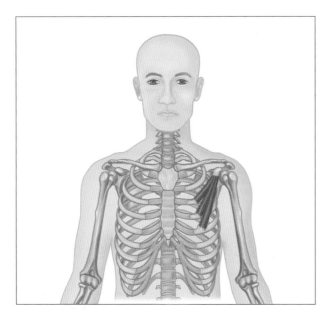

Origin: Outer surfaces of third, fourth and fifth ribs, and fascia of the corresponding intercostal spaces.

Insertion: Coracoid process of scapula.

Action: Draws scapula forwards and downwards. Raises ribs during forced inspiration (i.e., it is an accessory muscle of inspiration if the scapula is stabilized by the rhomboids and trapezius).

Nerve: Medial pectoral nerve with fibers from a communicating branch of the lateral pectoral nerve (C6, C7, C8, T1).

Biceps brachii

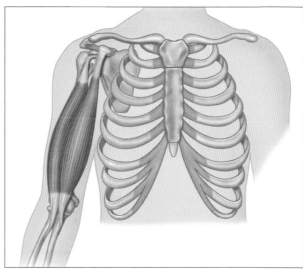

Origin: *Short head*: Tip of coracoid process of scapula. *Long head:* Supraglenoid tubercle of scapula (area just above socket of shoulder joint).

Insertion: Radial tuberosity (on medial aspect of upper part of shaft of radius). Deep fascia (connective tissue) on medial aspect of forearm.

Action: Flexes elbow joint. Supinates forearm. (It has been described as the muscle that puts in the corkscrew and pulls out the cork.) Weakly flexes arm at the shoulder joint.

Nerve: Musculocutaneous nerve (C5, C6).

Coracobrachialis

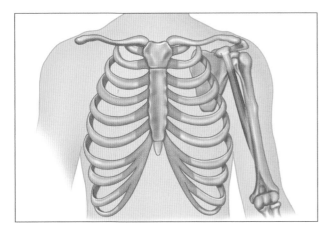

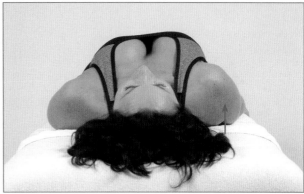

Figure 10.14: *Observing the position of the anterior aspect of the glenohumeral joint. The arrow shows that the distance is greater on the right side*

Origin: Tip of coracoid process of scapula.

Insertion: Medial aspect of humerus at mid-shaft.

Action: Weakly adducts shoulder joint. Possibly assists in flexion of the shoulder joint (but this has not been proven). Helps stabilize humerus.

Nerve: Musculocutaneous nerve (C6, C7).

Observational assessment of pectoralis minor

The test for the length of the pectoralis minor is carried out by observation (figure 10.14). The patient is supine as the therapist observes the position of the anterior aspect of the glenohumeral joint. If one shoulder appears to be more anterior, one would suspect a shortened pectoralis minor. (When I refer to the shoulder being anterior, the correct position is where the scapula is protracted.)

Coracoid muscles and differential diagnosis

Concluding that the relative shortness of the pectoralis minor is responsible for the anterior position, however, might not be correct, as the coracobrachialis and the short head of the biceps brachii also have attachments on the coracoid process.

To try to establish which structure is responsible for the perceived tightness, the therapist controls the patient's

right elbow and slowly flexes it (figure 10.15); if the shoulder is seen to return to its neutral position, the biceps brachii short head is the shortened structure.

Figure 10.16 shows the therapist again cradling the patient's right arm, but this time they are slowly flexing the shoulder. If the shoulder appears to return to the neutral position, the coracobrachialis is the muscle that is responsible for the anterior position of the shoulder.

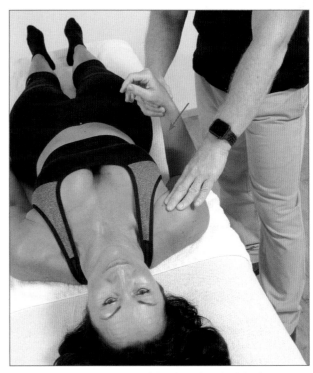

Figure 10.15: *Assessment of the short head of the biceps brachii. The elbow is passively flexed and the distance is observed. If it changes, the biceps brachii is short*

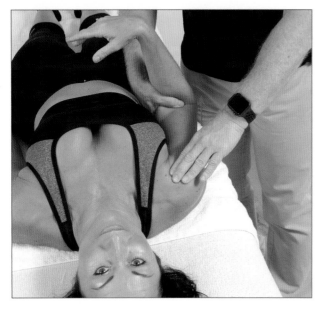

Figure 10.16: *Assessment of the coracobrachialis. The shoulder is passively flexed (arrow) and the gap is observed. If it changes, the coracobrachialis is tight*

If neither of these tests is positive then one can assume that the muscle responsible for the position of the shoulder is the pectoralis minor.

■ Subscapularis

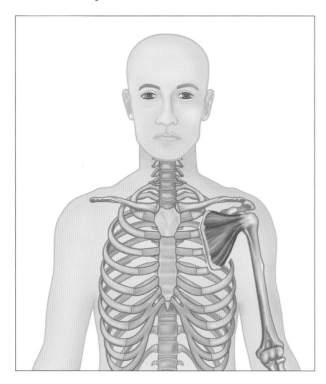

Origin: Subscapular fossa (anterior surface of scapula).

Insertion: Lesser tubercle at the top of humerus. Capsule of shoulder joint.

Action: As a rotator cuff, stabilizes shoulder joint; mainly prevents the head of the humerus being pulled upwards by the deltoid, biceps brachii and long head of triceps brachii. Medially rotates humerus.

Nerve: Upper and lower subscapular nerves (C5, C6, C7), from the posterior cord of the brachial plexus.

Assessment of subscapularis

The therapist takes the patient's arm to 90 degrees of abduction and 90 degrees of elbow flexion – an assessment in this position is known as the 90/90 test. From this position, the therapist supports the patient's elbow with their right hand and the patient's forearm with their left hand (figure 10.17).

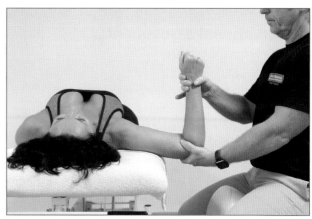

Figure 10.17: *Assessment of the subscapularis, starting from the 90/90 position*

The therapist then takes the patient's arm into external rotation until a bind is felt. For normal range of motion of the subscapularis, the external rotation should achieve 90 degrees, i.e., the patient's forearm should be parallel to the couch, as can be seen in figure 10.18a. If there is shortness of the subscapularis, the range of motion will be less than 90 degrees (figure 10.18b).

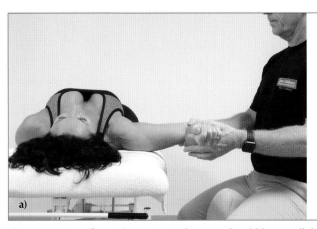
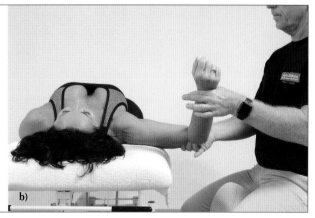

Figure 10.18a & b: *a: The patient's forearm should be parallel to the couch; b: the subscapularis is held in a shortened position as demonstrated by the limited range of motion in external rotation*

■ Infraspinatus

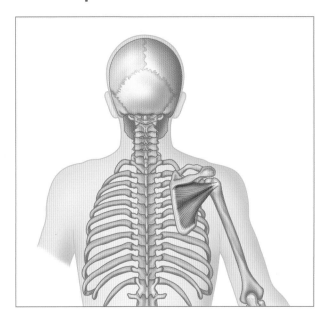

Origin: Middle two-thirds of dorsal surface of scapula, below spine of scapula.

Insertion: Greater tubercle at the top of humerus. Capsule of shoulder joint.

Action: As a rotator cuff muscle, helps prevent posterior dislocation of the shoulder joint. Laterally rotates humerus.

Nerve: Suprascapular nerve (C4, C5, C6), from the upper trunk of the brachial plexus.

Assessment of infraspinatus

From the 90/90 position, the therapist takes the patient's arm into internal rotation until a bind is felt (figure 10.19a). For normal range of motion of the infraspinatus, the internal rotation should achieve 70 degrees (figure 10.19b). If the range of motion is less than 70 degrees, the infraspinatus is classified as short.

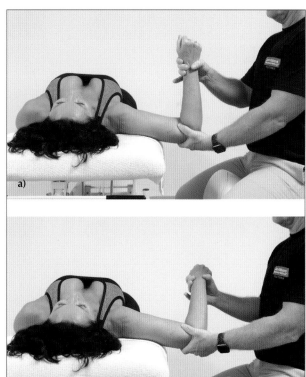

Figure 10.19a & b: *a: Start position for the assessment of the infraspinatus. b: Infraspinatus normal length position; internal rotation achieving 70 degrees*

11

Treatment of the shoulder and cervical spine using Muscle Energy Techniques (METs)

In this book I have several chapters that focus just on the 'treatment' aspect of the shoulder complex, rather than just one chapter like most other texts out there. By now you have probably realized this fascinating area might actually need many angles and various thought processes for you to truly understand it and be effective in your approach to what it is that is actually going on with your patients, especially in terms of considering implementing treatment strategies.

The previous chapter focused on how to assess the length of the associated muscles for the shoulder and cervical spine so in this chapter we will be focusing on using METs to lengthen these tissues so that a normal resting length can be achieved and, hopefully, any dysfunctional postural positions corrected.

■ MET treatment of right upper trapezius

The therapist places the right upper trapezius in a position of bind, asks the patient to either side bend the cervical spine to the right or elevate the right shoulder. Alternatively, the patient may be requested to perform both of these actions at the same time against a resistance from the therapist (figure 11.1a). Another way of communicating the technique is to ask the patient to bring

the ear to the shoulder, or the shoulder to the ear, against a resistance, holding for 10 seconds.

After the 10-second contraction, the patient is asked to relax, take a breath in and on the relaxation phase the cervical spine is taken further into a left side bend (figure 11.1b). If the side bending causes any discomfort, the shoulder can be taken into further depression, as this will also have the effect of lengthening the upper trapezius.

If a reciprocal inhibition (RI) technique is desired, the therapist takes complete control of the patient's cervical spine and shoulder as described above. From this position the patient is asked to reach slowly towards their lower right leg with their right hand, until a point of bind is felt (figure 11.1c). This approach will activate the lower trapezius as the patient is causing a depression of the right shoulder girdle. This will induce an inhibition of the right upper trapezius, allowing a safe way of lengthening, as it will override the activation of the muscle spindles.

The upper trapezius has three fiber components: anterior, medial and posterior. If you decided that certain fibers were particularly short, a simple rotation of the cervical spine would target specific fibers. Figure 11.1d shows the patient's cervical spine in a half rotation to the left;

this targets the middle fibers of the upper trapezius. If you were to take the cervical spine into full rotation, this would target the posterior fibers, as seen in figure 11.1e. No rotation of the cervical spine would target the anterior fibers.

An alternative hand position for the treatment of the upper trapezius is illustrated in figure 11.1f. The therapist uses a cradle type of hold with their left hand and some patients find this position more comfortable.

TIP: The upper trapezius often develops trigger points that can be responsible for headaches.

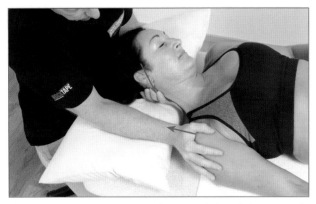

Figure 11.1a: *The patient is asked to side bend the cervical spine to the right or elevates the right shoulder, or both*

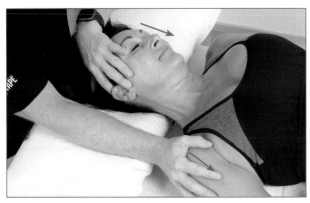

Figure 11.1b: *The therapist guides the cervical spine into left side bending to lengthen the upper trapezius*

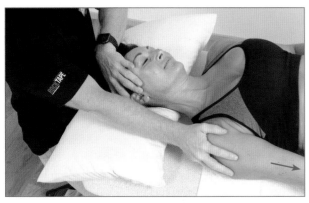

Figure 11.1c: *The patient is asked to depress the shoulder girdle activating the lower trapezius and this will relax the upper trapezius through reciprocal inhibition (RI)*

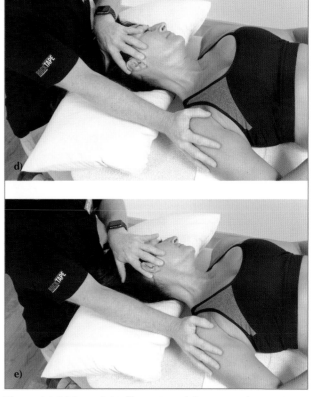

Figure 11.1d & e: *d: Half rotation of the cervical spine emphasizes the middle fibers of the trapezius. e: Full rotation of the cervical spine emphasizes the posterior fibers*

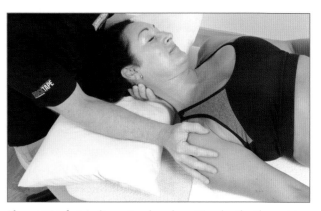

Figure 11.1f: *An alternative hand position by the therapist for the treatment of the upper trapezius*

■ MET treatment of levator scapulae

For this treatment the patient is supine. The therapist, while providing support, guides the patient's head into a side bend, followed by flexion. If a resistance is felt prior to the chin touching the chest, this indicates relative shortness of the levator scapulae.

Some therapists find it more appropriate to treat levator scapulae from the test position, rather than placing the patient in an alternative position. It will be a matter of choice, but in my opinion it is generally more comfortable to treat the levator scapulae from the supine position. However, there will be certain times when the patient is unable to adopt a supine position, as this can cause discomfort in some patients who present with cervical spine pain. In this case the seated position would be more appropriate for an MET treatment.

The hand positioning is similar to that for treatment of the upper trapezius, the difference being that the patient's cervical spine is held more into flexion to achieve the position of bind.

From the position of bind, the patient is asked to push their cervical spine into extension to initiate the contraction of the levator scapulae (figure 11.2).

After the appropriate time and on the relaxation, the patient's cervical spine is taken into further flexion, with an added left rotational movement (figure 11.3).

An alternative method can be achieved by the therapist adopting a standing posture rather than a sitting posture; standing is preferred by some because the head may be too heavy to control from the sitting position using only the arms.

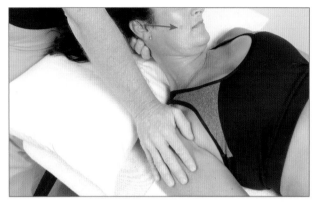

Figure 11.3: *The cervical spine is encouraged into further flexion to lengthen the right levator scapulae. The chin is taken towards the chest, with the therapist stabilizing the right scapula*

TIP: The levator scapula is working in an eccentric contraction when the cervical position is held in a forward head posture; this indicates that the muscle is in a lengthened position but still in a contracted state. The patient may experience pain at the insertion of the levator scapulae on the superior angle of the scapulae. If this is the case, an MET to lengthen an already lengthened structure might not be appropriate.

■ MET treatment of right sternocleidomastoid

The patient is asked to adopt a supine position, with their knees bent. Place a pillow between the patient's shoulder blades. The therapist then gently rotates the patient's cervical spine into full left rotation. The patient is asked to hold this position for about 10 seconds. You can see in

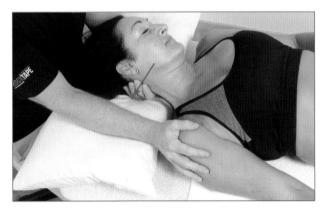

Figure 11.2: *The patient is asked to extend and side bend to the right to activate the levator scapulae*

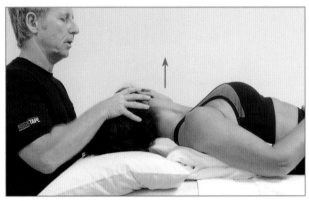

Figure 11.4: *The therapist rotates the cervical into left rotation and the patient is asked to isometrically contract their right SCM*

figure 11.4 that the patient is holding their head on their own with little contact from the therapist.

Once the patient has isometrically contracted the SCM muscle by holding their head in the rotated position for 10 seconds, the therapist then controls the position of the head, slowly lowering it down onto the couch (figure 11.5). In some cases, this will already have started to lengthen the SCM.

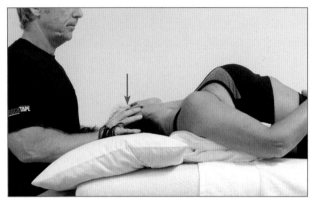

Figure 11.5: *The therapist is controlling the lowering of the patient's head towards the pillow*

To achieve an effective lengthening of the right SCM, the therapist places their right hand on the patient's temporal bone and their left hand on the patient's sternum (for females, the patient's hand is placed on their sternum, then the therapist's hand is applied on top). The patient is asked to breathe in, and on the relaxation phase the therapist encourages caudal pressure to their left hand while the right hand stabilizes the head (figure 11.6).

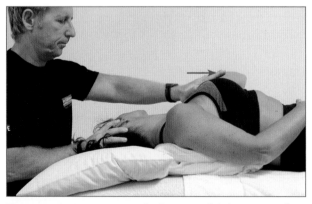

Figure 11.6: *Pressure is applied in a caudal direction with the left hand, while the head is stabilized with the right hand*

TIP: Bilateral contraction of the SCM will give the appearance of a forward head posture. Unilateral contraction of the SCM can result in torticollis, where the cervical spine flexes and rotates away from the side of contracture.

■ MET treatment of right scalenes

The patient adopts a position that is very similar to that for treatment of the SCM. A pillow is placed under their shoulder blades and their cervical spine is controlled by the therapist into full left rotation. (The SCM would also be influenced during the treatment of the scalenes.)

The therapist's left hand is placed over the patient's right temporal bone, and the patient's right hand is placed over their right clavicle. The therapist places their right hand on top of the patient's hand.

The patient is asked to breathe in, and the therapist resists the movement from the upper rib cage. The therapist stabilizes the position of the patient's head while applying pressure in a caudal direction; this will influence the posterior fibers of the scalene (figure 11.7).

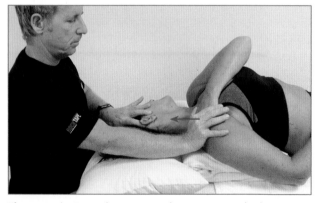

Figure 11.7: *From this position the patient is asked to breathe in against a resistance being applied by the right hand of the therapist*

After the patient has held the full contraction period and on the relaxing exhalation, the therapist applies a caudal pressure to the patient's left hand, which will induce a lengthening of the right scalenes (figure 11.8).

If you are aware of your anatomical origins and insertions, you will know that the scalenes comprise three groups of

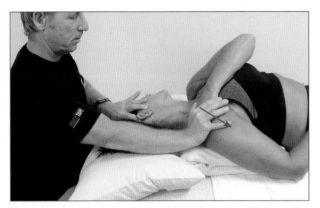

Figure 11.8: *Pressure is applied laterally and caudally, with the left hand stabilizing the head*

fibers, similar to the upper trapezius, as explained earlier in this chapter.

Due to the anatomical attachments of the scalenes, it is possible to apply a specific technique to influence the lengthening of individual fibers. The MET technique shown in figure 11.8 in which the patient has the neck in a full rotation will influence the posterior fiber of the scalenes. As the insertion of the posterior fibers is on the second rib, the hand position needs to be slightly adjusted. The hand placement is on the second rib, just below the center of the clavicle. The technique for lengthening the middle fibers would have the cervical spine in half rotation and if you felt that the anterior fibers of the scalenes needed an MET, the same technique and position would be used, except that there is no rotation of the cervical spine.

TIP: Overactivity of the scalenes anterior (scalenus anticus syndrome) can result in thoracic outlet syndrome (TOS). The neurovascular bundle comes from the C5–T1 vertebrae, known as the brachial plexus, and passes through the fibers of the anterior and middle scalenes, to connect with the subclavian artery. This bundle then continues under the clavicle, over the first rib and under the pectoralis minor. Any compression of the neurovascular bundle can result in pain or altered sensations in the arm and hand.

■ MET treatment of right latissimus dorsi

The patient lies on their left side and the therapist interlocks their left hand through the patient's right arm.

The patient is asked to adduct their right arm to the lumbar spine (figure 11.9).

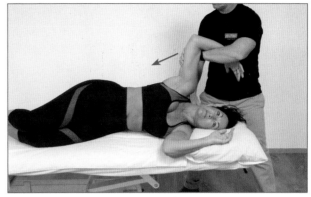

Figure 11.9: *The patient pulls their right arm towards the lumbar spine*

The therapist applies pressure to the patient's left iliac crest and after the contraction takes the patient's arm into further abduction; this will lengthen the shortened latissimus dorsi on the right side (figure 11.10).

Note: If there is underlying shoulder pathology – such as acromioclavicular sprain, impingement syndromes or adhesive capsulitis – the technique cannot be performed from this position, as it will generally exacerbate the presenting injury so the alternative technique below is recommended.

Alternative techniques for the latissimus dorsi can be performed with the patient in a sitting position and the patient is asked to place their arms together in horizontal flexion and to rotate to the left side until they feel resistance; from here the patient is asked to resist thoracic rotation to the right (figure 11.11a). After the contraction

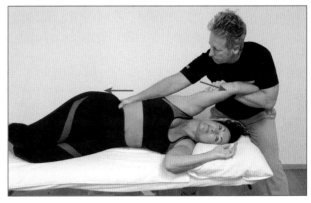

Figure 11.10: *Pressure is applied in the direction shown by the arrows to lengthen the right latissimus dorsi. The right hand of the therapist stabilizes the iliac crest*

the therapist encourages further thoracic rotation to the left (figure 11.11b).

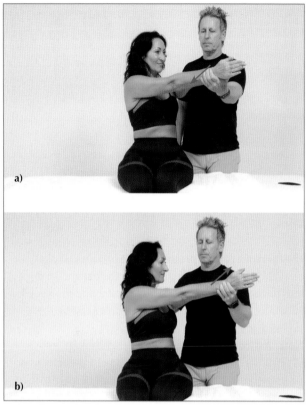

a)

b)

Figure 11.11a & b: *a: The patient horizontally extends against a resistance; b: the therapist takes both arms into thoracic rotation*

TIP: Overactivity, with resultant shortening of the latissimus dorsi, can be a result of gluteus maximus weakness on the contralateral side, due to the relationship of the posterior oblique sling through the thoracolumbar fascia.

■ MET treatment of pectoralis major

The arm is taken away from the body into the scapular plane to induce a lengthening of the sternal fibers of the pectoralis major. And the therapist will be palpating the muscle for the point of bind before they perform an MET.

From the point of bind, the patient is asked to pull their arm across the body (horizontal flexion) to induce a contraction of the right pectoralis major (figure 11.12).

Once the patient has contracted for 10 seconds, the patient (female) is asked to place her hand on her pectoralis major and the therapist places their hand on top of hers. The therapist then controls the patient's right arm and slowly takes the shoulder further away into the scapular plane. This will induce a lengthening of the sternal fibers of the pectoralis major (figure 11.13).

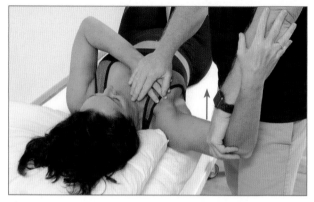

Figure 11.12: *The therapist palpates for the point of bind and the patient is asked to resist the pectoralis major muscle*

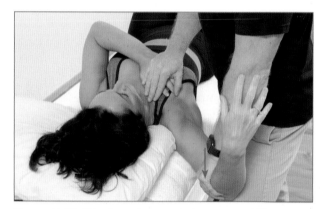

Figure 11.13: *The therapist uses their arm to stabilize over the female patient's arm. Pressure is applied in the direction of the left arrow to lengthen the right pectoralis major*

Clavicular fibers

The following technique is used to lengthen the clavicular fibers of the right pectoralis major. The patient's arm is gently taken from approximately 90 degrees of abduction and taken away from the midline to induce a bind of the clavicular fibers of the right pectoralis major. From the position of bind, the patient is asked to lift their arm against a resistance applied by the therapist. After a 10-second contraction, the clavicular fibers are then taken to their new position of bind (figure 11.14).

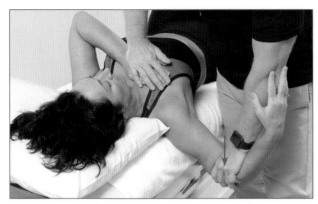

Figure 11.14: *Lengthening the clavicular fibers of the pectoralis major. Pressure is applied by the therapist in the direction of the arrow*

Alternative techniques for the pectoralis major can be done with the patient in a sitting position. The patient is asked to place their arm in 90 degrees of abduction and elbow flexion, and to horizontally flex against a resistance (figure 11.15a). After the contraction the therapist encourages horizontal extension (figure 11.15b).

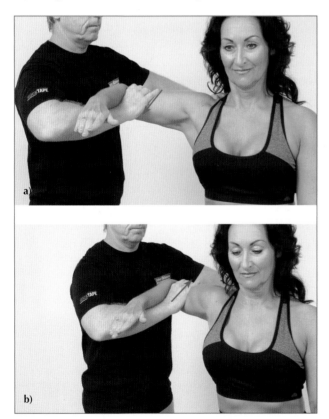

Figure 11.15a & b: *a: The patient horizontally flexes against a resistance; b: the therapist takes the arm into horizontal extension*

An alternative is to ask the patient to sit, place their hands on their hips, and then resist protraction against the therapist (figure 11.16a). After the contraction the therapist then takes the arms into further retraction (figure 11.16b).

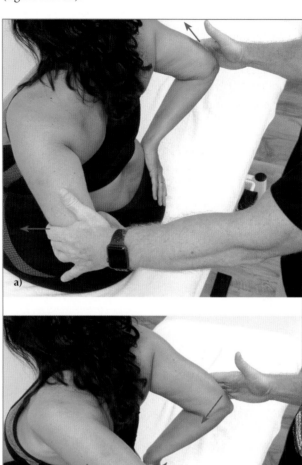

Figure 11.16a & b: *a: The patient is asked to protract; b: the therapist takes the patient's arms into further retraction, thus lengthening the pectoralis major muscle*

TIP: *Protraction of the scapula by the shortening of the pectoralis minor will result in the glenoid fossa rotating medially; this can ultimately place the pectoralis major in a shortened position.*

■ MET treatment of pectoralis minor

The patient adopts a supine position and the therapist places their left hand under the patient's right shoulder blade. The therapist then controls the anterior aspect of the patient's right shoulder. The patient is asked to protract the right scapula for the appropriate time (figure 11.17a). After the contraction, the therapist encourages the right scapula into a retraction position (figure 11.17b); this will encourage a lengthening of the right pectoralis minor.

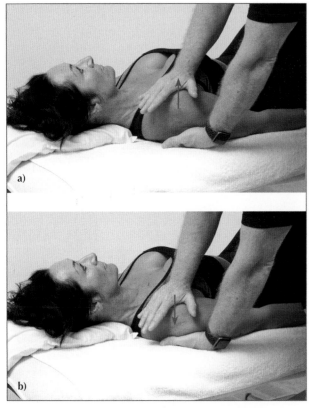

Figure 11.17a & b: *a: The patient protracts their right scapula – supine position. b: The therapist then slowly retracts the scapula*

An alternative MET for the treatment of the pectoralis minor can be performed with the patient in a side-lying position The therapist cradles the patient's right scapula as demonstrated in the figure below. The patient is asked to protract the right scapula against a resistance applied by the therapist (figure 11.17c).

After the 10-second contraction, the therapist gently encourages the right scapula into a retracted position (figure 11.17d), which will induce a lengthening of the right pectoralis minor.

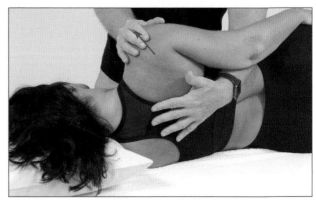

Figure 11.17c: *The patient protracts their right scapula – side-lying position*

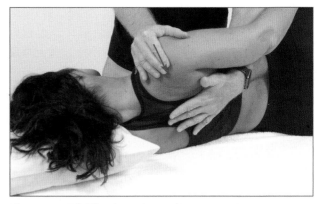

Figure 11.17d: *The therapist applies a retraction movement to encourage lengthening of the right pectoralis minor*

RI method

We can employ an RI technique for the pectoralis minor after the initial post-isometric relaxation (PIR) method shown in figure 11.17c, then we can ask the patient to imagine squeezing a coin between the shoulder blades and to reach across their body as the therapist applies the same pressure to the anterior shoulder, as this activates

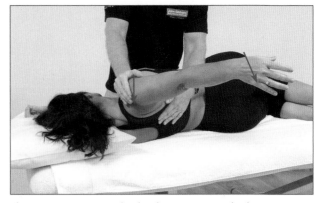

Figure 11.17e: *RI method – the patient is asked to squeeze the shoulder blades together as the therapist is still applying retraction pressure*

the rhomboid muscles and causes inhibition to the pectoralis minor (figure 11.17e).

TIP: *The neurovascular bundle travelling from the thoracic outlet contains the brachial plexus and artery. These structures travel underneath the pectoralis minor, so any hypertonicity of this muscle could result in a brachial neuritis or a vascular compromise to the arm/hand.*

■ MET treatment of subscapularis

PIR method

The therapist takes the patient's shoulder into external rotation until a bind is felt, and from this position, the patient is asked to contract the subscapularis by internally rotating their shoulder (figure 11.18a).

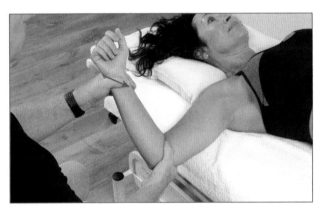

Figure 11.18a: *MET treatment of the subscapularis – PIR method. Position of bind of the subscapularis and the patient internally rotates the shoulder to activate the subscapularis*

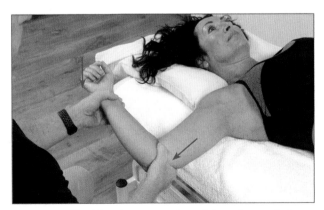

Figure 11.18b: *After the contraction of the subscapularis, the therapist applies traction to the humerus and encourages further external rotation*

After 10 seconds and on the relaxation phase, the therapist applies traction to the shoulder joint (to prevent an impingement) and slowly encourages the shoulder into further external rotation (figure 11.18b).

RI method

If the patient has discomfort activating the subscapularis, the antagonistic muscle of the infraspinatus can be activated instead. From the position of bind (explained above), the patient is asked to resist external rotation; this will contract the infraspinatus and allow the subscapularis to relax through RI (figure 11.19). On the relaxation phase, a lengthening procedure of the subscapularis can then be performed.

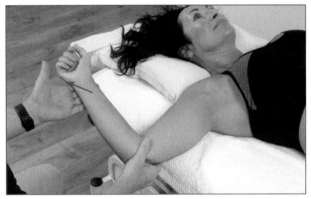

Figure 11.19: *RI method for the subscapularis by externally rotating the humerus causes the subscapularis to relax*

TIP: *The subscapularis is one of the rotator cuff muscles and is the main medial rotator of the glenohumeral joint. A subscapular strain can result in referred pain to the area of the deltoid tuberosity.*

■ MET treatment of infraspinatus

PIR method

The therapist takes the shoulder into internal rotation until the position of bind is felt and from this position, the patient is asked to externally rotate the shoulder (figure 11.20a), which will activate the infraspinatus. After the 10-second contraction, the therapist applies traction to the shoulder and slowly encourages the shoulder into further internal rotation (figure 11.20b).

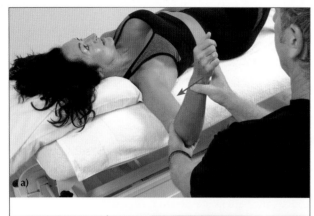

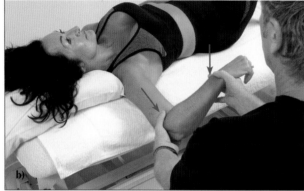

Figure 11.20a & b: *MET treatment of the infraspinatus – PIR method. a: Position of bind for the infraspinatus and the patient is asked to resist external rotation; b: the therapist applies a traction technique to the humerus and encourages further internal rotation to lengthen the infraspinatus*

RI method

If the patient has discomfort activating the infraspinatus, the antagonistic muscle of the subscapularis can be activated instead. From the position of bind (explained above), the patient is asked to resist internal rotation. This will contract the subscapularis and allow the infraspinatus to relax through RI (figure 11.21). On the relaxation phase, a lengthening procedure of the infraspinatus can then be performed.

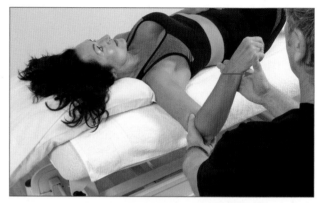

Figure 11.21: *RI method for the infraspinatus by internally rotating the humerus causes the infraspinatus to relax*

TIP: *Trigger points located within the infraspinatus commonly refer pain to the anterior part of the shoulder.*

12

Pathologies of the shoulder and cervical spine

In this chapter I would like to discuss some of the most common shoulder and cervical pathologies found in my clinic, using my own experience as context. There are of course many other possible medical conditions but for this text I will only consider the most common conditions, as otherwise this chapter would probably never come to an end. The pathologies are:

- Rotator cuff tendinopathies and subacromial impingement
- Throwing injuries
- Acromioclavicular joint (ACJ) sprain
- Anterior dislocation
- Bicipital tendinopathies
- SLAP lesion (superior labral tear from anterior to posterior)
- Adhesive capsulitis – frozen shoulder
- Axillary nerve palsy
- Long thoracic nerve palsy
- Cervical disc prolapse
- Facet joint syndrome
- Cervical spondylosis
- Thoracic outlet syndrome (TOS).

■ Rotator cuff tendinopathies and subacromial impingement

Think back to earlier chapters, as the rotator cuff comprises the supraspinatus, infraspinatus, teres minor, and the subscapularis muscles. These are thought of as active ligaments because of their role providing stability to the glenohumeral joint. In reality, specific pathologies of these muscles tend to relate to the supraspinatus rather than the other three muscles of the cuff, even though we can still strain/tear those muscles. Many years ago I attended a course with Dr Jeremy Lewis, who is one of those people I consider to be on top of their game, especially regarding the shoulder complex. You will probably come across numerous studies done by Dr Lewis and his colleagues regarding current methodologies relating to the shoulder complex. I remember one of his fascinating lectures where he discussed rotator cuff tendinopathy as a cause of the patient's pain rather than specifying each individual muscle of the cuff, even though the supraspinatus was mentioned.

Lewis (2009) mentioned that there are at least three reasons why the clinical assessment procedures for rotator cuff tendinopathy/impingement cannot isolate individual tendons and other structures and inform an accurate diagnosis. These are: the morphology of the rotator cuff; the lack of correlation between symptoms and contemporary methods of imaging; and the position and innervation of the subacromial bursa (SAB). Any test designed to assess the integrity and pain response from any of the rotator cuff tendons would involve bursal tissue.

Ide et al. (1996) also mention that the SAB is innervated and appears to have a central role in the presentation of pain to the shoulder.

The role and function of the rotator cuff muscles have been examined in earlier chapters so I will not go over these topics again here. However, if I were to say that the majority of rotator cuff tendinopathies involve the supraspinatus then I would not be far wrong. I have had the pleasure of sitting in on many seminars by top orthopedic consultants, the majority of which have been on shoulder impingement syndromes. The main structure of concern is the supraspinatus and the subacromial bursa as well as potential thickenings of soft tissues or various shapes of the acromion process (figure 12.1).

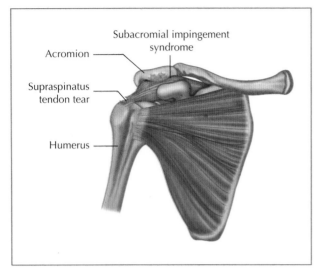

Figure 12.1: *Supraspinatus tendon and impingement within the subacromial space*

In terms of assessment and diagnosis, then an ultrasound (US) or better still a magnetic resonance type of imaging (MRI) will be classified as the gold standard way of diagnosing and will be of great value to determine if the rotator cuff is involved. This diagnosis can clarify the structures that are potentially responsible for the patient's presenting symptoms. Regarding manual therapy, there are numerous tests one can use to determine if the cuff is involved; however, manual testing does not confirm the extent of the underlying pathology as the tests are used simply as a guide to assist the therapist into coming up with a diagnosis.

Neer (1972, 1983) argued that 95% of rotator cuff tears are initiated by impingement and that trauma may enlarge a tear but is rarely the principal factor. Neer described three stages of the impingement process. The first occurs in people under 25 years of age and is associated with tendinous edema and hemorrhage; this does not require surgery. The second involves tendinitis and occurs in people aged 25–40; for this, bursectomy and coracoacromial ligament division should be considered after 18 months of conservative treatment. Neer stated that in this group an acromioplasty is not

usually required. The third stage occurs in people over 40 years of age and is associated with bone spurs and tendon rupture; this requires anterior acromioplasty. Neer stated that the reason rotator cuff tears develop in some people and not in others is principally due to the shape of the acromion.

Bigliani et al. (1986) also argued the shape of the acromion was more likely to be the cause of subacromial impingement syndrome and a rotator cuff tear.

If the hypothesis put forward in the two studies by Neer and Bigliani et al. was correct, and most pathologies sustained to the rotator cuff were because of the shape of the acromion, then one would expect to find a lot of irritation to the superior part of the rotator cuff tendons and the bursa. However, a study done by Ozaki et al. (1988) examined 200 shoulders from 110 cadavers. They reported that a partial thickness tear was observed in 69 specimens and that the majority involved the deeper articular side of the tendon. They argued that the prevalence of tears increased with age and occurred due to intrinsic degeneration and not external (acromial) irritation.

At the present time subacromial decompression is extremely popular and is generally recommended in terms of surgical intervention for shoulder pathology. This was discussed by Judge et al. (2014), who reported the number of patients undergoing this type of surgery to have increased by 746.4% from 2523 in 2000/1 to 21,355 in 2009/10. This has now reached a point where we have a dilemma: basically you can argue about the simple fact that if the patient has an altered shape to the acromion and this is deemed to be causing the patient's shoulder pain, then in this particular case, surgery would be recommended and would be of real value; however, if the causative factor of the patient's pain *is not* the shape of the acromion then surgery would fail. Another study, by Colvin et al. (2012), demonstrated a 600% increase of arthroscopic repair of the rotator cuff across all age groups in the US between 1996 and 2006.

Throughout each of the chapters in this book I will continually be discussing, assessing, treating and rehabilitating rotator cuff injuries so I will leave this topic for you to consider as you continue through the chapters, and turn to the subject of injuries that can happen while throwing.

■ Throwing injuries

Throwing an object such as a ball is not as simple as it looks. We have probably all thrown stones into the river to see if they skim across the water, but can you actually repeat this action many times without feeling discomfort in your shoulder? And how many friends do you know who have thrown a ball and felt discomfort after the first throw! The majority of us are capable of throwing something over our heads but how many of us do it well enough for it to become our sport of choice? This is another matter altogether. To throw an object over our head and achieve some distance requires most, if not all, of our entire musculoskeletal framework and all of the components need to work together in harmony to achieve this relatively simple skill, especially if you want to throw the ball accurately.

It is commonly understood that the further the shoulder can be externally rotated then the greater the potential for the ball to be thrown further, although obviously we are all different in terms of range of motion of our joints and there are many other factors to consider.

We have to remember and consider that throwing injuries in athletes are completely different to throwing injuries sustained by the older population, even though the pathology and mechanism (kinesthetics) of the injury will be roughly the same. This is obviously due to the mechanical and structural changes that occur with the inevitable aging processes.

Calliet (1991) says that the older person has pre-existing degenerative changes. The overhanging acromion process may be eburnated, causing overgrowth of the anterior margin of the acromion and a thickening of the coracoacromial ligament. There are postural changes that alter the alignment of these structures. The rotator cuff may have already undergone degenerative changes from the narrowing of the suprahumeral (subacromial space). This narrowing compresses the normal vascular supply to the conjoined rotator cuff tendon, which predisposes to further degeneration, partial tearing and even complete tearing.

Typically, the younger athlete will tend to be a lot fitter and stronger and have a tendency to throw harder and for longer: this in itself, in one respect, is a diagnosis for a disaster of shoulder pathologies due to the fact of the repeated movements.

Jobe et al. (1983) discussed five stages or phases of the throwing and pitching motion.

- Stage 1 – Wind-up
- Stage 2 – Cocking (early and late)
- Stage 3 – Acceleration
- Stage 4 – Deceleration
- Stage 5 – Follow through.

Wind-up

While the whole throwing motion takes approximately 2 seconds from start to finish, the wind-up stage on its own can take almost 1–1.5 seconds of the overall time, so it is generally a slow process. However, the purpose of the wind-up phase is to place the thrower in the correct position, while preparing the body for the cocking phase. One has to imagine throwing a ball to comprehend these five stages. Think about the initial phase: you have, say, a ball in your hand and are just about to throw it to your friend (figure 12.2) This is the start of the throwing action.

Cocking

Stage 2 of the throw is known as the cocking phase and this can be subclassified into an early phase (figure 12.3a)

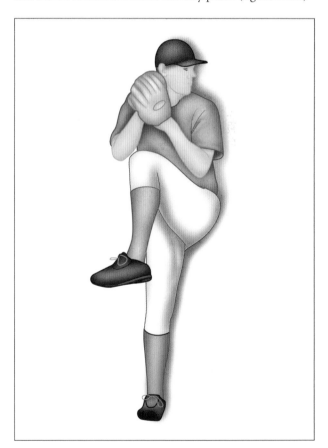

Figure 12.2: *Wind-up phase of throwing*

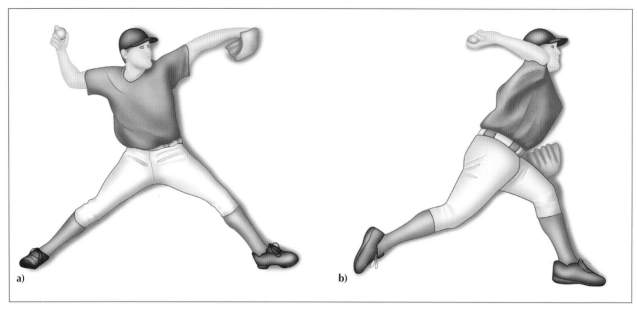

Figure 12.3a & b: *Cocking phase of throwing. a: Early phase; b: late phase*

and a late phase (figure 12.3b. If you look at the position of the right arm in the cocking stages, you will notice the shoulder is abducted to 90 degrees, horizontally extended to 30 degrees, and externally rotated to at least 90 degrees. This motion in the early cocking phase is mainly achieved through activation of the deltoid muscle with stabilization through the rotator cuff; in the late phase of the cocking motion the deltoids decrease their effect and it is now controlled primarily through activation of the rotator cuff. During late cocking the pectoralis major, subscapularis and latissimus dorsi muscles are all working eccentrically to control the stability of the humeral head and this position naturally places them on maximal stretch (as well as stretching the anterior joint capsule), which sets the muscles ready for the acceleration stage. The weight is now transferred to the rear right leg and the torso is right rotated. This is potentially where the rotator cuff tears occur due to the natural impingement process, especially if there is an inherent weakness or prior tears of the cuff to start with. The anterior oblique sling as well as the arm adductors of the pectorals and latissimus dorsi are on stretch and the shoulder is in a position of extreme external rotation as it is preparing for the next stage of throwing.

Acceleration

Stage 3 is the acceleration phase, during which you actually throw the ball, and this dictates the end of this stage (when you let go of the ball). The rotator cuff plays a minimal part here as the stronger pectoralis major and latissimus dorsi are contracting concentrically and these muscles will take the arm from a position of external

rotation into extension and internal rotation at maximal speed. The weight is now transferred to the left leg as the thorax is rotating to the left and this motion also utilizes the anterior oblique sling (figure 12.4).

Deceleration

Stage 4 is classified as the deceleration phase (figure 12.5). Once you have let go of the ball the rotator cuff now works exceptionally hard eccentrically to decelerate the motion of the humeral head; without this eccentric braking motion the humeral head would continue to rotate

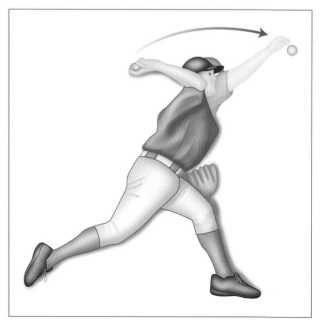

Figure 12.4: *Acceleration phase of throwing with the anterior oblique sling*

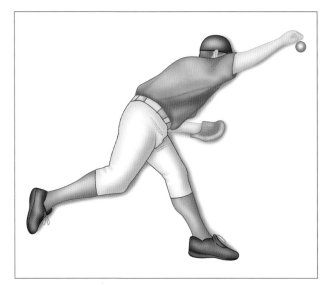

Figure 12.5: *Deceleration phase of throwing*

internally, hence this stage of the throwing motion can be the most traumatic phase and is a very common source of impingement syndromes and tearing that can often occur to the musculature of the cuff.

Follow through
Stage 5 is the last stage of the throwing motion and is called the follow through (figure 12.6). This is simply where the body is coming to a resting position and the muscle activation has reduced to a normal level.

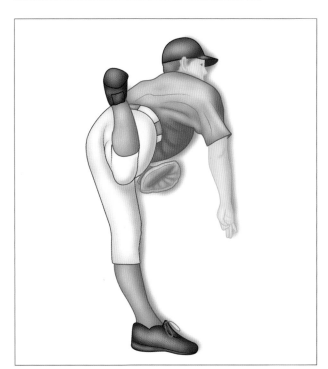

Figure 12.6: *Follow through phase of throwing*

■ Acromioclavicular joint (ACJ) sprain

The AC joint is a structure within the human joint system that I would call a *strut* or even a *hinge mechanism*. It is located within the shoulder complex and I consider this to be one of the most commonly sprained joints. We can sprain this joint not just in sport but also in day-to-day life. I wrote about this injury at the beginning of this book as I have personally sustained many injuries to this small but complex joint through different types of sporting events.

When I am in clinic and see a sprain of this joint, I have come to a conclusion that the worse the sprain looks the better it feels in terms of how much pain the patient experiences. It sounds a bit strange, but I do think what I am saying is true as I have seen some very 'disfigured'-looking AC joints where the patients have relatively little pain. The opposite is also true – a small sprain with no obvious displacement can cause a surprisingly substantial amount of pain. I believe this is because, in a case where the clavicle and acromion have been displaced far away from each other, there are simply no bones to rub against each other; conversely, if the sprain is very minor and with a small displacement, then the bones are not quite sitting correctly and hence can easily contact each other and subsequently rub together and ultimately cause pain, with eventual restriction.

In one respect, I believe that physical therapy treatment of the AC joint is sometimes a very difficult process to follow as every patient we see is individual and unique, so a treatment protocol for patient A might not work for patient B, and vice versa. Typically, overhead movements during the rehab process can sometimes be recommended; however, for some patients this motion can easily irritate the joint, especially if weights are included in the routine. From personal experience, I know that this joint can naturally take a very long time to settle down before no pain or instability is felt. Unfortunately it is relatively common practice in therapy to rehabilitate these AC joints way too quickly, before they are ready to perform certain motions.

Grades of AC joint sprain are shown in figure 12.7.

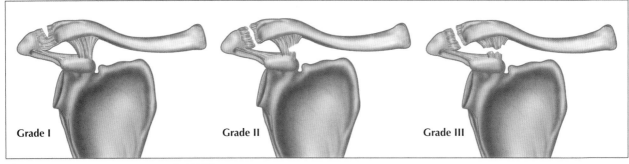

Figure 12.7: *AC joint sprain – grade I/II/III*

■ Anterior dislocation

Before I discuss luxations or dislocations of the glenohumeral joint, think back to the chapter where, in relation to the stability of this joint, it was likened to a golf ball sitting on a tee and it was said that it is a naturally unstable joint. Having said that, I have not seen that many fully dislocated glenohumeral joints, especially notable given all the time I have spent looking after athletes in a sporting context. With a full dislocation the shoulder joint is generally relocated within a hospital environment by a trained medical team. A partial dislocation tends to relocate itself on its own with a bit of persuasion from the patient with some general mobilizations.

However, I do want to discuss one case study that you might find of interest.

CASE STUDY

I was the therapist for a local rugby team and during a Saturday game one of the team members went in for a tackle and ended up dislocating his shoulder. When I ran over to him to provide first aid the first thing he said to me was to ask if I could relocate his shoulder. At the time I was tempted to assist; however, the hospital was close by so a friend took him there and the shoulder was subsequently relocated. I saw him later that evening in the clubhouse and I said to him that realistically, with the time it would take for the rehabilitation protocol, for him the rugby season was probably over. Three weeks later I was providing medical cover for the Saturday game and saw this chap just about to start a game and asked him what was going on. He said sorry, but the coach had told him to play. I said that was rather a silly thing to do and advised against it. However, he played and at the first tackle he dislocated his shoulder for the second time and had to be taken to hospital. The consultant was rather annoyed that he had to relocate his shoulder again. He told the

player that because he had sustained another dislocation in a short period he would probably need stabilizing surgery at some point in the near future and advised that he should refrain from playing any sport at all for the next few months.

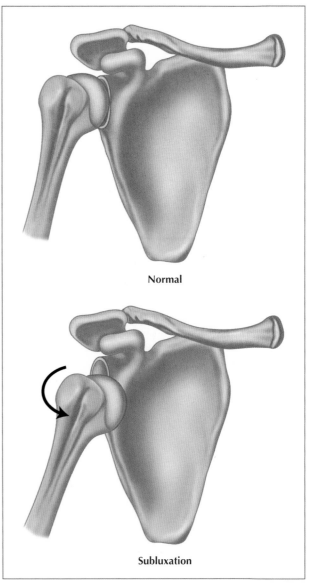

Figure 12.8: *Anterior dislocation*

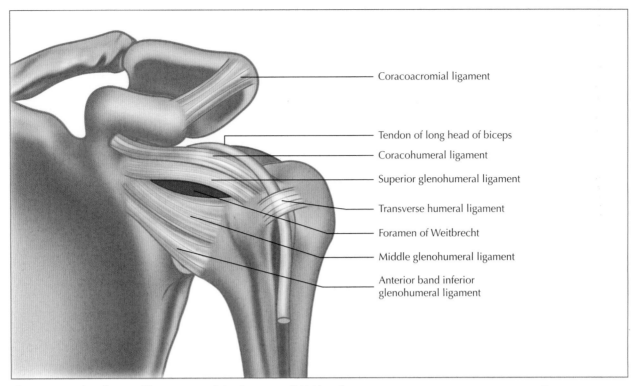

Coracoacromial ligament

Tendon of long head of biceps

Coracohumeral ligament

Superior glenohumeral ligament

Transverse humeral ligament

Foramen of Weitbrecht

Middle glenohumeral ligament

Anterior band inferior glenohumeral ligament

Figure 12.9: *Glenohumeral ligaments and the foramen of Weitbrecht*

The natural problem one has with a dislocation of the shoulder joint is the structures and soft tissues that will become damaged. This is also the case when the shoulder is relocated as the relocation maneuver itself can be very traumatic for the body, especially since it can take a while for the medical team to relocate the humerus within the glenoid fossa (shoulder socket). The axillary nerve is particularly vulnerable when this procedure is performed.

I remember the first time I dislocated my shoulder I was advised to keep it in a sling for at least four weeks with no movement. I was in the army at the time so I did what I was told and it did improve but it took many months of physiotherapy. In fact, I can still feel a weakness or even instability in my shoulder in certain positions and that injury happened many years ago.

I believe that one of the reasons the shoulder dislocates anteriorly is due to a design fault (figure 12.8). This is because of the anterior ligaments of the shoulder, the glenohumeral ligaments, which are basically folds of the capsule. They have three separate bands to them, superior, middle, and inferior, as shown in figure 12.9. You will notice that there is a gap in-between the bands. The space between the superior and middle portion, called the

foramen of Weitbrecht, is of particular concern and to me is a potential weak spot that can allow the humeral head to dislocate anteriorly.

■ Bicipital tendinopathies

Pain in the anterior aspect of the shoulder might be from the long head tendon of the biceps brachii and some form of tendinopathy (figure 12.10). I have had many therapy treatments over the years. Some therapists have poked and prodded the biceps long head tendon in an aggressive way while others have used massage type of friction work over the tendon of the long head, to the point that it has irritated the soft tissues for many days afterwards. The tendon is located within a sensitive synovial sheath as it penetrates the joint capsule to its attachment onto the supraglenoid tubercle; the structure is overall pretty delicate and it definitely does not like too much massage work, so my suggestion is to leave it alone! My experience tells me that if a patient presents with pain to the anterior shoulder which has been present for a long time, and the long head of the biceps tendon is tender to palpate, then I should investigate further as it could be an underlying SLAP lesion.

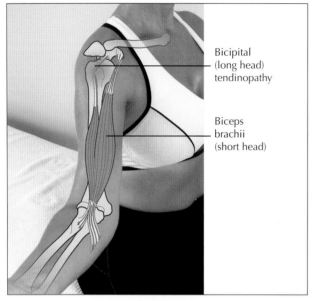

Figure 12.10: *Bicipital tendinopathy*

Labels in figure:
- Bicipital (long head) tendinopathy
- Biceps brachii (short head)

■ SLAP lesion or tear

SLAP stands for Superior (top) Labrum (rim of cartilage) Anterior (front) to Posterior (back). The superior part of the glenoid labrum (supraglenoid tubercle) has the long head of the biceps tendon attaching to it and if the shoulder is forced into an unnatural motion like a dislocation, or more commonly in sporting activities such as rugby or throwing, where force can be applied to the arm, then the humeral head will act like a lever and tear the tendon and labrum in an anterior to posterior direction (hence the name SLAP).

SLAP lesions, like other injuries such as sprains and strains, are classified into four types (figure 12.11):

Type I SLAP lesion

Involves some roughing or fraying of the labrum but it is still intact to the glenoid. It is related to the aging process so a type I is normally seen in the older patient.

Type II SLAP lesion

This lesion is generally thought of as the most common type. The tendon with the superior labrum is completely detached from the glenoid so that a space appears under the labrum and the articular cartilage, which causes instability of the biceps-labral anchor point.

Type III SLAP lesion

This is similar to a meniscus tear in the knee. It is called a bucket handle tear of the labrum. The biceps tendon will still be attached and will drop into the shoulder joint. This lesion will probably cause locking or clicking within the joint.

Type IV SLAP lesion

This is also a bucket handle tear of the labrum but now this lesion also extends and involves the biceps tendon as well so the stability mechanism of the biceps-labrum anchor point is compromised.

Patients generally complain of deep shoulder pain, especially when performing certain activities, such as weight training or throwing objects. Some mention a reduction in the range of motion and others find it difficult to pinpoint the exact source of their pain. Weakness and decreased function in sports performance is also common with a SLAP lesion.

If a SLAP lesion has been diagnosed through an MRI (even though small tears can be missed) and is

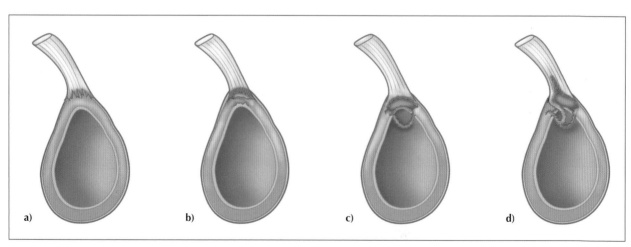

Figure 12.11a–d: *Four types of SLAP tear. a: Type I; b: type II; c: type III; d: type IV*

a)   b)   c)   d)

affecting the patient's day-to-day activities then surgical intervention of an arthroscopy is normally recommended as the preferred and realistic choice of treatment.

■ Adhesive capsulitis – frozen shoulder

Unfortunately, even now this condition is not truly understood. Over the years it has had many names: one of the first was Duplay's disease, named after Duplay in 1906, when he discussed a shoulder condition that he described as a periarthritis, which is now recognized as the typical frozen shoulder. There are many other terms for this condition, for example, adhesive bursitis and pericapsulitis. It is considered that the synovial tissues associated with the subacromial and subscapularis bursa, also the conjoined tendon of the rotator cuff, the biceps long head and the glenohumeral capsule are potentially involved in some way or another with this type of pathology as they are all interconnected with each other. It was Codman in 1934 who made the most extensive study of this condition. He initially considered it was due to adhesions to the subacromial bursa and later related the condition to a tendinopathy of the rotator cuff.

Typically, frozen shoulder is not seen in patients under the age of 40 and it usually occurs between the ages of 50 and 65, with women being more prone to this condition than men.

CASE STUDY

A 54-year-old female came into the clinic with general restriction and pain to her to right shoulder, which had been getting worse over the previous few weeks. The issue had begun around 4 weeks earlier when the patient participated in a 'bodypump' exercise class, as she wanted to loose some weight. She was squatting to music as directed by the instructor, with a light barbell over her shoulders. When the exercise sequence finished she went to lift the bar off the upper part of her back and immediately felt a sharp pain to her right shoulder. Initially she was concerned, but the pain settled down over the next few days, assisted by some painkillers, and she thought nothing more of it. Over the next few weeks she noticed she was having difficulty doing simple things, such as unclipping her bra strap at the back, reaching for the seatbelt in the car, and even placing tins of beans on the

top shelf of her cupboard. Even at night she noticed that it was starting to become painful to lie on her right side and to move her arm in certain positions.

I asked my patient to simply place her elbows by her side and to bend them to 90 degrees and then I asked her to externally rotate both her shoulders as far as comfortable. The right side was very limited and painful (shown in figure 12.12), thus indicating a capsular pattern or a capsular restriction, as external rotation is generally the first movement to be lost with adhesive capsulitis.

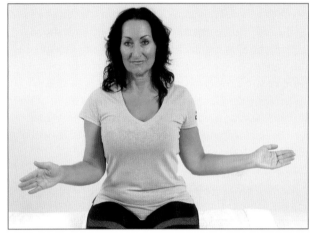

Figure 12.12: *External rotation restricted to the right side demonstrates a capsular restriction*

I have what you might think rather a strange analogy for this type of pathology, which I relate to *lighting of gunpowder*, though I consider the concept works. When the lady in question felt the initial pain lifting the bar off the head, she 'lit' a very thin trail of gunpowder so that it is now appears as a slow-burning long line of powder and in the distance there is a large pile of gunpowder. My theory is that if the large pile of gunpowder goes *boom* then she will likely achieve a frozen shoulder (not through choice) that will last a considerable amount of time (possibly 1–2 years), so the plan must be to extinguish the flame and this can be achieved by physical therapy intervention. However, there is a *window of opportunity* to achieve this and by that I mean we probably have a limited amount of time, this being a few weeks and not months, to extinguish the flame. If this burning flame is left to continue and reach its end goal, the large pile of powder, then this will be indicative of a chronic pathology and adhesive capsulitis now ensues.

Sometimes, we need to think about treatments of specific body parts like the shoulder complex in a less complicated way. What I mean by that is the following: if the patient has what we suspect to be a frozen shoulder then obviously the main objective has to be to return function and mobility as well as trying to reduce pain.

There are potentially numerous reasons why one might present with an adhesive capsulitis with no obvious underlying causative factor. However, the majority of patients that present to my clinic with capsulitis are female and they are normally between the ages of 48 and 58 years old. It is an interesting fact that women between these ages are more susceptible to this type of condition and there needs to be more research conducted on why this should be the case. Currently, studies do not truly understand or explain the why and the how of the pathophysiology of this condition. We know there is a link between diabetic patients and a frozen shoulder and this may be due to a systemic metabolic vascular component as a result of the diabetes, as discussed by Bridgman (1972), who found a 10.8% incidence of a frozen shoulder in a series of 800 diabetic patients.

The condition generally starts off insidiously with pain usually felt over the insertion of the deltoid muscle to the tuberosity of the humerus; the bicipital tendon and the supraspinatus attachment onto the greater tubercle can also be tender to touch. Specific motion, particularly into abduction and flexion, will exacerbate the pain. In the early phase, active and passive range of motion become limited to approximately 10–15 degrees at certain end ranges and by now the patient is probably aware of the shoulder discomfort at night because it will naturally interfere with their sleep patterns.

In terms of treatment for this type of condition, it has been said many times to me by medical practitioners that this condition will resolve itself within 18 months to 2 years. I presume this is one answer to a chronic problem; however, my patients might not want to wait that long for it to resolve, and I can perfectly agree with them. If we think of the *keep it simple* analogy then the primary goal is to try and improve mobility and functionality because the motion has simply been lost, so the physical therapist has to devise a plan to promote and encourage mobilizations without increasing the pain. I know this process is not as straightforward as one might think because I have seen numerous patients with a frozen shoulder and they are all unique so that treatment for patient A might not work for patient B. Unfortunately, therefore, I cannot give you a set treatment protocol. However, that said, what I can add is this: for every one of those patients I have

seen (and will see), I endeavor to try my best to work on *improving the mobility* because to me that has to be the primary goal.

■ Axillary nerve palsy

This is an interesting one as the axillary nerve originates from the C5 and C6 nerve root and innervates the deltoid and the teres minor muscles. If one has been shown how to perform myotome (muscle area) testing then it would be relatively easy to see why the practitioner would suspect a C5 nerve root pathology rather than an axillary nerve palsy, because the myotome for C5 is mainly abduction of the glenohumeral joint and we know that the deltoid muscle abducts the humerus.

I would like to discuss a case with you that I feel is of value when looking at this particular pathology. It might clarify what it is I am trying to discuss, especially as this patient presents with a potential shoulder problem, and it makes sense in the context of this book to cover all possible avenues, including the area of the cervical spine and nerves.

CASE STUDY

A 45-year-old male likes to do 50 press ups every morning. Three weeks ago, after performing only five of the 50 presses, he felt a sudden pain within the right shoulder and had to stop. He comes to see me a week later and is unable to fully abduct and flex the shoulder joint; this is mainly due to weakness rather than pain. Strangely, if the patient lies in a supine position (i.e., on his back) then he is able to abduct fully, but not consecutively – he would need to rest for 30 seconds before he could lift his arm again. The patient also complained of a strange feeling to the deltoid insertion. On examination, it was obvious that the deltoid muscle was unable to contract and other muscles such as the pectorals and supraspinatus were compensating. I told him that I suspected he had damaged the axillary nerve due to the push-ups as the nerve is located close to the humeral head and if there was excessive motion of the humerus for some reason (think of a dislocation), then the nerve might be implicated. I told him that the nerve normally regenerates at a rate of 1 mm a day so it will probably take him a few weeks to recover. The reason why he felt a strange feeling to the deltoid area is because the axillary nerve supplies the sensation

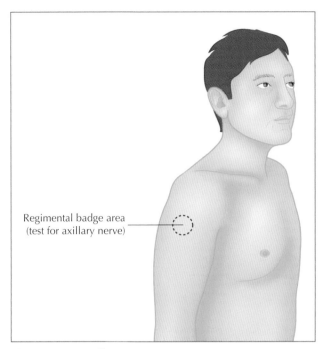

Figure 12.13: *Axillary nerve sensory innervation*

to that part of the arm called the regimental badge (figure 12.13) and if the nerve is damaged then the patient will perceive altered neurological sensations to this specific area.

Long thoracic nerve palsy

CASE STUDY – MYSELF

I consider myself to have damage to the long thoracic nerve, even though I have not had any nerve conduction tests done. You can see from figure 12.14 that my right scapula has excessive winging. The nerve originates from the level of C5, 6, 7 and innervates the serratus anterior muscle. This muscle is responsible for certain motions of the scapula and its main function is to protract and upwardly rotate the scapula (in combination with shoulder joint abduction), as well as to maintain the scapula in suspension with the thoracic cage. If for some reason there is a weakness of this muscle then the scapula will probably have a 'winging' appearance. In my case I reckon I have actually damaged the long thoracic nerve rather than having weakness. I believe this happened when I went waterfall kayaking, took the wrong route off a rather high waterfall, hit a large rock below with my right arm, and dislocated the right shoulder. It was relocated under general anesthetic and I woke up with damage to the

axillary nerve. I explained the consequence earlier as the nerve supplies the deltoid and teres minor muscle and that ceased to work correctly for many months. Unknown to me at the time, I probably sustained damage to the long thoracic nerve as well, and this was probably due to the initial shoulder dislocation.

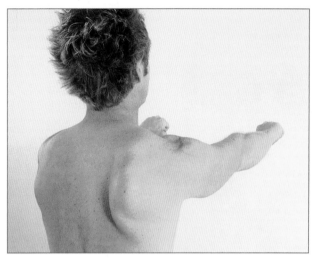

Figure 12.14: *Scapula winging*

Over the years I have tried to strengthen the serratus anterior to help correct the winging; however, if I am being honest, nothing seems to have helped and now I am resigned to the fact that maybe the muscle might never regain its strength because of the nerve damage. I am generally happy with that because I do not have any pain and never really had any. I now have a scapula that sticks out, and do you know what, I actually like it as it's my sort of party trick (even though I don't go to many parties these days!).

Cervical spine pathologies, discs, facet and degeneration (OA)

It is considered that the majority of shoulder pain is directly or indirectly related to the cervical spine and in this text I would like to discuss some very common musculoskeletal structures that can be responsible for the patient's symptomology of pain perceived in the upper limb.

Disc prolapse

The most common disc disturbance, as I like to call it, are the following: disc bulge, protrusion, extrusion, prolapse, herniation or even sequestration (this is where the nucleus actually detaches off the annulus) (figure 12.15). These pathologies happen mainly at the disc level of C4/5, C5/6 and C6/7. Remember there is no such thing as an actual slipped disc even though it is mentioned often. It is the inner fluid called the nucleus pulposus (located within the outer shell called the annulus fibrosis) that is generally responsible for the pain and this sensation is only perceived (pain that is) when a pain-sensitive structure has been contacted, e.g., posterior longitudinal ligament or exiting nerve root, that can refer to the specific dermatome region (figure 12.16). Think of a tube of toothpaste – if you squeeze one end of the tube, the other end tends to 'bulge', and vice versa, so the paste (nucleus) is pushing against the outer shell covering (annulus) from the inside and causing it to change shape but there is no actual slippage of the disc.

Intervertebral discs are amazing structures. They have cells, called proteoglycan aggrecans, located within them that are like tiny sponges and can carry approximately 500 times their own weight of water. Over time these unique cells eventually die so the water content within will naturally reduce. This process will eventually lead to a condition called degenerative disc disease (DDD). The disc is kept living by the vertebral end plates. These structures have been likened to parts of a tire – the inner nucleus is the 'air' within the tire, the annulus is the tire's strong walls and the tread of the tire is the end plates. The discs are mainly avascular structures; however, discs are hydrated through diffusion by the vertebral bodies and subsequent end plates (figure 12.17). The nerve supply is mainly from the sinuvertebral nerves and it is only innervated to the periphery of the disc.

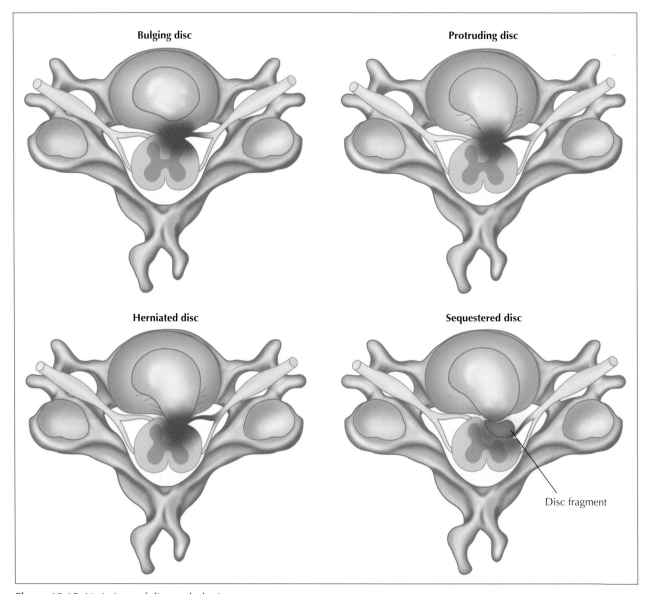

Bulging disc

Protruding disc

Herniated disc

Sequestered disc

Disc fragment

Figure 12.15: *Variations of disc pathologies*

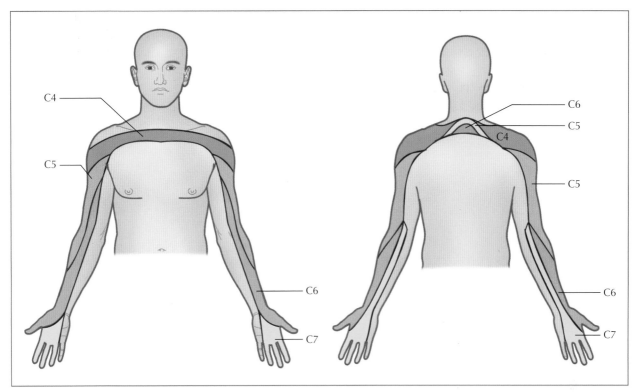

Figure 12.16: *C4, C5, C6 and C7 dermatome pain pattern*

Cervical spine facet joint

These are highly sensitive structures (figure 12.18) and neurologically innervated through pain receptors – so much so that the facets have the probability of causing ongoing chronic neck, shoulder and arm pain. Many of my previous patients have had cervical facet joint injections (guided through ultrasound) in spinal pain clinics before they have come to me to see if these structures are responsible for their shoulder pain. In one way to have an injection is considered as a sort of diagnostic procedure, even though this is debatable as a correct treatment protocol. In a positive way, if the patient does have a reduction of symptoms in their shoulder after the injection, then the doctor confirms a facet joint as the possible causative factor. To me, however, the whole musculoskeletal issue has been missed; remember the saying that where the pain is the problem is not? I consider that these cases, where the patient has ongoing neck and

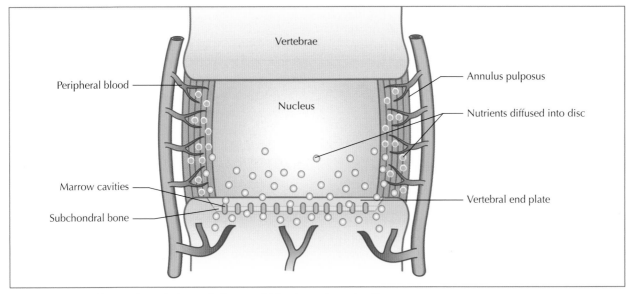

Figure 12.17: *Hydration through the end plates and blood supply to the disc*

shoulder pain, are probably the result of lots of small musculoskeletal manifestations that have caused long term dysfunctional changes over the preceding years and now the small inconsequential changes have slowly manifested themselves and become a larger problem for the patient.

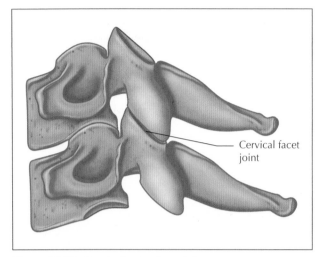

Figure 12.18: *Cervical spine facet joint*

I have another analogy that might fit these and other patients. I say that everyone has a *reservoir of compensation*; for some people it is the size of a huge lake and will never run out of water, or in this case your body will always be able to compensate, no matter what the problem. You will know friends and athletes like this who can participate in every sport, do all daily tasks and never complain of pain anywhere. However, for the majority of patients the lake is a lot smaller and is slowly starting to dry up, so now the body is struggling to compensate, and this could be the reason for their presenting symptoms. For example, a friend of yours has been a runner for 20 years, running three times a week every week, and suddenly in the last two months says their knee, or hip, or foot (it doesn't really matter what body part hurt) is becoming painful. Why? Because maybe, just maybe, their reservoir of compensation is starting to dry up.

■ Cervical spine spondylosis (OA)

Unfortunately, sooner for some than others, age comes with some naturally degenerative changes and certain areas of the human body, such as the hip and knee, can especially suffer. That is also true for the lower three components of the cervical spine (C4/5, C5/6 and C6/7) as these areas can also become degenerative. In the spine we call it spondylosis (*spondy* relates to spine and *osis* relates to degeneration). Spondylosis generally affects the vertebral bodies as well as the facet joints (figure 12.19).

The spaces where the nerves will exit are called the intervertebral (neural) foramina and these spaces can eventually narrow due to the underlying pathology and cause painful symptoms.

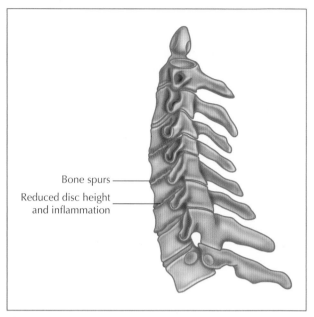

Figure 12.19: *Spondylosis (OA) of the cervical spine*

CASE STUDY

A 72-year-old female came to the clinic with generalized aching to both her shoulders, especially in the morning when she woke up. This ache would settle down after about 20 minutes, and she found some relief from having a hot bath or shower, which would reduce some of her symptoms. Her active range of cervical rotation was limited, especially to the left, and she kept saying that her neck 'just feels stiff all the time'. When I performed passive rotation to her cervical spine in a supine position, her motion was still very restricted and uncomfortable. Surprisingly, the deep tendon reflexes and (myotome) power all tested normal. Her trapezius muscles felt exquisitely tender and very rigid on palpation; however, she felt a good massage would be of benefit. I mentioned to her that I considered she had degenerative changes and a week later a MRI proved that she had multilevel disc dehydration and degeneration to the vertebral bodies and facet joints with osteophytic changes (bony spurs), especially to the lower three bodies of the cervical spine.

With regards to treatment strategy, the patient asked me if I was going to manipulate her neck (using a high velocity thrust technique, called HVT) and I said that under the circumstances, and especially since there are bony spurs and multilevel degenerative changes present, these techniques were not appropriate and even potentially very dangerous. I said that soft tissue techniques, gentle mobilizations and muscle energy techniques to correct some of the shortened muscular tissues, and some postural re-education exercises would be my recommendations.

I told the patient that I would never be able to *fix* her neck because of what was shown on the scan; however, I did say to her that I would be able to *help* her in terms of improving some of her mobility and pain relief through soft tissue techniques and gentle mobilizations. Some of the techniques I performed on her are covered in later chapters.

■ Thoracic outlet syndrome (TOS)

I have already covered this condition briefly when I discussed pain associated with the superior angle of the scapula. However, this topic needs to be covered from another perspective as textbooks have been written about this subject matter. The history of TOS started back in 1861 when a 26-year-old female had a painful and ischemic left arm. The diagnosis of a cervical rib was made (there were no X-rays available at this time) and Mr Holmes Coot successfully performed the surgical excision.

There are three different types of TOS and these are:

1. arterial
2. venous
3. neurological.

The arterial type is caused by compression of the subclavian artery, the venous is caused by compression of the subclavian vein and the neurological type is caused by compression of the brachial plexus.

Rob and Standeven in 1958 reported 10 cases of arterial occlusion as a complication of what they termed *thoracic outlet compression syndrome* and thus introduced the term to the surgical literature.

According to Vanti et al. (2007), non-specific neurogenic TOS makes up the bulk of diagnosed cases as most patients have neurological symptoms and they suggest it may account for up to 85% of TOS and often follow an ulnar nerve (C8/T1) distribution.

Just to recap from an earlier chapter, the thoracic outlet comprises the brachial plexus (C5–T1) and the subclavian

artery with the returning subclavian vein. These soft tissue structures exit at the root of the neck on their journey to the upper extremity, hand and arm, and exit through a small space called the thoracic outlet. The brachial plexus and subclavian artery pass through the natural space formed between the anterior and middle scalenes and this area is called the 'interscalene triangle' (figure 12.20). Please note that the subclavian vein does not normally pass through this interscalene triangular space; it passes adjacent to the anterior scalene muscle and there is a natural groove formed over the first rib for the passage of the vein (figure 12.20). These three structures now continue their journey and pass over the first rib and under the clavicle as well as passing under the pectoralis minor, and there is no doubt that these delicate tissues can be compressed anywhere along their continued pathway. Because the structures are neural as well as vascular, the patient's symptoms can be anything from pain, numbness, tingling, paresthesia or weakness to temperature changes and even swelling to the area of the shoulder, arm, forearm, hand and fingers.

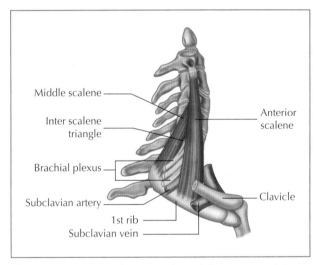

Figure 12.20: *Interscalene triangle and the passage of the brachial plexus and subclavian artery, and subclavian vein passes adjacent to anterior scalene and over the groove in the first rib*

It is typically the lower medial cord of the brachial plexus that is affected and the symptoms are generally related to the nerves from the levels of C8 and T1. The ulnar nerve is formed from this level as well as the cutaneous (sensory to the skin) nerves that subdivide from these levels; these are the medical brachial and medial antebrachial nerves. The C8 and T1 dermatome will affect mainly the medial aspect of the arm and forearm, the hypothenar eminence of the hand, the fifth and half of the area of the ring finger.

If the subclavian artery is compressed (please note that this pathology is very rare), the condition is normally associated with a cervical rib or first rib anomaly and this causes a narrowing of the artery with a potential to form an aneurysm just beyond the site of compression. The patient might perceive the following symptoms: a sudden onset of hand pain and weakness, arm fatigue with numbness and tingling in the fingers. The fingers will feel cold and pale with diminished sensation and the patient will mention that if wounds are present in the arm and hands that are very slow to heal. If this condition is suspected, then an immediate medical referral is recommended. If the capillary refill test is applied to the nail bed, the blood flow to the nail will be slow to refill and if it is used, the Allen test (tests the speed of blood flow to the hand – see below) will be positive.

TOS – special tests

Allen test
This test is designed as an arterial vascular test to rule out distal arterial disease in patients with hand symptoms of tingling and numbness.

The patient adopts a seated position. The therapist passively lifts the arm of the patient and the patient is asked to quickly clench their fist several times (3–5 times is normal) (figure 12.21, as this maneuver will remove the blood flow to the hand.

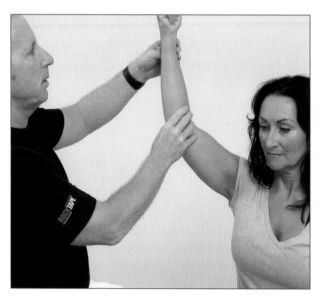

Figure 12.21: *The patient is asked to clench the fist many times*

Next, with the patient's fist still clenched, the therapist compresses both radial and ulnar arteries of the wrist (figure 12.22).

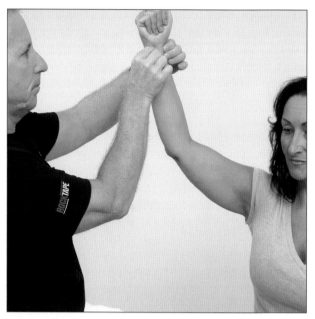

Figure 12.22: *The therapist compresses both the radial and ulnar artery*

The patient's arm is then lowered and the fist is opened, but with pressure still applied to each of the arteries. First the radial artery is released (figure 12.23) and the time it takes for the capillary refill is noted; then the whole procedure is repeated but this time the ulnar artery is released and the capillary refill time is again measured.

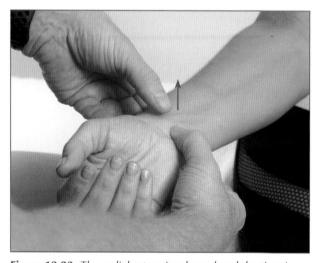

Figure 12.23: *The radial artery is released and the time is noted for the blood to refill*

By compressing both distal arteries and pumping the fist, blood is effectively eliminated from the hand. Then, by releasing one artery, the hand perfusion time can be measured and compared to normal values, thus ascertaining the effectiveness of each artery.

Adson test

The patient is asked to take a seat and the therapist locates the radial pulse in the symptomatic arm. The patient is asked to rotate the head *toward* the affected side and to extend the head and neck back.

The shoulder is externally rotated, abducted to 90 degrees and horizontally extended 10 degrees. From this position, the patient is asked to take a deep breath and hold it as shown in figure 12.24, while the therapist continues to monitor the patient's pulse. The therapist asks the patient to mention if they feel any changes in their arms or hands.

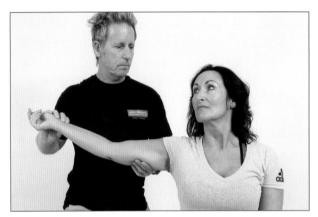

Figure 12.24: *The therapist externally rotates, abducts and horizontally extends the shoulder and the patient is asked to take a breath in, while maintaining contact with pulse*

Adson's test increases the tension of the scalene muscles, potentially compressing the neurovascular bundle. Gillard et al. (2001) reported that Adson's test was one of the better performing tests of those commonly used for TOS, having a positive predictive value of 85%. In this particular study, either loss of the radial pulse or reproduction of symptoms was considered to be positive. A positive Adson's test suggests that the scalene muscles should be assessed and treated for hypertonicity and trigger points.

Roos test

The patient is asked to adopt a sitting position and is instructed to externally rotate and abduct their shoulder to 90 degrees and also to flex their elbows to 90 degrees (figure 12.25a). This is known as the *I surrender* position (figure 12.24a).

In this position the patient is instructed to clench and open the hand at a slow rate (every 2–3 seconds). The test should continue for 3 minutes or until the patient can no longer continue due to pain (figure 12.25b).

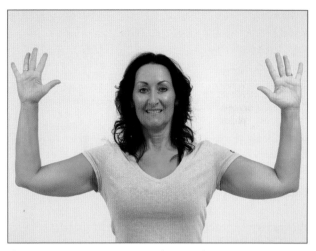

Figure 12.25a: *Roos position of external rotation at 90 degrees*

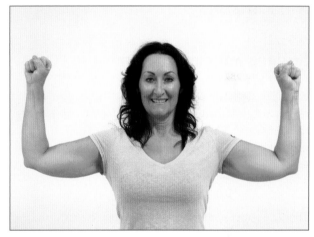

Figure 12.25b: *The patient is asked to open and clench fists for 3 minutes*

According to Gillard et al. (2001), a positive test is reproduction of pain in the arm, shoulder, chest or neck, numbness or tingling in the extremity or the inability to keep up the fist clenching. Roos (1996) suggested that the best positive result is the inability to continue the fist clenching for the full 3 minutes due to pain.

Cervical ribs and TOS

The ribs naturally start at the first thoracic vertebra of T1 and finish at T12, hence 12 pairs of ribs. If there is an extra rib present, then typically it will be at the level of the seventh cervical vertebra and this has been suggested as a cause of neurovascular compression at the thoracic outlet (figure 12.26). The rib can basically be anything from a small stump to a full size rib that projects from

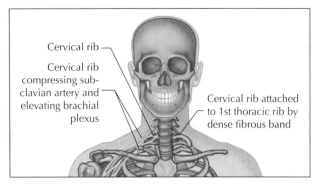

Cervical rib

Cervical rib compressing sub-clavian artery and elevating brachial plexus

Cervical rib attached to 1st thoracic rib by dense fibrous band

Figure 12.26: *A cervical rib causing TOS*

the transverse process of C7 and can even connect with the first rib by way of a fibrous cartilaginous connection. Some of these extra ribs can be seen on standard X-ray; unfortunately some cannot be seen because not all of these extra ribs calcify and they are normally only found through a surgical procedure.

Scalene anticus syndrome and TOS

Naffziger (Naffziger and Grant 1938), who was chief of neurosurgery at the University of California, considered the anterior scalene muscle to be the key to the neurovascular compressive abnormalities with patients with *cervical rib syndrome* and thus used the term *scalenus syndrome*.

Thoracic outlet syndrome was attributed to spasm and shortening of the anterior scalene muscle. TOS was considered to develop as a result of a contraction, fibrosis or hypertrophy of the anterior scalene muscle.

Another chief of neurological services at the Mayo Clinic named Adson (Adson and Coffey 1927) started to surgically remove the anterior scalene muscle in patients diagnosed with a cervical rib. He said the compression originated superiorly and compressed the neurovascular structures against the bony structure below and he felt that this operation was safer than resection of the cervical rib.

We use our scalene muscles all the time so it is easy for them to become tight; if we are a bit anxious we end up breathing from our upper chest instead of using the diaphragm. I talked about posture earlier in this text. If one has developed a forward head posture with rounded shoulders then the thoracic outlet can become compromised with subsequent trigger points forming within the shortened scalene muscles.

Costoclavicular compression syndrome and TOS

The position of the clavicle is parallel to the position of the first rib and the space formed between these two bony structures will be limited. One relatively quick way to test if the clavicle is compressing the underlying rib is through adopting a military, or 'policeman on parade', posture: shoulders back and down with chest out and both arms extended (this stretches the neurovascular bundle) (figure 12.28). The therapist can also palpate the radial pulse at the same time if they wish. If this military position exacerbates the patient's symptoms by compressing the neurovascular bundle then one can ascertain the clavicle is compressing against the first rib. However, on the odd occasion the pectoralis minor can also be involved in the compression. If a patient has had a previous clavicle fracture and it has been allowed to heal conservatively rather than being surgically repaired, then the extra bone callous that forms might be one reason why the patient is experiencing TOS symptoms.

In 1998, Plewa and Delinger mentioned that positive test results can be seen as being on a continuum: loss of pulse is the least specific finding (and the most likely to be positive even in asymptomatic subjects), followed by production of paresthesia, followed by the most specific finding, which is pain production in the upper extremity.

Hyperabduction and TOS

The movement of shoulder abduction with end range flexion (figure 12.29) can be very relevant to TOS because this position might be where the patient needs to place their arm on a daily or regular basis because of their work and it might well be this continual end range position that is compromising the neurovascular bundle.

Think about an electrician working on a building site all day every day. He is responsible for placing and wiring all of the ceiling lights in every room, in every house, and this means his arms will be placed above his head for many hours a day on a regular basis. Even though this shoulder position causes the patient's symptoms, we can use this to our advantage as a way of an assessment to decide if the TOS symptoms are exacerbated by the position of hyperabduction.

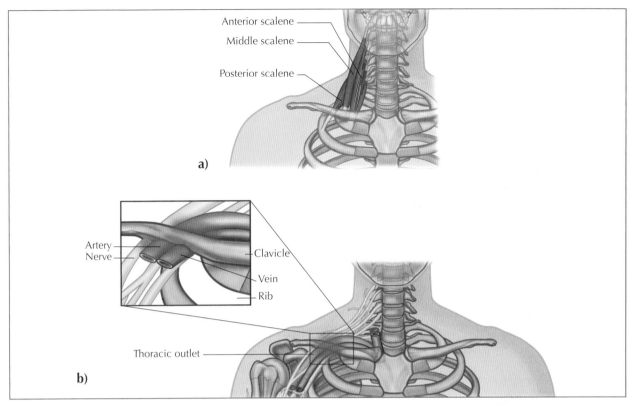

Figure 12.27a & b: *a) Scalene anticus syndrome; b) Costoclavicular compression syndrome*

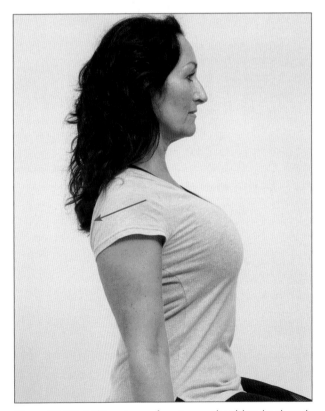

Figure 12.28: *Military type of posture – shoulders back and down, with chest out*

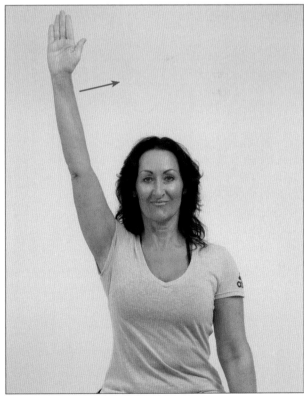

Figure 12.29: *Abduction with end range flexion can compromise the neurovascular bundle*

In this position the clavicle can approximate the first rib and it is considered that the pectoralis minor is also involved in this position due to the neurovascular structures passing directly underneath this muscle and the underlying ribs. The position causes these structures to compress.

Test procedure

The patient is sitting and the therapist palpates the wrist while they are holding the patient's arm in the hyperabduction position (figure 12.30). The therapist asks the patient to let them know if they feel any symptoms, and the pulse is also monitored for any changes. This position is typically held, while the pulse is monitored, for at least 30 seconds.

When the arms become abducted, the pectoralis minor tendon is stretched and may compress the axillary artery (continuation from the subclavian artery), reducing the strength of the radial pulse and potentially reproducing the presenting symptoms. Malanga et al. (2006) suggest that this test can close down the costoclavicular space, compressing the neurovascular bundle.

Novak et al. (1996) suggested that the test could be enhanced with directing downward pressure on the brachial plexus by digitally pressing just above the clavicle between the scalene muscles (figure 12.31).

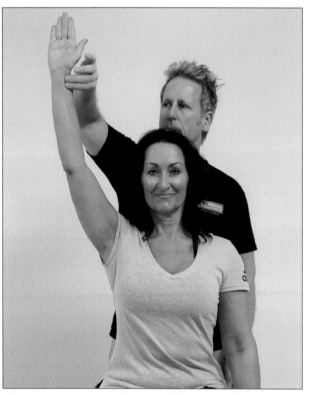

Figure 12.30: *Hyperabduction position of the patient, while the therapist palpates the radial pulse*

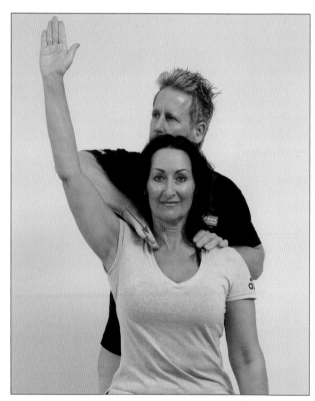

Figure 12.31: *Pressure applied downward to the brachial plexus*

13

Assessment of the shoulder complex

The general consensus (with which I agree) is that the majority of patients presenting with shoulder complaints are suffering from shoulder impingement syndromes of the rotator cuff and the subacromial bursa (SAB), and this accounts for anywhere between 50% and 60% of these complaints, if not more.

Shoulder impingement was first described by Neer (1972) and has been classified into two types: structural and functional. Subacromial impingement can be caused by narrowing of the subacromial space (SAS) due to bony growth or soft tissue inflammation (structural) or superior migration of the humeral head caused by weakness and/or muscle imbalance (functional), as described by Brossman et al. (1996) and Ludewig and Cook (2002). It is possible that some subacromial impingement results from a combination of both structural and functional factors.

The natural space formed within the SAS is approximately 9–10 mm or 1 cm. This space has been shown to be greater in men than in women. If the subacromial space is less than 5–6 mm it is considered pathological. Subacromial impingement happens when the structures located within the subacromial space and the coracoacromial ligament get compressed. The structures in question are the rotator cuff, long head of biceps and the subacromial bursa, the most common tissue of concern being the rotator cuff muscle group and in particular the supraspinatus. This is mainly due to the fact that the supraspinatus gets caught underneath the acromion, especially when the shoulder is abducted to approximately 90 degrees and internally rotated to 45 degrees.

Page et al. (2010) mentioned in the literature that Dr Janda suggested subacromial impingement results from a characteristic pattern of muscle imbalance, including weakness of the lower and middle trapezius, serratus anterior, infraspinatus and deltoid, coupled with tightness of the upper trapezius, pectorals and levator scapulae. This particular pattern is often referred to as part of Janda's upper crossed syndrome.

It has been clinically proven using MR imaging that the subacromial space is reduced with patients with impingement syndrome on the symptomatic side during abduction, compared to the asymptomatic (non painful) side.

From a functional perspective, we know that the shoulder complex utilizes muscles to provide the necessary dynamic stability and that this is a requirement to perform continual overhead movements, such as throwing a cricket ball. However, if this function is impaired in any way through muscle imbalances, structural damage may result.

The assessment procedure I will present in this chapter is very similar to the examination protocol that I follow with my own patients at my clinic in Oxford; however, you are not expected to initially follow every single process, especially during the first consultation. It could take a lot of time for you to gather all the information from the individual tests; moreover, once that has been done, you would need to assimilate all that necessary information in order to come up with a plan of action.

I am sure that there are numerous therapists out there who can help patients with only one session, and I believe that is the same for me. That said, I believe that it takes a few physical therapy sessions to truly have a good understanding of the patient's individual musculoskeletal biomechanical framework. That is why I might not include all the tests I demonstrate in this chapter during my initial consultation, as some of the specific testing criteria might be more relevant in the second, or even third or fourth follow-on session.

I hope that you will use this text, and specifically this chapter, time and time again as a reference point, especially when you first meet a patient that presents with shoulder and cervical spine pathology. I would love to think that this book over time would assist you greatly in trying to understand this fascinating area of the shoulder complex as well as helping you to reduce any presenting pain pathologies that your patients and athletes might present with.

■ Assessment procedure: part 1

The following assessment criteria will be covered in this section:

- Standing balance
- Active range of motion (AROM)
- Passive range of motion (PROM)
- Resisted/strength testing.

Table 13.1 is replicated in the Appendix and will be useful for noting down the relevant positional landmarks for your patient in the standing position. Similarly, all the tables in this chapter can be used to record the clinical findings for any type of shoulder or cervical complex dysfunction that exists.

Standing balance test

With the patient standing, the comparative levels of the landmarks listed in Table 13.1 are noted.

Table 13.1: Anatomical landmarks checklist

Landmarks	Left side	Right side
Pelvic crest (posterior view)		
Posterior superior iliac spine (PSIS)		
Greater trochanter		
Gluteal and popliteal folds		
Leg, foot, and ankle position (anterior/posterior view)		
Lumbar and thoracic spine		
Inferior angle of scapula (T7)		
Medial border of scapula		
Superior angle of scapula		
Position of acromion (levels)		
Position of cervical spine		
Pelvic crest (anterior view)		
Anterior superior iliac spine (ASIS)		
Sternoclavicular joint		
Acromioclavicular joint		
Glenohumeral position		

Posterior view

The patient is asked to stand with their weight equally distributed on both legs. The therapist sits or kneels behind the patient and places their hands on the top of the iliac crest to ascertain the level (figure 13.1).

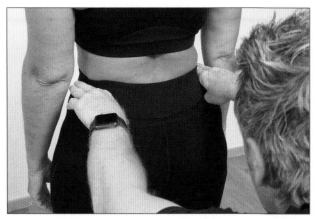

Figure 13.1: *Pelvic balance test: posterior view of the pelvic crest – hand position for ascertaining the level*

Before we look at the area of the shoulder and cervical complex, we need to ascertain the position of the pelvis. Why is this necessary? Because, as often I mention, this area (the pelvis) is the structural foundation of the body and everything else is built on this structure. If the foundation is not level then everything else will be in a state of compensation, and the fact that the pelvis is not balanced correctly could be a reason why the patient has shoulder and neck pain.

For example, in standing, it is very common to find the right iliac crest of the pelvis slightly higher, especially if there is a presentation of a right-sided anterior rotation (the most common finding) or an iliosacral upslip. (These pelvic dysfunctions will not be discussed in this book and the reader is directed to John Gibbons, *Functional Anatomy of the Pelvis and Sacroiliac Joint*). Be careful, though – the right side innominate could actually appear lower in standing even though the innominate is still in an anterior rotation: this could be because of an overpronation of the subtalar joint (STJ) of the ankle and foot. In the lying prone positions, on the other hand, the iliac crest might actually be higher on the right side that is fixed in an anteriorly rotated position, because of the effect on the pelvis of the shortened right quadratus lumborum – in other words; it might not be as straightforward as you initially think.

If one does find the iliac crests are not level then this needs to written down in the patient's notes and it will probably require further investigation at some point, especially if the presenting symptoms are not reducing, particularly in the region of the shoulder complex.

Next, the therapist places the pads of their thumbs under the PSIS and compares the levels (figure 13.2).

From the PSIS the therapist places their hands (fingertips) on top of the greater trochanters, again to determine the height (figure 13.3).

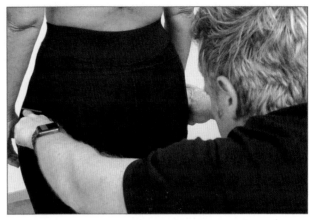

Figure 13.3: *Hand position for ascertaining the height of the greater trochanter*

The therapist observes the position of the shoulders, scapula, thoracic spine, lumbar spine, gluteal and popliteal (knee) folds for asymmetry, then observes the relative position of the leg, foot, and ankle (figure 13.4), looking in particular for an external rotation of the lower leg, and also observes the position of the foot and looks for overpronation (pes planus), supination (pes cavus) or a neutral position (pes rectus).

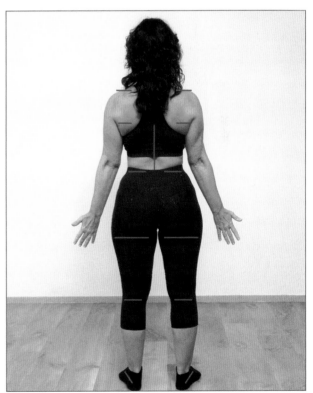

Figure 13.4 *Observation of the anatomical landmarks that are highlighted in red*

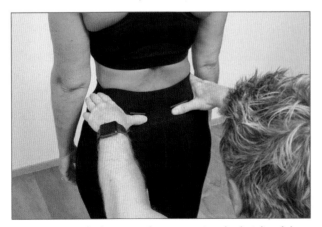

Figure 13.2: *Hand position for comparing the height of the PSIS on the left and right sides*

Anterior view

The patient is asked to stand with their weight equally distributed on both legs. The therapist sits or kneels in front of the patient and places their hands on the top of the iliac crest to ascertain the level (figure 13.5).

The therapist then places the pads of their thumbs under the ASIS and compares the levels (figure 13.6)

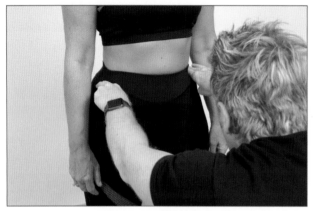

Figure 13.5: *Anterior view of the pelvic crest – hand position for ascertaining the level*

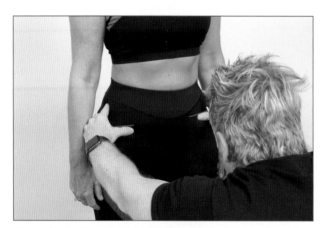

Figure 13.6: *Hand position for comparing the height of the ASIS on the left and right sides*

The therapist observes the position of the shoulders, the sternoclavicular (SCJ) and acromioclavicular (ACJ) joints, the relative position of the cervical spine, and then observes the anterior position of the leg, foot and ankle (figure 13.7).

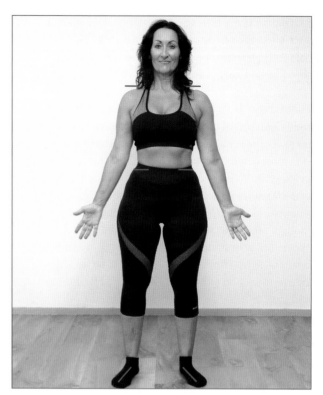

Figure 13.7: *Observation of the anatomical landmarks highlighted in red*

■ Active range of motion (AROM)

We now ask the patient to perform functional range of motion tests that include the glenohumeral joint (Table 13.2), scapula thoracic articulation and the cervical spine.

Table 13.2: Normal range of motion for the glenohumeral joint

Glenohumeral joint	Left side in degrees	Right side in degrees
Flexion	180	180
Extension	60	60
Abduction	180	180
Adduction	45	45
Internal rotation	70	70
External rotation	90	90
Horizontal flexion (adduction)	130	130
Horizontal extension (abduction)	50	50

1. Glenohumeral motion

a. Flexion – normal range 180 degrees

Ask the patient to lift both arms forward as far as possible. Look for the range of motion and compare left and right shoulder movements (figure 13.8).

Note: End range of shoulder flexion is controlled by thoracic extension; for example, if you have a patient who has a slight kyphosis of the thoracic spine (flexion deformity) then you will notice the motion of end range of flexion will be limited because the thoracic spine is unable to extend fully. This can place extra pressure on the shoulder joint and eventually cause pain. If this is the case then the thoracic kyphosis will need addressing.

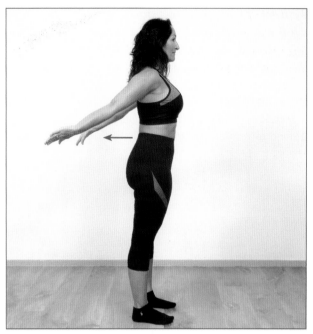

Figure 13.9: *Active extension*

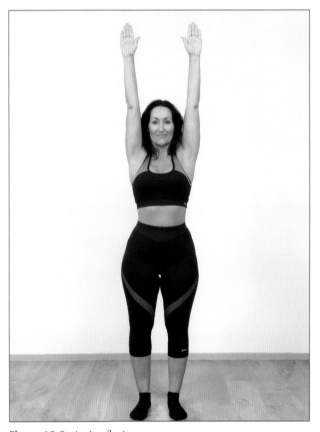

Figure 13.8: *Active flexion*

b. Extension – normal range 60 degrees

From the position of full flexion ask the patient to go as far as possible into extension (figure 13.9).

c. Abduction – normal range 180 degrees

Ask the patient to place their arms by their side and with the thumbs facing towards the ceiling; ask them to abduct their arms as far as possible and can they touch the thumbs (figure 13.10). Look for the range of motion and compare left and right shoulder movements.

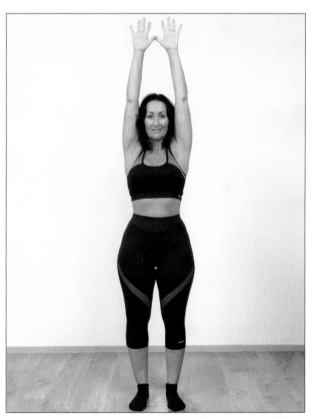

Figure 13.10: *Active abduction and thumbs to touch at end range*

d. Adduction – normal range 45 degrees

Ask the patient to place their arms in front of their body and to adduct their arms as far as possible, as shown by arrows in figure 13.11.

e. Internal (medial) rotation – normal range 70 degrees

Ask the patient to stand against a wall and to place their shoulders into an abducted position and also their elbows flexed at 90 degrees to the wall (figure 13.12).

The patient is then asked to internally rotate their arms as far as possible; 70 degrees would be the normal range (figure 13.13).

If they have less than 70 degrees (figure 13.14), then this is called a GIRD (glenohumeral internal rotation dysfunction).

Alternative position for internal rotation: the patient is standing and places the back of their hands onto their lower back; the patient is asked to push away as this motion induces internal rotation (figure 13.15).

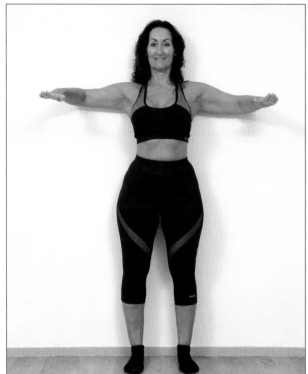

Figure 13.12: *Patient places their arms against a wall*

Alternative position: the patient is standing and places their elbows by their hip and is asked to actively externally rotate the shoulder; a range of 90 degrees is normal (figure 13.17).

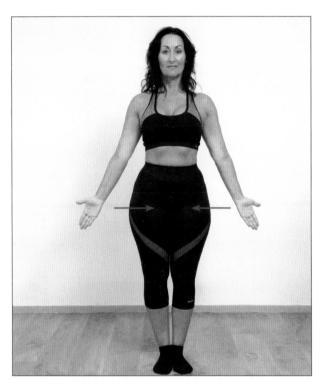

Figure 13.11: *Active adduction*

f. External (lateral) rotation – normal range 90 degrees

The patient is asked to adopt the same position as in figure 13.12 and now is instructed to externally rotate the shoulder as far as comfortable; a range of 90 degrees (as in figure 13.16) is classified as normal. Any restriction less than 90 degrees is to be noted down.

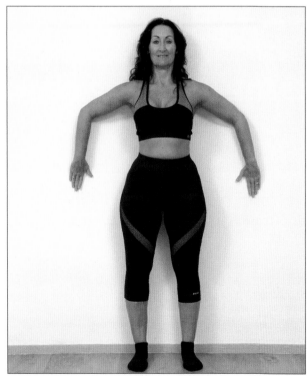

Figure 13.13: *Normal range of 70 degrees for internal rotation*

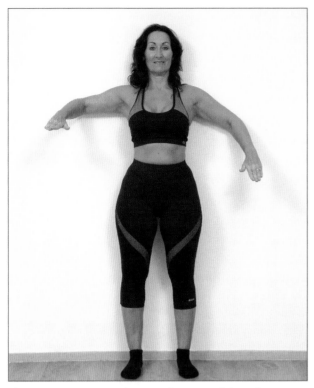

Figure 13.14: *Restricted range of motion of the right shoulder for internal rotation (GIRD)*

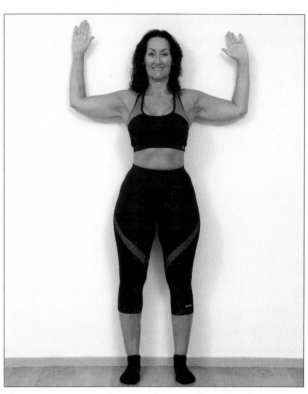

Figure 13.16: *Normal range of motion for external rotation of 90 degrees*

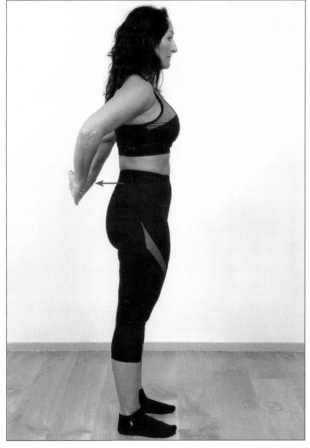

Figure 13.15: *Normal range of motion for internal rotation*

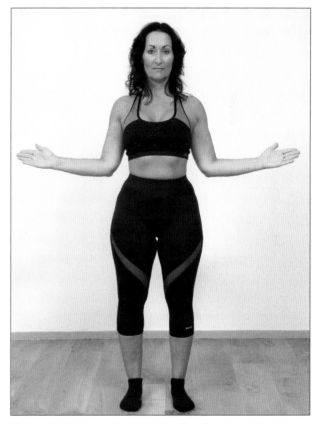

Figure 13.17: *Normal range of motion for external rotation*

g. Horizontal flexion/adduction – normal range 130 degrees

The patient is now asked to abduct their arms to 90 degrees (figure 13.18) and then to horizontally flex or adduct the shoulder as far as possible; a range of 130 degrees is classified as normal (figure 13.19).

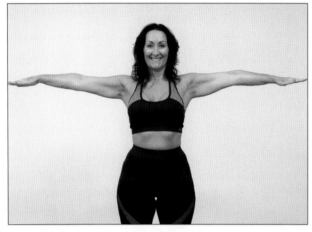

Figure 13.18: *Shoulder abducted to 90 degrees*

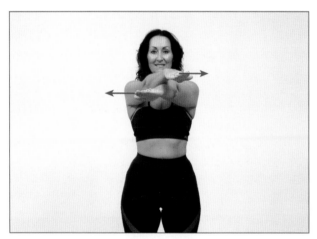

Figure 13.19: *Normal range of motion for horizontal flexion*

h. Horizontal extension/abduction-normal range 50 degrees

From the position of figure 13.18, the patient is asked to horizontally extend or abduct their shoulder as far as comfortable; a range of 50 degrees is classified as normal (figure 13.20).

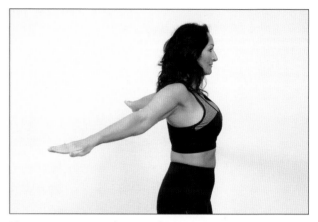

Figure 13.20: *Normal range of motion for horizontal extension*

2. Scapula motion

The patient is asked to perform the following four scapula motions (shown in figures 13.21 to 13.24): elevation, depression, protraction (scapula abduction) and retraction (scapula adduction).

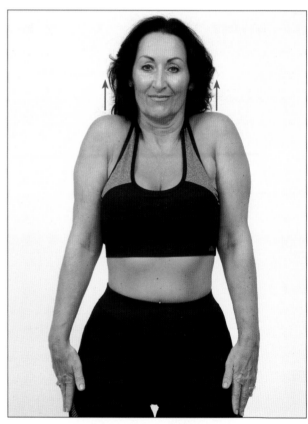

Figure 13.21: *Elevation of the scapula*

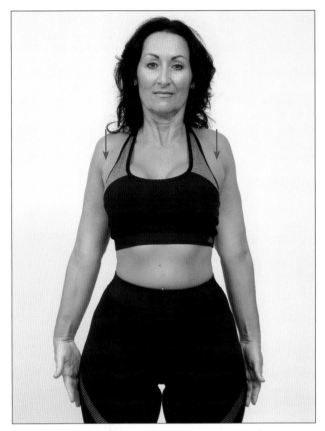

Figure 13.22: *Depression of the scapula*

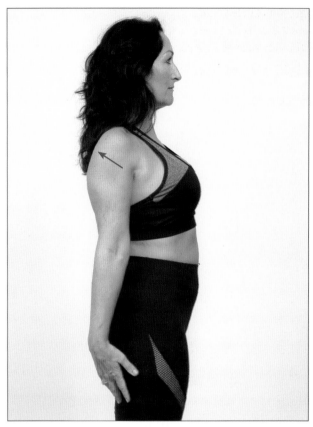

Figure 13.24: *Retraction of the scapula*

3. Cervical spine motion (Table 13.3)

The patient is asked to perform the following motions of the cervical spine (shown in figures 13.25–13.27).

The patient is asked to rotate to the right, then to the left (figure 13.25).

Next the patient is asked to flex and to extend (figure 13.26).

Finally, the patient is asked to side bend to the right and then to the left side (figure 13.27).

Table 13.3: Normal active range of motion (AROM) for the cervical spine

Cervical spine	Degrees
Rotation (left and right)	80
Flexion	50
Extension	60
Lateral flexion (left and right)	45

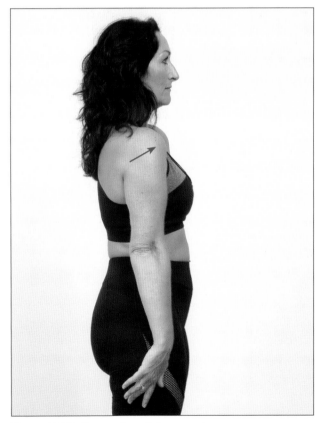

Figure 13.23: *Protraction of the scapula*

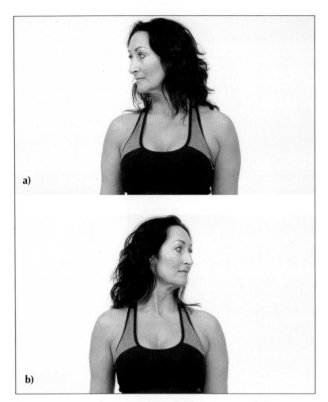

Figure 13.25a & b: *a: Rotation right; b: rotation left*

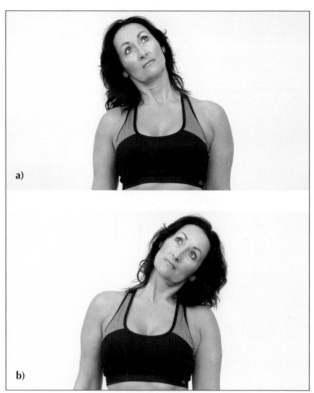

Figure 13.27a & b: *a: Lateral flexion right; b: lateral flexion left*

■ Passive range of motion (PROM)

These passive ROM tests are simply used as guidelines in screening for any underlying pathology that might be associated with the shoulder joint as well as cervical spine. The tests I will be demonstrating for these areas are taken from my own experiences of treating thousands of patients, so much so that I have included some of my own thoughts on the way one might apply some of the tests. There are numerous other tests that can be used to screen the shoulder joint and some of these will be covered later in this chapter under *special tests*, but that will be the choice of the therapist at that time in their own clinic with their own patients; as I have said already, the tests I am demonstrating here have been selected on the basis of my own personal experience and preferences.

The specific *passive* ROM tests given in this chapter for screening the shoulder and cervical spine for pathology are used in particular for identifying the awareness one would feel through one's hands at the end range of the

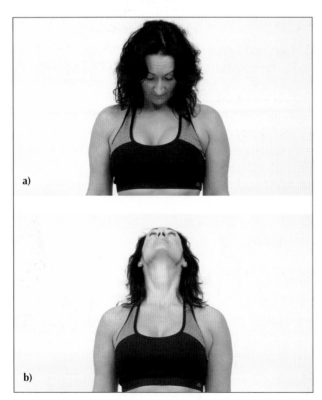

Figure 13.26a & b: *a: Flexion; b: extension*

joint that is being tested; this technique is called the *joint end feel*. The end feel of a joint is basically the quality of movement that is perceived by the therapist at the very end of the available ROM. The joint end feel can reveal a great deal about the nature of various pathologies located within the joint that is being tested.

There are four common classifications of what is considered to be a 'normal' joint end feel (or joint end range) and which are typically present within any synovial joint:

- soft end feel, e.g., elbow flexion
- hard end feel, e.g., knee extension
- muscular end feel, e.g., hip flexion (hamstrings)
- capsular end feel, e.g., external rotation of the shoulder joint.

When you are assessing your patients/athletes, and especially when you are performing the passive ROM tests, you may experience (through your hands) a different type of joint end feel to what has already been described as a 'normal' end feel. In this case you can assume that there is what is called a *pathological end feel* present within the architecture of the joint; this positive test should be noted down, and further investigation, or even a referral to a specialist, might subsequently be necessary.

Please remember that patients have two arms and one should perform a comparison between the two, just to make sure that an actual pathology is indeed present. For example, if you passively take the patient's *left* shoulder into full abduction, with a range of at least 170–180 degrees being achieved with no pain or stiffness, and your patient is comfortable at the end of the available range, then one can assume that this movement is normal and no pathology is present. Suppose, on the other hand, only around 60–70 degrees of abduction or less can be achieved when the same movement (abduction) is performed passively on the *right* shoulder, and the end range of the joint also becomes particularly painful and/or feels restrictive to your patient (especially in the deltoid insertion area). From these findings, you can safely say that the ROM of the right shoulder is not normal; moreover, because of the restrictive/painful barrier, the end feel would be classified as *pathological*, meaning that the test is positive and further investigation is required.

I will include only some of the passive testing pictures below for the shoulder and cervical spine rather than every single one because a lot of the passive motions have already been covered in other chapters. For example, the MET chapter on the assessment of the rotator cuff was when I tested the length of the infraspinatus muscle, I passively guided the shoulder into full internal rotation and looked for 70 degrees and the same for the subscapularis as I passively took the shoulder into external rotation and was looking for 90 degrees of motion; these ranges would be classified as normal ROM.

Some of the following passive testing can be done while your patient is standing, seated or lying, so the choice can be yours. The option of lying is sometimes easier as the patient often feels more relaxed as compared to sitting or standing.

Passive ROM
a. *Shoulder abduction*
b. *Flexion*
c. *Extension*
d. *External rotation*

The therapist takes control of the patient's arm with their right hand and palpates the shoulder joint with their left hand and slowly abducts the right shoulder as far as comfortable (figure 13.28a). A normal joint range of 180 degrees should be achieved. Next the therapist brings the patient's arm back to the side and then passively flexes their shoulder to full range of flexion and 180 degrees is classified as normal (figure 13.28b). From here the therapist takes the arm into full extension and 60 degrees is classified as normal (figure 13.28c) and figure 13.28d shows the arm taken into an externally rotated position.

Passive ROM
a&b. *Cervical spine – rotation*
c&d. *Cervical spine – lateral flexion*

The patient is supine and the therapist takes control of the patient's cervical spine with both their hands and places them over the ears (open fingers). The therapist then gently rotates the patient's neck to the left and then to the right and a range of 80 degrees is normal (figure 13.29a&b).

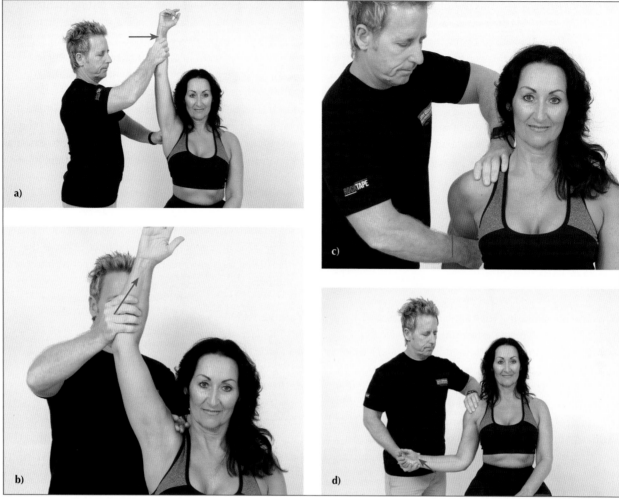

Figure 13.28a–d: *Passive ROM tests: a: The right shoulder is abducted to 180 degrees; b: flexion to 180 degrees; c: extension to 60 degrees; d: external rotation to 90 degrees*

Next the therapist brings the patient's cervical spine into left and right lateral flexion (figure 13.29c & d) and a normal range of 45 degrees is seen.

■ Resisted testing

When one is testing the integrity of the muscular and tendinous components of the body then a resisted testing procedure is generally the rule of thumb because if, for example, a patient has torn or strained a muscle or tendon then one would expect the pain or discomfort to naturally increase or the patient will be more aware of the injury on activation of these contractile soft tissues and yes, of course, that is and should be the case.

The only problem I envisage is the way the physical therapist performs the resisted testing maneuvers, because one therapist will perform their resisted tests in a particular way and notes that their patient has strained the rectus femoris muscle, while another therapist might say the opposite by saying they have not strained the muscle. This might be because they conducted completely different resisted tests or because of the way they performed the test; perhaps the patient felt no pain, even though a muscle still might have been strained. Let me explain, we have lots of choices in our toolbox of using *resisted tests* and some of these methods of testing are from the following; we have an *isometric* way of resisted testing (patient is static so no motion) or/and an *isotonic concentric* way of resisting (shortening of the tissue, while still contracting) and finally an *isotonic eccentric* (lengthening of the tissue, while it is still in a state of contraction). We can even place

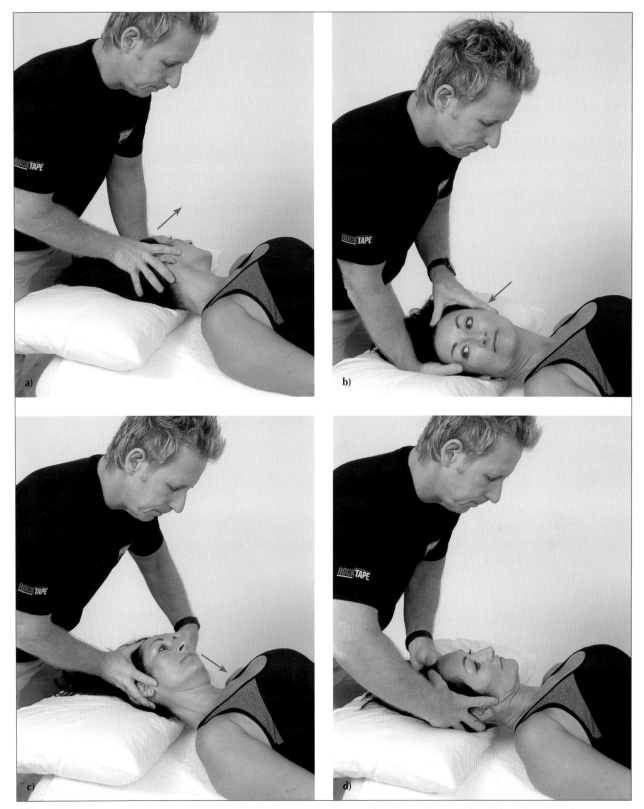

Figure 13.29a–d: *Passive ROM test for cervical: a: The therapist rotates the cervical spine left and b: right to 80 degrees; c: the therapist takes the cervical spine into lateral flexion to 45 degrees to the left and d: to the right)*

the contractile tissue being tested in various functional motions or we can alter the joint position, like inner or outer range (tissue is positioned and tested in a shortened or lengthened position); we can even rotate the joints, like the hip to specify the lateral or the medial hamstrings, and so it goes on. The simple explanation for this change of position is because the patient might have torn their hamstring while rotating their leg, so does it not makes sense to test the contractile tissues in various positions. Unfortunately, it is not in the scope of this book to go through every single variation and I just wanted to make you aware of some of the choices you have when testing the contractile tissue.

Resisted tests for the GH joint

a. *Shoulder abduction – supraspinatus and deltoid muscle*
b. *Flexion – anterior deltoid, pectoralis major (clavicular) and biceps brachii*
c. *Extension – latissimus dorsi, teres major, pectoralis major (sternal), triceps long head*

d. *Adduction – latissimus dorsi, teres major, subscapularis, pectoralis major (sternal), triceps long head*
e. *Internal rotation – subscapularis, latissmus dorsi, anterior deltoid, teres major and pectoralis major*
f. *External rotation – infraspinatus, teres minor and posterior deltoid*
g. *Horizontal flexion – pectoralis major and anterior deltoid*
h. *Horizontal extension – infraspinatus, teres minor and posterior deltoid*

The therapist takes control of the patient's arm with their right hand and palpates the shoulder joint with their left hand and asks the patient to resist against a resistance being applied by the therapist to all the various positions shown in figures 13.30a to 13.30h. The patient is asked to say if they feel any pain during the tests.

Resisted tests for the shoulder girdle

a. *Shoulder girdle elevation – upper trapezius, levator scapulae and rhomboids*

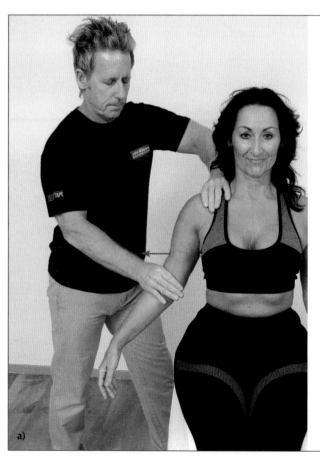
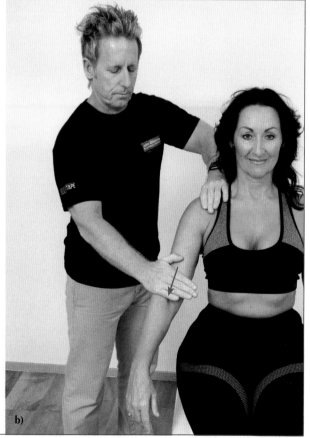

a)   b)

Figure 13.30a–h: *(Continued)*

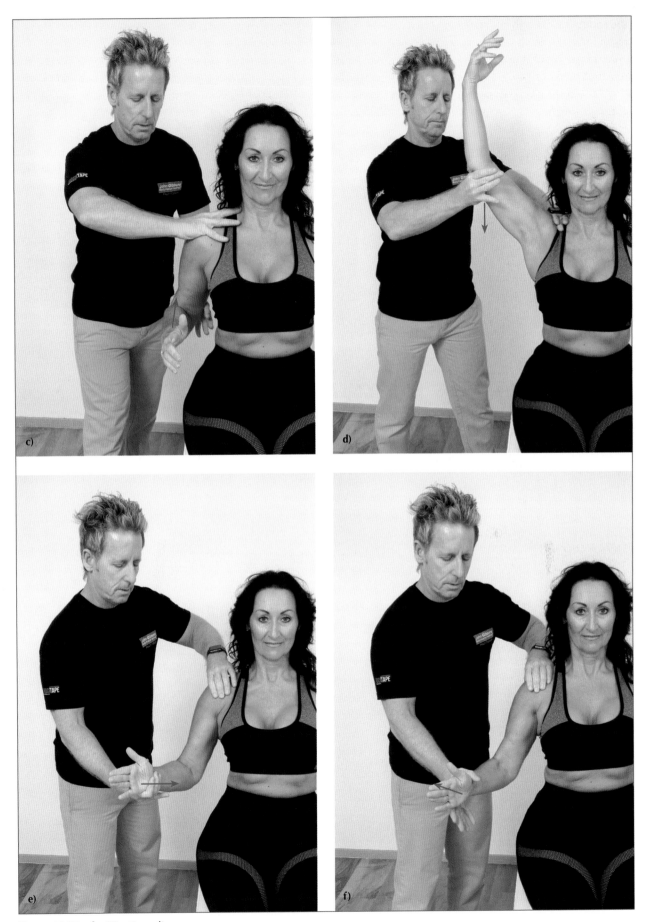

Figure 13.30a–h: *(Continued)*

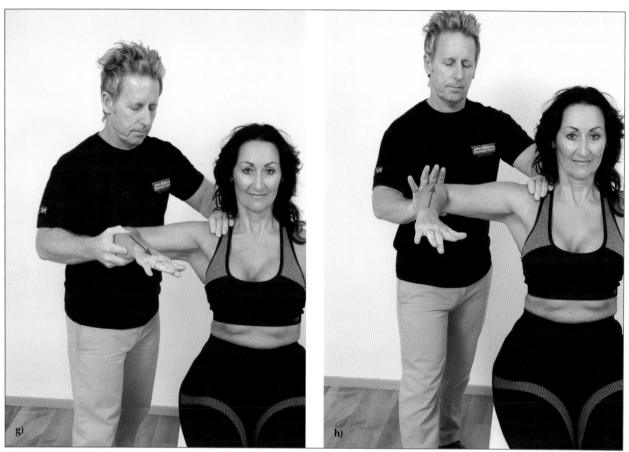

Figure 13.30a–h: *Resisted tests: a: Abduction; b: flexion; c: extension; d: adduction; e: internal rotation; f: external rotation; g: horizontal flexion; h: horizontal extension*

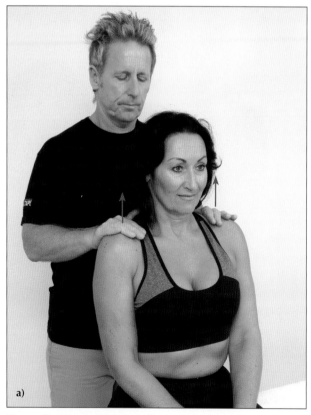

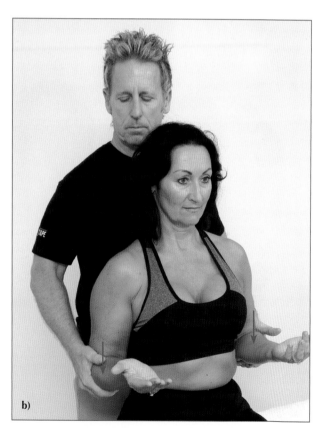

Figure 13.31a–d: *(Continued)*

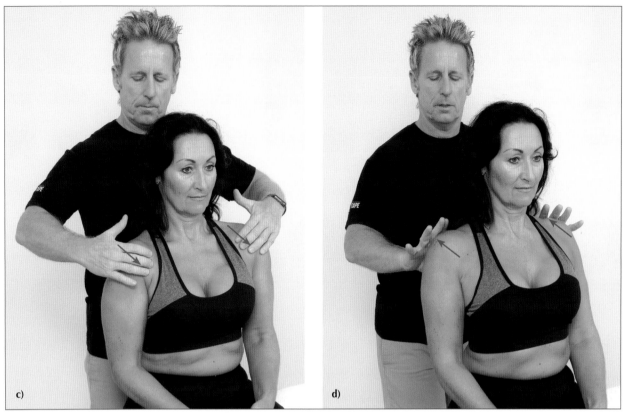

Figure 13.31a–d: *a: Shoulder girdle elevation; b: depression; c: protraction; d: retraction*

b. *Shoulder girdle depression – lower trapezius, pectoralis minor*
c. *Shoulder girdle protraction – serratus anterior and pectoralis minor*
d. *Shoulder girdle retraction – rhomboids and middle trapezius*

The therapist controls the patient's shoulder girdle with both their hands and asks the patient to resist against a resistance being applied by the therapist to all various positions of the shoulder girdle (figure 13.31a to figure 13.31d). The patient is asked to say if they feel any pain during the tests.

14

Special tests associated with the shoulder complex

There are an unbelievable number of special or orthopedic tests for the shoulder complex. In this chapter I list and describe some of the more popular ones used by physical therapists:

a. O'Brien active compression test
b. Neer sign
c. Hawkins–Kennedy test
d. Jobe's/Empty and full can test
e. Speed's test – SLAP lesion
f. Yergason's test
g. Gerber's lift-off test
h. Apley's scratch tests
i. Shrug and Prayer tests

■ a. O'Brien active compression test

O'Brien et al.'s (1998) active compression test was primarily developed for assessment of acromioclavicular joint (ACJ) pathology following a patient's demonstration of what reproduced their shoulder pain. The O'Brien test is also considered in certain patients to detect glenoid labral pathology, for example a SLAP lesion.

Procedure
The patient is asked to adopt a sitting or standing position and they are asked to flex their arm to 90 degrees with the elbow fully extended and from this position to then adduct (horizontally) the arm 10–15 degrees with full internal rotation (figure 14.1).

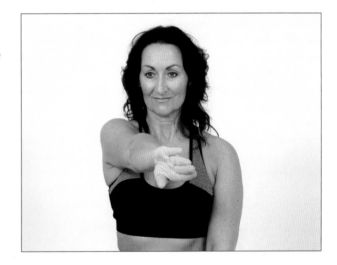

Figure 14.1: *Flexion to 90 degrees then 10–15 degrees of horizontal adduction and full internal rotation*

The therapist applies downward pressure towards the floor and the patient resists the applied pressure (figure 14.2).

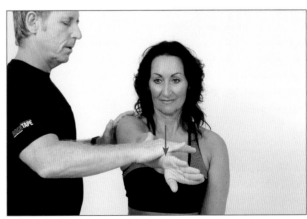

Figure 14.2: *Pressure applied by the therapist towards the floor, with the patient's arm in internal rotation*

The procedure is repeated in external rotation (figure 14.3).

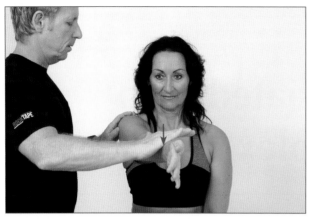

Figure 14.3: *Pressure applied by the therapist towards the floor, with the patient's arm in external rotation*

The O'Brien test is designed to maximally load and compress the ACJ and superior aspect of the glenoid labrum. For positive results the patient should have symptoms (pain or clicking, if labrum) on the internal rotation resisted test but no symptoms on the resisted external rotation test.

■ b. Neer impingement test or sign

Charles Neer in 1972 proposed that impingement was due to the anterior third of the acromion and the coracoacromial ligament and suggested surgery should be focused on these areas. The test was based on his findings during shoulder surgery and he considered that the critical area for degenerative tendonitis and tendon ruptures was focused on the supraspinatus tendon and occasionally the infraspinatus and the long head of biceps. Elevation of the arm in external or internal rotation causes critical areas of the soft tissues to pass under the acromion or/and the coracoacromial ligament.

Procedure

The patient is asked to adopt a sitting or standing position and the therapist takes the patient's arm into internal rotation (figure 14.4a) with passive abduction in the scapular plane, while at the same time stabilizing the scapula (figure 14.4b). Any increase of symptoms during this maneuver is classified as positive for an impingement syndrome.

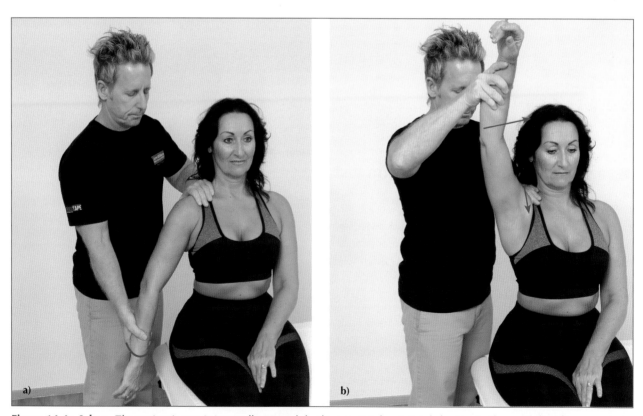

Figure 14.4a & b: *a: The patient's arm is internally rotated; b: the arm is taken into abduction in the scapular plane*

c. Hawkins–Kennedy impingement test

This test came about from the work of Hawkins and Kennedy (1980) and is used to interpret impingement syndrome between the greater tuberosity of the humeral head and the overhanging coracohumeral ligament.

Procedure

The patient is ask to adopt a sitting position and the therapist controls the patient's symptomatic arm and guides the motion of the upper limb to 90 degrees of flexion with their elbow flexed to 90 degrees (figure 14.5).

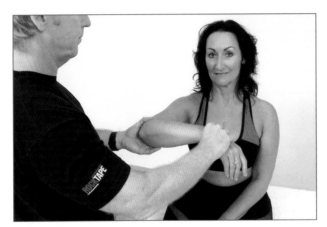

Figure 14.5: *The patient's arm at 90 degrees of shoulder flexion and 90 degrees of elbow flexion*

Next, the therapist stabilizes the elbow with their hand and with the other holds the patient's wrist. The therapist then guides the arm into internal rotation (figure 14.6) and the patient is asked to say if the movement exacerbates their symptoms.

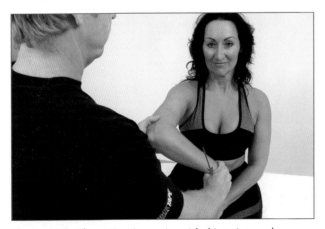

Figure 14.6: *The patient's arm is guided into internal rotation*

d. Jobe's empty can (EC) test

Jobe and Moynes (1982) reported that the function of the supraspinatus muscle can be isolated and then assessed to some degree with the shoulder near 90 degrees of elevation (abduction), 20 degrees of horizontal adduction, and full internal rotation, a position they named the empty can (EC) test. It is also very common to assess isometric strength in this position and is commonly referred to as the supraspinatus test. Holtby and Razmjou (2004) found the sensitivity of the supraspinatus test to be high (88%) for large to massive tears but lower for less severe injuries to the tendon; specificity was less (70% or less) for any injury to the supraspinatus tendon.

Procedure

The patient is asked to externally rotate their shoulder and to abduct their arm to 90 degrees with their thumb facing towards the ceiling and horizontally adduct 20–30 degrees (figure 14.7). From this position the patient is to imagine holding a can of water or beer and is then asked to empty the can (figure 14.8). If the patient perceives pain during this motion then the supraspinatus is suspected.

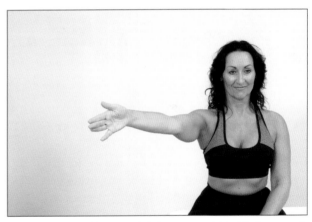

Figure 14.7: *90 degrees of abduction and 20–30 degrees of horizontal adduction*

Empty can (EC) with overpressure

The same test can be performed by overpressure, as this ascertains an isometric contraction and is considered more specific for isolating the supraspinatus tendon. From the test position above, the therapist applies pressure towards the floor and the patient resists this motion (figure 14.9); if pain is perceived then the supraspinatus is involved.

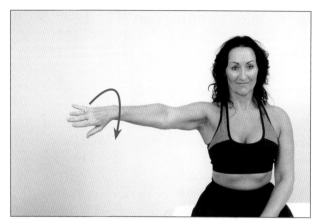

Figure 14.8: *Emptying the can*

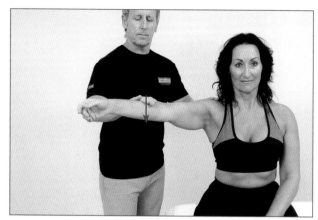

Figure 14.10: *Full can (FC) test with arm at 90 degrees*

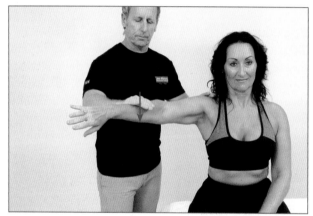

Figure 14.9: *Emptying the can with overpressure applied by the therapist*

■ Alternative: full can (FC) test

Kelly et al. (1996) proposed a resistance test for assessment of the function of the supraspinatus muscle and tendon with the shoulder below 90 degrees of abduction, also in the plane of the scapula, and 45 degrees of external rotation. The called this the full can test (FC) (figure 14.10). They suggested the empty can (EC) position caused subacromial impingement of the shoulder at 90 degrees of abduction and suggested the full can (FC) position was less irritating to the supraspinatus as it passes within the subacromial area.

Yasojima et al. (2008) reported EMG activity of the supraspinatus was significantly greater than those of the infraspinatus or teres minor muscles in the FC position at 45–60 degrees of abduction in the scapular plane when loaded with a set resistance and this 45–60 degree position was considered a better position to reduce impingement and compensatory motions.

■ e. Speed's test

SLAP (superior labrum anterior posterior) lesions are probably more common than one thinks and to diagnose this without the appropriate scans might be difficult. The Speed's test in my opinion works well; however, my modified version seems to work better to isolate this area.

Procedure

The patient is asked to externally rotate the humerus and to apply an isometric resistance against the therapist (figure 14.11). The patient is then asked to concentrically contract and overcome the resistance applied by the therapist (figure 14.12).

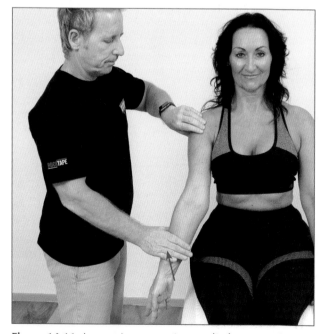

Figure 14.11: *Isometric contraction applied – no motion*

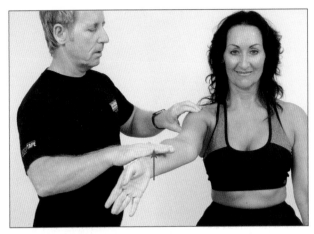

Figure 14.12: *Concentric contraction – the muscle is allowed to shorten against a resistance*

Modified version

With the patient's arm at 90 degrees of flexion and external rotation, the patient is asked to resist the pressure applied from the therapist; however, the therapist WILL overcome the resistance from the patient so it now becomes a modified eccentric contraction (figure 14.13). This maneuver, as compared to the other two, confirms a SLAP lesion, especially if the patient complains of pain deep within the shoulder joint.

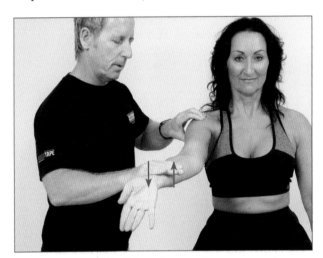

Figure 14.13: *Modified Speed's test using an eccentric contraction – the patient contracts concentrically and the therapist overcomes the resistance eccentrically*

■ f. Yergason's test – bicipital instability/tendinopathy

If a patient has pain or clicking to the anterior aspect of the shoulder then the long head of the biceps tendon might be the involved tissue in the pathology; this could

also be from a SLAP lesion or if there is an audible 'click' on motion then the transverse humeral ligament might have been torn and be causing the biceps tendon to flick out of its natural groove (intertubercular sulcus or bicipital groove).

Procedure

The patient is asked to sit or stand and to place their elbow at 90 degrees and with the forearm pronated. The therapist palpates the bicipital grove with one hand and the other is applied to the distal forearm of the patient (figure 14.14a)

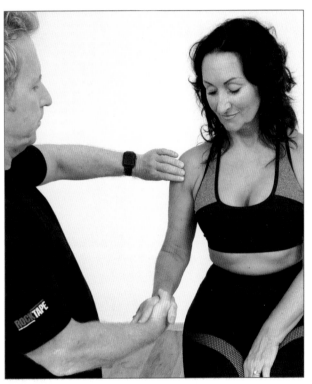

Figure 14.14a: *The patient's elbow at 90 degrees and pronated*

Next the patient is asked to supinate their forearm and at the same time to externally rotate their shoulder and flex the elbow as the therapist applies a resistance (figure 14.14b). With biceps tendonitis the patient will exhibit pain, snapping or both within the bicipital groove. Pain with no snapping might indicate bicipital tendinopathy; snapping only might indicate a tear or laxity of the transverse humeral ligament. Pain at the superior glenohumeral region indicates a SLAP lesion.

Gleason et al. (2006) found through MRI and dissection that the transverse humeral ligament (THL) might not actually exist and that the long head of the biceps tendon sits between the deep and superficial fibers of the subscapularis tendon. They found that when the biceps dislocates it is commonly found in conjunction with tears to the subscapularis.

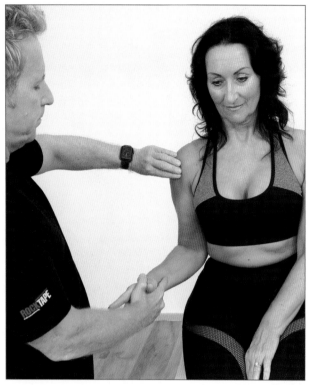

Figure 14.14b: *The patient is asked to supinate their forearm, externally rotate the shoulder and elbow flex against a resistance applied by the therapist*

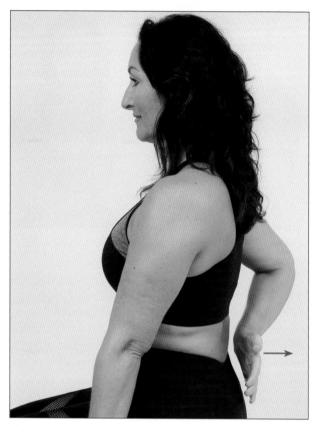

Figure 14.15: *The patient is asked to lift their arm off the lower back*

■ g. Gerber's lift-off test – subscapularis

Gerber and Krushell (1991) designed this test. The maneuver is considered to be an effective way to assess for the subscapularis muscle, especially full thickness tears.

Procedure

The patient is asked to fully internally rotate their arm and then to place the dorsum (back) of their hand onto their lower back and to 'lift' off their hand, away from the lumbar (figure 14.15). We can also apply a resistance to test the strength of the subscapularis (figure 14.16).

The ability to actively lift the dorsum of the hand off the back suggests a normal lift-off test. However, the inability to move the dorsum off the back is suggestive of an abnormal lift-off test and indicates a rupture of the subscapularis tendon.

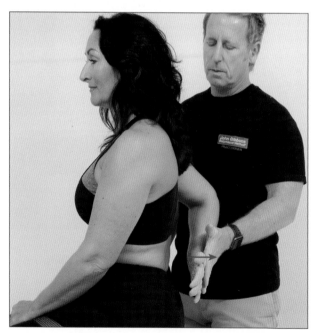

Figure 14.16: *The patient is asked to resist the motion; this induces a contraction for the subscapularis muscle*

■ h. Apley's scratch tests – mobility

We can specify the scratch tests into two separate motions:

1. adduction with internal rotation
2. abduction with external rotation.

These are simple mobility tests and basically test four motions for the glenohumeral joint.

Procedure

We ask the patient to internally rotate the humerus and then to adduct and to see how far up the thoracic spine they can touch (scratch) with a finger. The motion is then compared with the opposite side (figure 14.17).

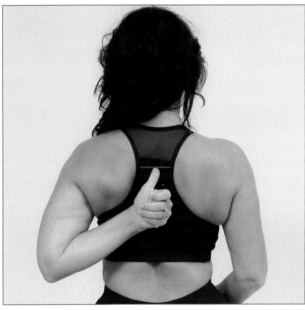

Figure 14.17: *Internal rotation with adduction*

Next, we ask the patient to externally rotate the humerus and then to abduct and to see how far down the thoracic spine they can touch (scratch) with a finger. The motion is then compared with the opposite side (figure 14.18).

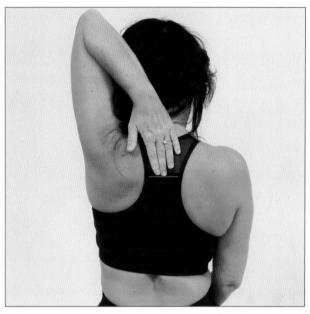

Figure 14.18: *External rotation with abduction*

■ i. Shrug and Prayer tests

These two tests are used to identify dysfunction within the sternoclavicular joint (SCJ).

Shrug test

The patient is supine and the therapist places their index finger on the superior aspect of both of the SC joints, located on the proximal end of the clavicle (figure 14.19a). The patient is then asked to shrug (elevate) their shoulder girdle; the proximal clavicle should be seen to inferiorly glide (figure 14.19b).

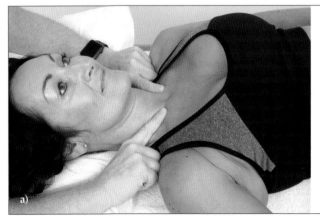
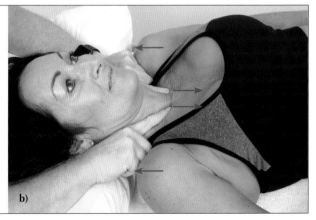

Figure 14.19a & b: *a: The therapist palpates the superior left and right proximal clavicle. b: The patient shrugs their shoulder girdle – an inferior glide of the proximal clavicle is normal*

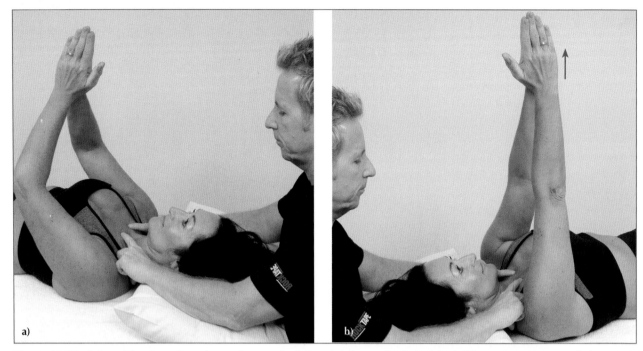

Figure 14.20a & b: *a: The therapist palpates the anterior left and right proximal clavicle. b: The patient protracts their shoulder girdle – a posterior glide of the clavicle is classified as normal*

Prayer test

The patient is supine and is asked to place their hands together in front of their body at 90 degrees. The therapist places their index finger on the anterior aspect of both of the SC joints, located on the proximal end of the clavicle (figure 14.20a) and the patient is asked to protract their shoulder girdle; the proximal clavicle should be seen to posteriorly glide (figure 14.20b).

Note: The treatment of the SC joint is shown in the next chapter under the treatment protocols. This joint is such an important *hinge* in relation to the mechanics of the shoulder complex and simply needs normal inferior and posteriorly gliding motions to allow normal function of the glenohumeral (GH) and scapulothoracic (ST) joints.

15

Treatment protocols for the shoulder complex

From a realistic perspective, what would you consider to be our main goal with the patient or athlete that presents with shoulder pain? My own goal is to try my utmost to reduce the patient's pain or discomfort and to improve their movement and functionality. Quite simple really! How we go about achieving that goal is a completely different story. Let me give you a quick example. Let us say for a moment that you are an actual patient with shoulder pain; this pain has been present for many months and you have now been referred from your local doctor to an orthopedic surgeon because the MRI showed a tear of the supraspinatus with some calcification and a reduced subacromial space. Let us be realistic about orthopedic shoulder surgeons – surgery is their main (often their only) option. I believe that the toolbox of possible techniques and treatment protocols available to the physical therapist is actually a lot more extensive than that of the surgeon. We might well need the assistance of the surgeon in the near future; however, a good starting point might be to first take out one or two tools at a time from your own personal therapy toolbox and see whether they work or not. If the tool you choose does not work then it is not a problem – you can simply place that tool back in the box and look for another tool, then another one, and so on until there is one that actually does work! Sounds feasible, would you not agree? Only after you have exhausted all of the tools in your bag would you consider referring to the surgeon.

I hope in this chapter to give you some ideas about how to decide which tools to choose. In an earlier chapter I discussed muscle energy techniques (METs) These unique techniques would be one of the tools you could use initially to assess and subsequently treat your patients with shoulder pain. Soft tissue techniques using a fascial wax as a medium, as described in a later chapter, is another set of tools one could use. There is a chapter on various types of taping techniques, using Kinesiology tape as well as athletic taping products such as zinc oxide; these would also be classified as treatment tools you could utilize. You can see therefore that this is not the only chapter on treatment protocols for the shoulder complex. What we are doing here is trying to decide what tools to use and when to use them to have the greatest effect on patients presenting with pain to the shoulder complex.

Remember the primary treatment goal, which is to reduce the patient's shoulder symptoms and improve their functionality. Naturally we need to address the underlying causative factor for their pain, and hopefully we can achieve some of our aims within the first few treatment sessions. I have a devised a strategy using what I call a *symptom-reducing protocol or SRP*. This set of tools can be applied to all areas of the body of patients who present with pain and not just to the region of the shoulder.

■ Symptom-reducing protocol (SRP)

Think about these words just for a minute: the focus of *any* treatment protocol is to reduce the painful symptoms that the patient is presenting with and as long as you achieve this to at least some degree or improve their functionality then it will be a win–win situation for everybody concerned.

The main treatment protocols are from the following techniques:

1. Alignment of the humerus
2. Alignment of the scapula
3. Soft tissue techniques (Chapter 16)
4. Specific taping techniques (Chapter 17)
5. Mobility for the thoracic spine (Chapter 18)
6. Strength activation with specific exercise (Chapter 18).

Lewis (2008) has a similar concept to myself, which he calls the *shoulder symptom modification procedure* (SSMP). He uses a series of four mechanical techniques, while the patient performs the movement that reproduces their symptoms. The techniques Lewis uses are: (1) a humeral head procedure; these techniques are applied to the humeral head through the use of manual pressure, mobilization belts, resistance tubing or neoprene slings; (2) changing the scapular position through manual therapy or taping techniques; (3 and 4) cervical and thoracic spine procedures through the use of manual therapy, as well as taping techniques focusing on the thoracic spine to see if the patient's symptoms reduce during movements. Lewis says a 30% change through the use of SSMP represents a substantial and meaningful change for patients.

Lewis is a true specialist when it comes to problematic shoulder dysfunction and the reader is encouraged to look through his research articles in the bibliography at the end of this book. Some of the following therapy techniques will overlap with Lewis's SSMP approach to the shoulder complex.

■ Alignment of the humerus into abduction

The following techniques are designed to reduce the patient's pain and improve mobility, especially when the patient actively abducts and flexes their shoulder.

Accessory inferior gliding technique

If we are looking at whether the shoulder can fully abduct and flex, it is easy to measure this specific motion (and all other joint motions of the body) by using a device called a goniometer. We can also simply use our eyes and say the joint motion has achieved 90 or 120 degrees. However, for these simple shoulder motions (abduction and flexion) to occur we need the assistance of what is called an *accessory* motion. Typical examples of accessory motions are those known as *spin*, *roll* and *glide*. In the particular case of

shoulder motion, we need to promote inferior *gliding* of the humeral head only by a few millimeters, as this small motion will allow the humerus to achieve full abduction and flexion. Figure 15.1 shows the humeral head gliding inferiorly down the glenoid fossa as the shoulder is abducted.

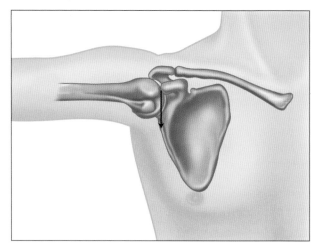

Figure 15.1: *Humerus inferiorly glides as the shoulder is abducted*

So just to recap, for a gross (large) range of motion (180 degrees) to occur, such as abduction, we only need a very small amount (mm) of inferior gliding to take place at exactly the same time to allow the natural motion of abduction. It is actually very difficult to measure this accessory gliding motion and if this fine-tuning motion of the accessory glide is not permitted for some reason, then you can probably guess the consequence, namely that an impingement type of syndrome will ensue.

Assess, treat and re-assess

This is a very simple concept because we ask our patient to perform a movement of abduction until they feel discomfort and we are able to measure the achieved range of motion. Next, we treat the patient's shoulder using the following techniques. After the treatment we re-test to see if the presenting pain has reduced and/or the motion has improved.

Technique 1
The patient is asked to adopt a side lying position on the couch and then asked to abduct their arm and to mention when it becomes painful. For this example let us say the shoulder pain is perceived around 80–90 degrees (figure 15.2).

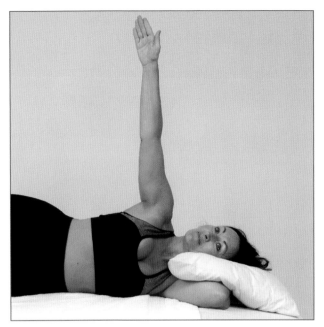

Figure 15.2: *The patient abducts their shoulder and perceives pain between 80 and 90 degrees*

The therapist controls the patient's arm and simultaneously initiates passive abduction, while applying traction and external rotation (figure 15.3a).

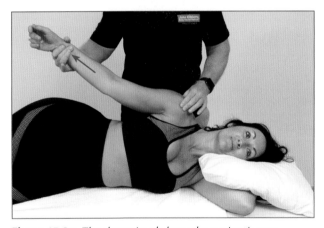

Figure 15.3a: *The therapist abducts the patient's arm passively with traction and external rotation*

Next, as the patient's arm is reaching approximately 70–80 degrees of abduction the therapist gently applies a caudal (inferior) pressure with their fingers to the humeral head to induce an inferior gliding motion (figure 15.3b), while the arm is still being abducted (figure 15.3c). Please bear in mind that pain is perceived at about 80–90 degrees so the therapist has to be in tune with the motion as the goal is to improve the overall range and reduce their pain. It is difficult to say how many times I perform this technique as my focus is on improving the motion

rather than thinking about the repetition but in reality it is somewhere between 6 and 10 repetitions.

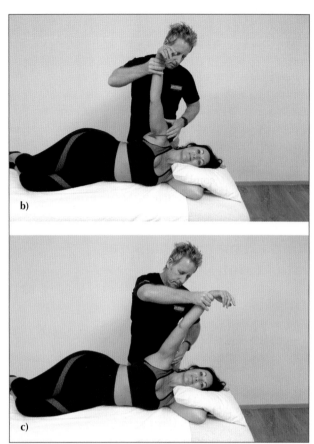

Figure 15.3b & c: *b. The therapist applies a caudal pressure to the humeral head at approximately 80 degrees during abduction. c. The therapist continues passive abduction*

Technique 2 – MET

From time to time I use a muscle energy technique to assist the accessory glide to improve abduction. I passively take the patient's arm to 45 degrees and

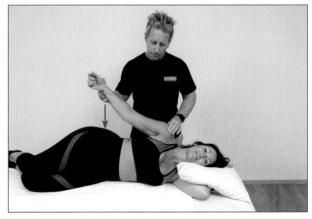

Figure 15.4: *The patient is asked to adduct their shoulder against a resistance*

I ask them to ADDUCT against a resistance for 10 seconds at approximately 30–40% effort (figure 15.4); this is repeated three times.

This technique is a post-isometric relaxation (PIR) of MET and is used to activate the adductor muscles of the humerus as well as the inferior rotator cuff muscles. This contraction with a subsequent relaxation has the effect of causing an inferior gliding motion to the humeral head and on the relaxation phase the arm is passively taken into further abduction by the therapist (with simultaneous traction, external rotation and inferior gliding to the humeral head). A combination of inferior gliding and METs provides a very effective tool to improve abduction.

Re-positioning of humerus into flexion

Technique 3

This is similar to technique 1 as the patient is ask to adopt a side lying position on the couch and the therapist controls the patient's arm and simultaneously flexes the patient's elbow and initiates passive flexion (figure 15.5a) of their shoulder.

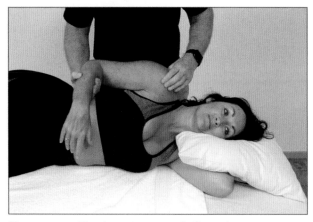

Figure 15.5a: *The therapist passively flexes the patient's elbow and shoulder*

Next, the therapist gently applies a posterior caudal (inferior) pressure with their fingers to the anterior aspect humeral head to induce a posterior inferior gliding motion, while the arm is still being flexed (figure 15.5b). I perform this technique somewhere between 6 and 10 repetitions.

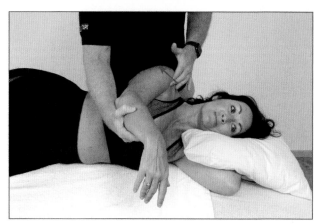

Figure 15.5b: *The therapist applies a posterior caudal pressure to the humeral head during flexion*

Technique 4 – MET

This technique will improve flexion. I passively take the patient's arm to 45 degrees of flexion and I ask them to EXTEND against a resistance for 10 seconds at approximately 30–40% effort (figure 15.6). This is repeated three times.

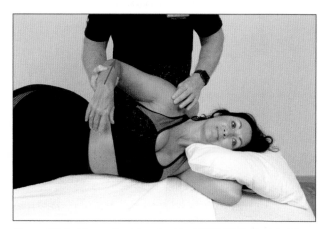

Figure 15.6: *The patient is asked to EXTEND their shoulder against a resistance*

This technique is a post-isometric relaxation (PIR) of MET and is used to activate the extensor muscles of the humerus as well as the inferior cuff muscles. This contraction has the effect of causing the extensors to go through a relaxation phase, and then the arm is passively taken into further flexion by the therapist, with simultaneous posterior inferior gliding to the humeral head.

Technique 5 – reciprocal inhibition (RI) of MET

I like the following technique because it uses the analogy of reciprocal inhibition of MET but with a slight twist.

This simply works on the concept of inducing a relaxation into the antagonistic (opposite) muscle group while the agonist is contracting.

As per technique 1, the patient adopts a side lying position and the therapist holds the patient's arm just off the level of their hip. The patient has to imagine that there is a small fly or insect between their arm and the fingers of the therapist and is instructed to gently push into adduction but not too much, as that will squash the fly, but to gently push down as the therapist slowly abducts their arm (figure 15.7). This induces an RI effect into the antagonistic (abductors) muscles because the agonist (adductors) muscles are contracting, while the arm is being passively abducted.

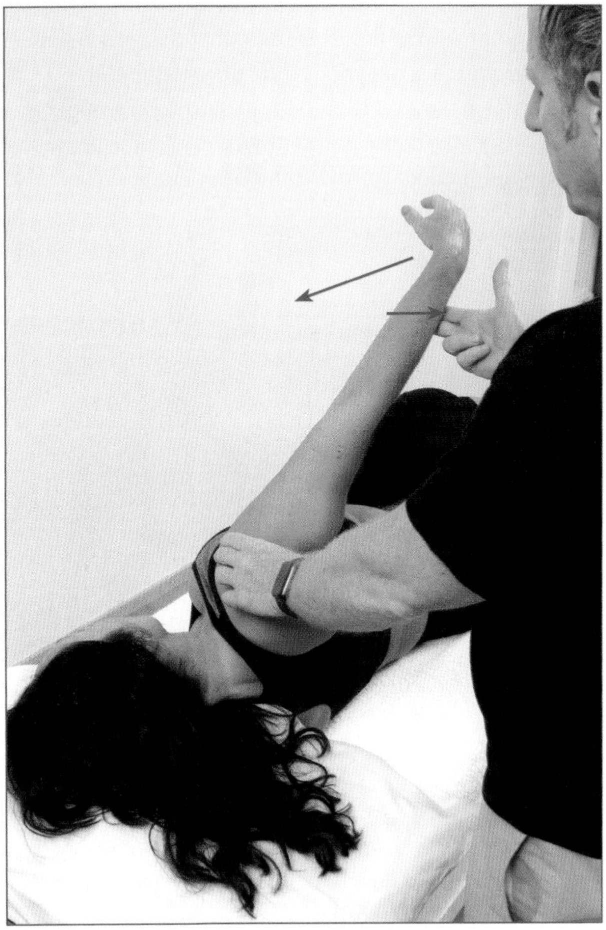

Figure 15.7: *RI technique is induced because the patient is adducting against a 'fly' as the therapist passively abducts their arm*

Technique 6 – active – passive – active

This technique sounds a bit strange; however, it utilizes the active motion of the patient with passive assistance from

the therapist and the two working together is exceptionally effective.

As per technique 1, the patient adopts a side lying position and the therapist takes control of the patient's arm. They are then instructed to assist the motion of abduction by only 10% to start with, about 90% being controlled by the therapist. Hopefully, the range of motion gradually passes 90 degrees with the patient perceiving less pain, because of all the previous techniques performed. However, if they

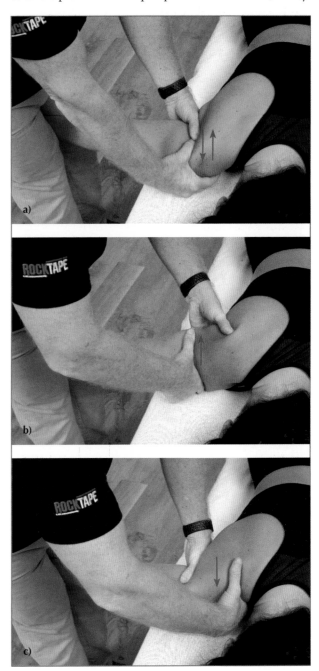

Figure 15.8a–c: *The therapist mobilizes the shoulder in all directions. a: Anterior-posterior glide; b: inferior glide; c: superior glide*

still have pain during this motion then the technique is best left alone for another day. From 10% the patient is asked to assist abduction a bit more (around 30% with 70% from the therapist) and so on until they are basically abducting their arm on their own without any assistance from the therapist. If the patient is able to do this on their own side lying without any pain and with full range of motion, then it would make sense that on standing they to could perform the same motion pain free.

Some of the other techniques I use are described and subsequently located in other chapters, for example, the taping techniques.

In 1999 Boyle described manual therapy techniques to the upper thoracic spine that helped reduce shoulder impingement pain.

Technique 7 – prone mobilizations to glenohumeral (GH) joint

These techniques are very effective at improving the overall mobility of the glenohumeral joint as one can focus on one restriction at a time or the patient can perform a combination of techniques in various planes of motion.

The patient is prone on the couch and the therapist straddles the patient's arm with their legs to stabilize its position. The therapist cradles the whole of the GH joint with both hands and applies a technique that they feel is applicable to the restriction plane. The therapist can mobilize in an anterior or posterior direction (figure 15.8a) or in an inferior (caudad) or superior (cephalad) direction (figure 15.8b and c). The same techniques can also be performed to the patient's shoulder with traction applied from the contact to the arm by the therapist's legs (figure 15.9).

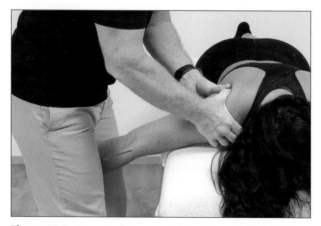

Figure 15.9: *Same techniques with traction applied by the therapist's leg*

■ Scapula mobilizations

I would say that most therapists only mobilize the GH joint and this is a very common procedure in any treatment protocol for shoulder pathology; however, it goes without saying that the scapulothoracic (ST) articulation would also need some treatment as well as the GH joint; it too is part of the shoulder complex and so it cannot be neglected. It is possible that it is the ST joint that is the bigger part or piece that is missing in the jigsaw puzzle.

Technique 1

From the position of technique 7 above, the scapula can be mobilized instead of the GH joint even though the technique looks very similar. The therapist has to control the GH joint with both hands but rather than performing gliding techniques in various directions to the GH the motion is induced to the scapula instead. Example motions are retraction, protraction, elevation, depression, and circumduction clockwise and then anticlockwise. Some of these motions are shown in figure 15.10.

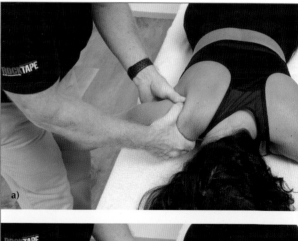

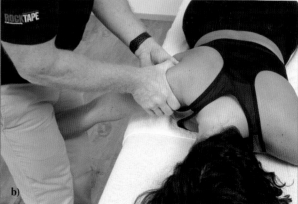

Figure 15.10a & b: *a: Prone mobilization to scapula – protraction/elevation; b: retraction/depression*

Technique 2

The next technique is probably one of my favorite techniques, especially for the upper limb. It is near impossible for the patient to perform these movements on their own so they need some assistance and that is where the physical therapist steps in. All my patients (and students, when I demonstrate them) think these are very effective ways of encouraging mobilizations to the scapula. On occasion this single mobilization motion has reduced rotator cuff impingement pain within the first physical therapy session. I do feel the scapula motion is so important, especially in an upward and also a downward elevation, and any restriction can be partly or even wholly responsible for rotator cuff tendinopathies and subacromial bursitis. The following technique can even assist in mobilizing the acromioclavicular (AC) and sternoclavicular (SC) joints because these two are naturally involved with rotational motions of the scapula during flexion and abduction.

The patient is side lying and places their right arm to 45 degrees of abduction. The therapist places their left hand over the top of the GH joint and their right hand under the scapula so that the fingers of both hands are in slight contact (figure 15.11).

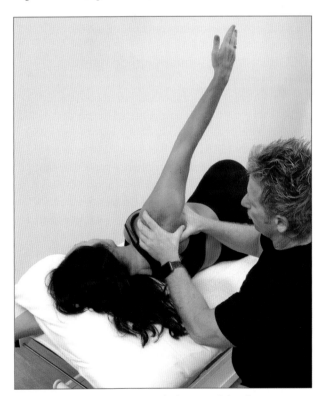

Figure 15.11: *The patient is side lying and the therapist cradles the right scapula*

The patient is now asked to slowly abduct as far as they comfortably can while the therapist maintains the contact with the scapula and controls the motion with overpressure at the end of motion (figure 15.12) as this will promote upward rotation of the ST joint. If the patient has some discomfort during this technique, they are asked to change the position slightly so that they horizontally flex or horizontally extend a few degrees while they are still abducting.

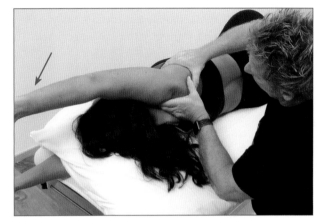

Figure 15.12: *The patient abducts fully as the therapist controls the motion of the scapula with some overpressure to end range*

From this position the patient is asked to adduct as far as they can, even to pass the level of the hip, as this specific motion will promote downward rotation of the ST joint.

Oscillatory/harmonic motion

I was shown some of these techniques many years ago by a colleague of mine called Dr Eyal Lederman. I have since modified my approach slightly but if you require further information on harmonics and Dr Lederman there is quite a bit available on the Internet.

I have used the following techniques over and over again with patients and athletes and taught them to thousands of my students. I believe they work very well as a mobilization tool for the shoulder complex. I will only show a few simple ideas in this text, as it is very difficult to write an explanation of movements while only showing static pictures of what I am trying to demonstrate. I mentioned earlier in the book that I have hundreds of YouTube videos that you are able to access for free and some videos will include most of the techniques shown throughout this text.

Technique 1

The patient is supine and the therapist takes control of the patient's wrist with their fingers and thumb; their other hand is palpating the patient's shoulder and abducts to 90 degrees with elbow flexed to the same angle. The therapist now performs a type of *rocking* motion to the wrist with their fingers and thumb, as this will induce abduction and adduction (figure 15.13).

From here the therapist can now induce a circular motion clockwise then a circular motion anticlockwise. The size of the circles can range from very small to bigger circles (figure 15.14).

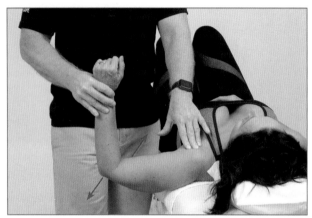

Figure 15.13: *The therapist controls the patient's arm and takes them into 90 degrees of abduction and elbow flexion. The therapist rocks the patient's arm into abduction and adduction*

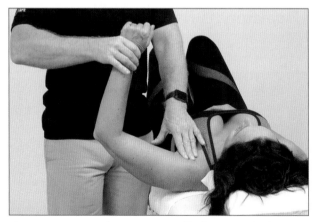

Figure 15.14: *Circular motion (small – big) in a clockwise and anticlockwise direction*

If the patient perceived pain during some or any of these motions because of, say, a capsulitis, then I would take the arm to less abduction, say 70 degrees, and perform these techniques, instead of 90 degrees, because this position might be causing an impingement syndrome and less abduction might be what is needed to improve the joint mobility without exacerbating the symptoms.

Note: The way I teach these techniques to my students is that I describe the GH joint as a ball and socket joint and say it is similar to an engine with oil. Why? Because the synovial fluid is like the oil in this example, and like all 'engines', every part needs motion and also lubrication and these harmonic types of motions allow that to happen.

When I use these techniques I have a tendency to perform the side-to-side motion (abduct/adduct) first then add in small circular motions one way, back to side-to-side, then small circular motions the opposite way, then back to side-to-side, then increase the size of the circles and so on. That seems to work very well for me in my practice.

Treatment of the sternoclavicular joint using METs

In the earlier chapter we discussed how to assess the SC joint through use of the shrug and prayer test. If on the shrug test the clavicle did not inferiorly glide then this would be one way to encourage the motion. Or if the clavicle were unable to posteriorly glide on the prayer test then the second treatment would be the option.

MET treatment 1 – inferior glide (positive shrug test)

The patient is supine and the therapist holds onto the patient's upper arm with one hand; the fingers of the other hand are gently cradling (or hooking) over the proximal clavicle (figure 15.15a). The patient is asked to depress the shoulder girdle against a resistance applied by the therapist for 10 seconds at 20% effort (figure 15.15b). After the relaxation phase the therapist elevates the shoulder girdle, at the same time encouraging the inferior gliding motion of the clavicle (figure 15.15c).

MET treatment 2 – posterior glide (positive prayer test)

The patient is supine and reaches their arm to the back of the therapist; then the therapist simultaneously holds onto the patient's upper shoulder with one hand while the palm of their other hand is gently placed over the proximal clavicle. The patient is asked to retract the shoulder girdle against a resistance applied by the therapist for 10 seconds at 20% effort (figure 15.16a). After the relaxation phase the therapist protracts the shoulder girdle, at the same

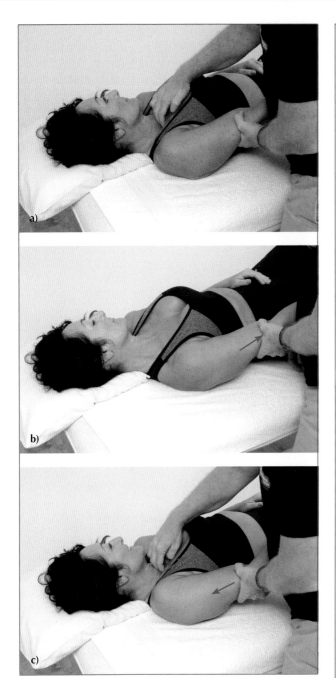

Figure 15.15a–c: *a: The therapist controls the patient's arm and gently hooks over the proximal clavicle. b: The patient depresses the shoulder girdle against resistance. c: The therapist takes the arm into further elevation and inferior glides the proximal clavicle*

time encouraging posterior gliding motion of the clavicle (figure 15.16b).

Note: There are countless other ways to treat the shoulder complex. I cover most of these complex treatment options throughout the book in various chapters rather than simply focusing only on treatment within this chapter.

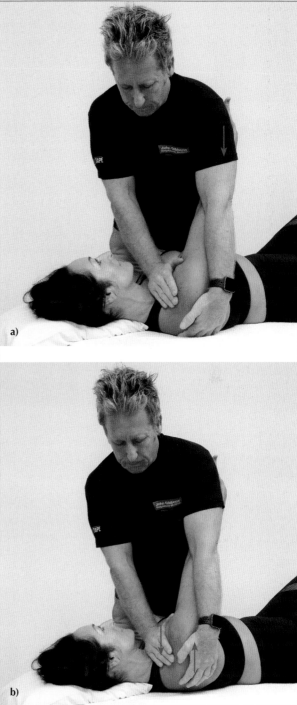

Figure 15.16a & b: *a: The therapist controls the patient's scapula and the patient is asked to retract their shoulder girdle against resistance. b: The therapist takes the shoulder girdle into further protraction and posterior glides the proximal clavicle*

Here I simply wanted to show you how I would personally treat the shoulder and describe some of the techniques I would incorporate into the treatment process.

16

Myofascial soft tissue treatment of the shoulder complex

I n this chapter I wanted to discuss with you what I consider to be a very effective way of treating the soft tissues of the cervical and shoulder regions. These techniques are classified under the umbrella of myofascial release. Over the many years of my ongoing studies in this field of manual therapy, I am exceptionally fortunate to have been taught by soft tissue therapists known as Rolfers (the concept is called Rolfing, after the founder, Ida Rolf), or another similar concept known as Structural Integration. These specialists have taught me some of the techniques I describe in this chapter.

I have many colleagues who teach many various forms of myofascial release techniques, and I am sure they would have their own views of some of the techniques I am demonstrating throughout this text. However, this book contains what I consider to be a variety or even a mix of techniques that I have accumulated over many years of lecturing as well as practicing as a manual therapist, specializing in osteopathy.

My company, the Bodymaster method®, is fortunate enough to be sponsored by many companies and one of these is Songbird Wax (figure 16.1), who kindly supply my soft tissue courses with a particular type of medium designed for myofascial release techniques. I think it is an excellent product and the students that have attended my courses in the past have also agreed with how good the product is.

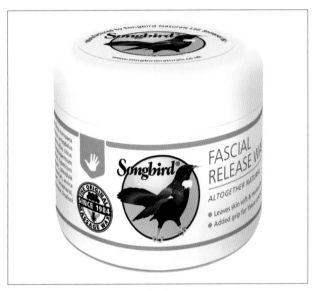

Figure 16.1: *Songbird Fascial Release Wax*

Rotator cuff treatment

It is relatively difficult to explain all of the soft tissue variations I include in this chapter, but I will try my best to convey to the reader how and when to apply them. It is of course much easier to show how it is done in a real situation, which is probably why most therapists attend my courses to learn the techniques first hand.

Pressure
I suggest that on your first contact with the patient you should use only light pressure with the placement of the

fingers on whatever bodily part you decide to use, such as pisiform, forearm, elbow and so on. If we press too firmly to start with then we will probably restrict the active motion from the patient because of the applied pressure and every single technique I demonstrate in this chapter is with motion, whether actively by the patient, passively from the therapist, or a combination of both. Some therapists say it is like 'massage with motion' and this is a good term that actually makes a lot of sense. My view is that it is potentially a lot more technical in its application and understanding than this description allows for. I will show you a quite a few variations of the theme, so follow closely!

■ Supraspinatus

Technique 1 – active gliding

The patient adopts a sitting position. The therapist crosses the middle finger over the index finger to use as reinforcement and then locates the supraspinous fossa of the scapula. The patient is asked to abduct their arm to 90 degrees and now the therapist applies gentle pressure initially to the supraspinatus, with the reinforced index finger that is located within the fossa (figure 16.2). The patient is asked to slowly lower their arm down to their side (this means the patient is actively lowering their arm on their own), while the therapist glides their reinforced finger along the fossa until they reach the medial border of the scapula (figure 16.3). This can be repeated many times until a release is felt.

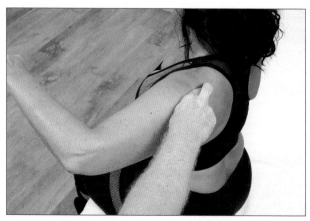

Figure 16.2: *The therapist palpates the supraspinatus muscle, which is located within the supraspinous fossa, with a reinforced finger*

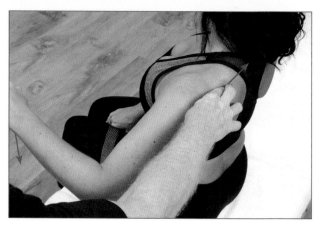

Figure 16.3: *The therapist glides along the supraspinous fossa with a reinforced finger as the patient lowers their arm (active gliding)*

Technique 2 – passive gliding

This technique is very similar to the one above; however, this time instead of the patient lowering their arm actively, the therapist controls the patient's abducted arm and lowers the arm for them passively, while at the same time the therapists reinforced finger, which is located within the fossa, continues to glide along the supraspinatus muscle (figure 16.4).

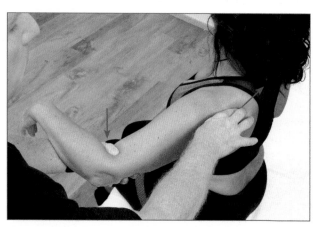

Figure 16.4: *The therapist glides along the supraspinous fossa with a reinforced finger; at the same time the therapist is lowering the patient's arm (passive gliding)*

Technique 3 – reciprocal inhibition (RI) gliding

The therapist controls the patient's abducted arm and asks them to contract gently by *adducting* (concentrically) against a resistance that is applied by the therapist. The goal of this technique is to 'switch off' or 'inhibit' the supraspinatus by contracting the antagonist muscles of the shoulder (adductors). This technique is especially effective if the upper trapezius is hypertonic and it is difficult to access the supraspinatus muscle due to the increased muscle tone. So basically, the patient is adducting their arm against an external force applied by the therapist, while at the same time the therapist applies gliding pressure along the supraspinous fossa (figure 16.5).

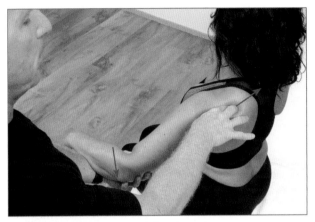

Figure 16.5: *The therapist glides along the supraspinous fossa with a reinforced finger as the patient lowers their arm against a resistance (inhibition gliding)*

Technique 4 – MET – combined post-isometric relaxation (PIR) and reciprocal inhibition (RI)

The therapist asks the patient to maintain the position of 90 degrees of abduction (isometric contraction) for at least 10 seconds; this is a muscle energy technique (MET) called post-isometric relaxation. After the contraction the patient is then asked to gently adduct (concentrically) against a resistance that is applied by the therapist. The goal of this technique is to initially 'switch on' the supraspinatus through isometric contraction (PIR). After the 10-second contraction there is a natural relaxation phase within the supraspinatus muscle due to the effect of the PIR that we can use to our advantage as we can encourage the supraspinatus to switch off even more by contracting the antagonist muscles (similar to above inhibition process) against a resistance into adduction, while we continue gliding along the fossa.

This combination technique is especially effective if the upper trapezius is hypertonic or if the supraspinatus is particularly tender to palpate.

Technique 5 – supraspinatus lock with active/passive motion

The following technique has many alternative names, for example, soft tissue release (STR), sliding STR, active release technique (ART), pin and stretch, to name just a few (though be careful what you call it as some of these names have trademarks and patents, etc.). The technique

I demonstrate can be likened to a key placed within a lock of a door: basically the therapist applies a pressure (key) through use of an applicator (finger, thumb, etc.) to the soft tissues and the patient is asked to open the door (active); another way is for the therapist to open the door for them (passively); and the third way is to get the patient to open the door with guided assistance from the therapist (active/passive).

These techniques are very effective at identify and treating potential adhesions. These restrictions can be related to a build up of continual micro trauma that eventually forms over time as scar tissue and they are found within all types of soft tissues. One thought process is that the applicator is applied as a *fixed* pressure *superior to* or *above* the level of the adhesion so that the tissue above the problem site is now fixed in a locked position. It is almost like saying a *new origin* of the muscle has been applied (think of an epicondyle strap for tennis elbow – the strap is applied below the pain site and fixes the extensor muscles in a locked position, subsequently offloading the painful area).

So with regards to the technique, if we are able to fix the tissue in a potentially locked position above the site of the restricted tissue, when the patient lowers the arm or the therapist lowers the arm for them, then it has the desired effect of lengthening the tissue directly below the applicator. Hopefully, if there is an adhesion present, then maybe this technique has the benefit of stretching that specific area and will improve the overall mobility and subsequent healing mechanisms of the involved tissues.

As above, the patient adopts a sitting position and is asked to abduct his or her arm to 90 degrees. The therapist can either cross the middle finger over the index finger to use as reinforcement or use a thumb, and then locates

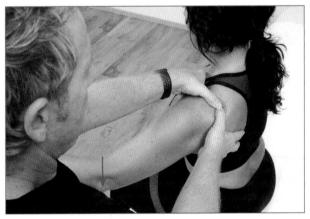

Figure 16.6: *The therapist locks into the supraspinatus as the patient lowers their arm (active lock motion)*

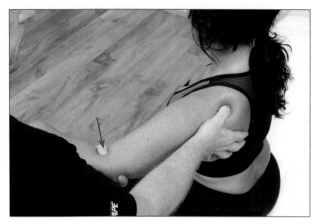

Figure 16.7: *The therapist locks into the supraspinatus and lowers the patient's arm for them (passive lock motion)*

the supraspinous fossa. This time they apply a sustained pressure to the supraspinatus muscle with no motion or gliding (lock or fixed) from the applicator. The patient is asked to slowly lower their arm down to their side actively with the therapist maintaining the fixed pressure within the fossa (figure 16.6).

An alternative is that the therapist can lower the arm for the patient (passively) (figure 16.7), using the thumb (reinforced) to lock the tissue, or the patient lowers their arm with assistance from the therapist (active/passive).

Please note: On occasion a thumb may be used, even though the thumb is not recommended, especially when used on a regular basis as over time the first carpometacarpal joint or even the first metacarpophalangeal (MP) joint that relates to the thumb (pollux) can eventually degenerate (osteoarthritis, OA) and this condition will cause stiffness and pain.

A combination of the 'lock' technique can be incorporated with the muscle energy techniques of PIR and RI as per the other techniques demonstrated above.

■ Infraspinatus and teres minor

These techniques can be performed either with the patient in a sitting position or side lying. For the demonstrations the patient will be sitting.

Technique 1 – active gliding
These soft tissue techniques naturally follow the treatment for the supraspinatus. The only difference is that the therapist uses reinforced fingers and the patient is

asked to horizontally flex their shoulder. The therapist places their reinforced fingers inferior to the spine of scapula to contact the infraspinous fossa; this is where the infraspinatus muscle is located. The patient is asked to abduct their shoulder to 90 degrees with 20 degrees of horizontal extension to shorten the infraspinatus (figure 16.8).

The patient is then asked to slowly horizontally flex their shoulder while the therapist maintains contact to the infraspinatus and glides along the infraspinous fossa (figure 16.9).

An alternative technique is to use the knuckles instead of the fingers (figure 16.10). Many therapists prefer this technique as some find it easier to perform and feel that it results in less pressure on the wrist and fingers.

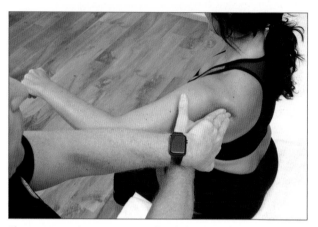

Figure 16.8: *The patient initially abducts and horizontally extends their shoulder as the therapist applies pressure to the infraspinatus with reinforced fingers*

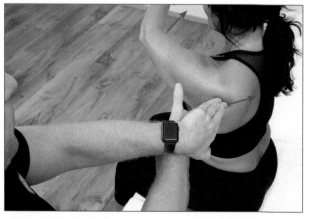

Figure 16.9: *The patient is asked to horizontally flex their shoulder as the therapist applies gliding pressure along the infraspinous fossa with reinforced fingers*

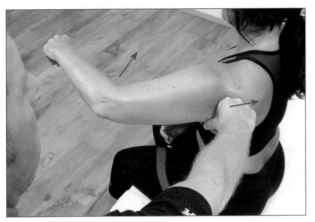

Figure 16.10: *Alternative techniques using the knuckles instead of the fingers*

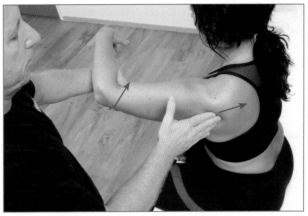

Figure 16.12: *The therapist glides along the infraspinous fossa with one hand as the as the patient is asked to horizontally flex against a resistance (RI)*

Technique 2 – passive gliding

The following applications are very similar to the treatment of the supraspinatus. We have done the active gliding one and technique 2 shows the passive gliding motion performed by the therapist (figure 16.11); the difference is that the therapist is not able to reinforce their fingers during the gliding technique.

Technique 3 – reciprocal inhibition (RI) gliding

In the RI technique, the patient is asked to horizontally flex against applied resistance from the therapist; at the same time the therapist applies a gliding technique with their fingers along the infraspinous fossa so that the infraspinatus muscle is treated.

Technique 4 – PIR and RI

This next technique is a combination of PIR and RI muscle energy techniques. The patient is asked to resist horizontal extension for 10 seconds (figure 16.13). After the relaxation phase the patient is asked to now horizontally

flex against a resistance applied by the therapist while they glide with their fingers along the infraspinous fossa (figure 16.14).

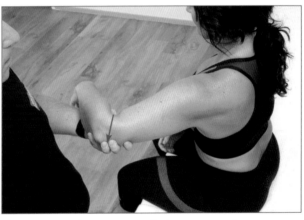

Figure 16.13: *The patient is asked to contract the infraspinatus isometrically (PIR) by horizontally extending for 10 seconds*

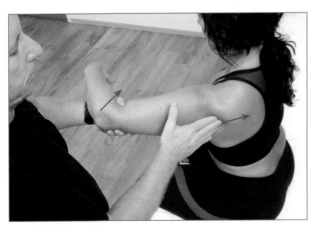

Figure 16.11: *The therapist glides along the infraspinous fossa while controlling the motion of horizontal flexion (passive gliding)*

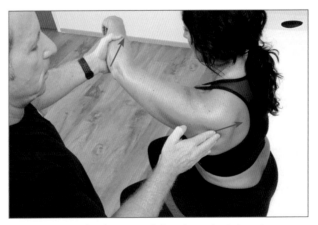

Figure 16.14: *The therapist glides along the infraspinous fossa with their fingers as the patient takes their arm forward against a resistance (inhibition)*

Technique 5 – infraspinatus/teres minor lock with active/passive motion

This technique is the lock motion and it is utilized while the patient horizontally flexes their shoulder actively (figure 16.15), or passively by the therapist.

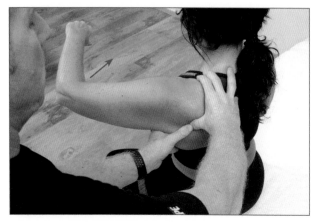

Figure 16.15: *The therapist applies a lock into the infraspinatus with fingers or reinforced thumb as the patient horizontally flexes their arm (active)*

Note: A combination of the 'lock' technique can be incorporated with the passive motion performed by the therapist, as well as the PIR and RI as per the other techniques demonstrated above for the supraspinatus.

■ Subscapularis

Technique 1 – lock

The patient adopts a supine position and the arm is placed in 90 degrees of elbow flexion and abduction. The therapist gently applies contact using their fingers (short nails) to the subscapularis fossa and the patient is asked to contract the medial rotator (subscapularis) to make sure anatomically they have located the correct muscle (figure 16.16).

With pressure gently applied through the contact fingers on the muscle, the patient is asked to slowly externally rotate the shoulder joint (figure 16.17).

Technique 2 – MET (PIR) and lock

The patient adopts same position as per technique 1; this time the patient is first asked to contract the subscapularis against a resistance for 10 seconds to initiate a PIR effect into the muscle (figure 16.16 above)

After the contraction the therapist applies pressure (lock) to the muscle and then the therapist slowly externally rotates the shoulder (figure 16.18).

Technique 3 – MET (PIR/RI) and lock

The patient adopts same position as per technique 2; this time the patient is asked to contract the subscapularis against a resistance for 10 seconds to initiate a PIR effect into the muscle. After the contraction the therapist now asks the patient to contract the infraspinatus by externally

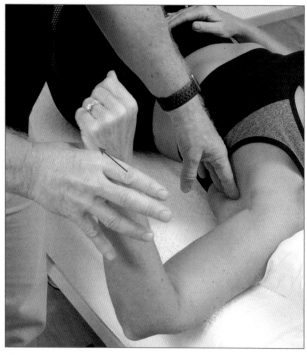

Figure 16.16: *The patient is supine and is asked to gently contract the subscapularis muscle while the therapist palpates the muscle*

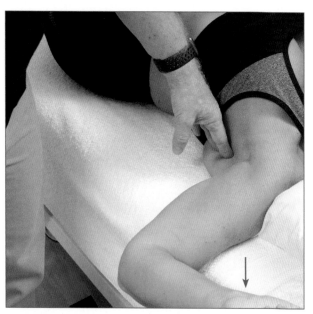

Figure 16.17: *The therapist contacts and applies pressure to the muscle as the patient is asked to slowly externally rotate the shoulder actively*

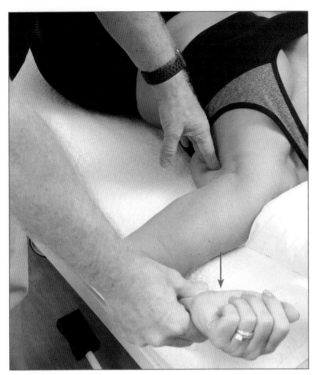

Figure 16.18: *The therapist contacts and applies pressure (lock) to the muscle and then passively externally rotates the humerus*

rotating the shoulder and to continue the contracting movement concentrically as this will cause inhibition into the subscapularis. At the same time the therapist applies pressure (lock) to the muscle, while the patient continues external rotation of the shoulder (figure 16.19).

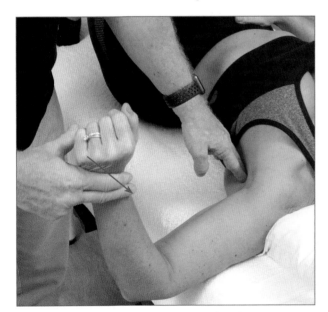

Figure 16.19: *The therapist contacts and applies pressure (lock) to the subscapularis muscle as the patient is asked to slowly externally rotate against a resistance (inhibition technique)*

■ Pectoralis major and minor

Pectoralis major is particular easy to treat because it is the most superficial of the two muscles; pectoralis minor is a deeper structure anatomically and is located underneath the major so it is not easily accessible. The following techniques will be applied directly to the major muscle; however, these techniques will still have a great effect on the deeper minor muscle because of its natural proximity. I have also covered an MET technique on the minor muscle in an earlier chapter so we have not neglected this very important, albeit small, muscle.

Technique 1 – active gliding

The patient adopts a supine position and is asked to place their arm into shoulder flexion of 120 degrees and the therapist applies contact to the patient's sternal fibers of the pectoralis major using the proximal phalanges of their hand (with reinforcement from the other hand)

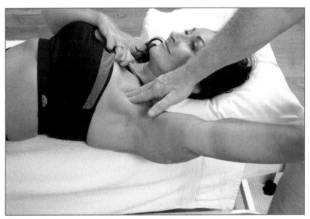

Figure 16.20: *The therapist applies pressure to the sternal fibers of the pectoral major muscle using their proximal phalanges of the straight arm*

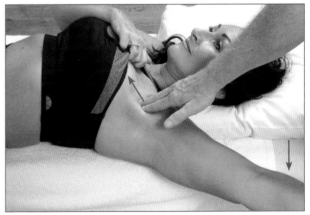

Figure 16.21: *The therapist applies inferior, medial gliding pressure to the pectoral major muscle, while the patient is actively lowering their arm*

(figure 16.20) and maintaining a straight arm the patient is asked to slowly take their arm away from the midline of the body, while at the same time the therapist glides their straight arm towards the sternum (figure 16.21). An alternative technique through the use of a relaxed fist could be utilized (figure 16.22).

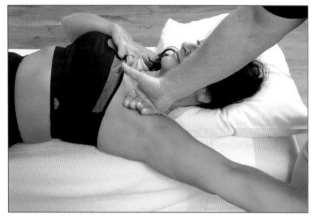

Figure 16.22: *Alternative technique using a relaxed fist to achieve the same outcome*

Technique 2 – MET (PIR) with active gliding

The patient adopts same position as per technique 1. This time the patient is asked to contract the pectoralis major muscle against a resistance for 10 seconds to initiate a PIR effect into the muscle (figure 16.23). After the contraction the therapist applies gliding pressure with either reinforced fingers or a relaxed fist to the muscle, while the patient moves into the scapular plane.

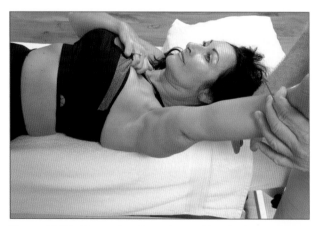

Figure 16.23: *The patient is supine and is asked to contract the pectoralis major muscle for 10 seconds*

The therapist contacts and applies gliding pressure to the muscle as the patient is asked to move into the scapular plane.

Technique 3 – MET (PIR/RI) and lock

The patient adopts same position as per technique 2. This time the patient is asked to contract the pectoralis major muscle against a resistance for 10 seconds to initiate a PIR effect into the muscle.

After the contraction the therapist now asks the patient to contract the antagonist (opposite) muscles by moving into the scapular plane against a resistance applied by the therapist and to continue the contracting movement concentrically as this will cause inhibition into the pectoralis major (agonist). At the same time the therapist applies gliding pressure to the muscle (figure 16.24).

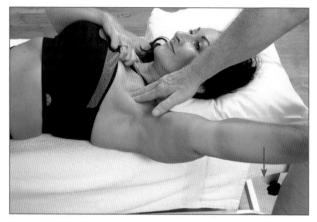

Figure 16.24: *The therapist contacts and applies gliding pressure to the pectoralis major muscle as the patient is asked to slowly resist the scapular plane against a resistance*

The therapist can now, if they wish to do so, apply a lock to the tissue of the pectoralis muscle as the patient is taking their arm towards the scapular plane (figure 16.25).

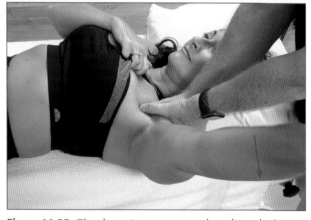

Figure 16.25: *The therapist contacts and applies a lock pressure to the pectoralis major muscle as the patient is asked to actively slowly take the arm towards the scapular plane*

The therapist can also guide the patient's arm into the scapular plane passively, while still applying the lock (figure 16.26).

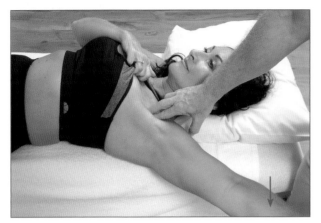

Figure 16.26: *The therapist contacts and applies a lock pressure to the pectoralis major muscle; at the same time their arm is guided passively towards the scapular plane*

■ Upper trapezius and levator scapulae

Out of all the treatment protocols ever designed, this area of the neck and shoulder region has to be one of the most popular areas to treat, so to me it makes sense to become very proficient in treating it. If you were to offer people a free 30-minute massage on any part of the body they would probably choose the neck and shoulders, or possibly the lower back.

You would expect the treatment for these two muscles to be very similar because of their location; however, the upper trapezius rotates the cervical spine contralaterally (opposite), while the levator scapulae rotates the cervical spine ipsilaterally (same side), so we can use this subtle information to treat these two muscles more effectively. For example, if we were to treat the right upper trapezius then rotation right would stretch the muscle and rotation left would shorten it. The opposite would apply to the right levator scapulae: right rotation would shorten the muscle and left rotation would lengthen it, as explained below.

Technique 1 – active gliding
The patient adopts a sitting position with their head in a neutral position and the therapist places the distal phalanges of their hand, with gentle reinforcement from their opposite hand, to apply and initiate contact to the base of the right side of the occipital bone, as this is close to the attachment of the trapezius muscle (figure 16.27).

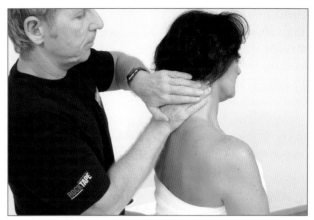

Figure 16.27: *The patient is sitting with head in neutral and the therapist applies pressure to the right side of the base of the occipital bone*

Trapezius
The patient is asked to slowly flex their head and then to side bend to the left and rotate to the *right* about 40 degrees (half rotation). The therapist applies a gliding pressure through the tissues with their fingers laterally towards the clavicle for the trapezius muscle (figure 16.28).

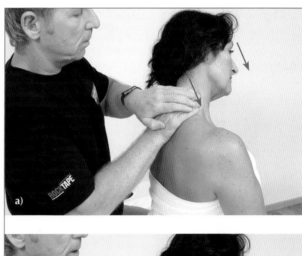

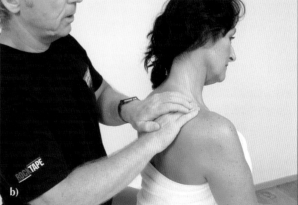

Figure 16.28a & b: *a: Upper trapezius (right). The patient is asked to flex, side bend left and rotate their cervical spine to the right side. b: Finish position*

Levator scapulae

The method is similar to the above but this time to treat the right levator muscle the patient is asked to slowly side bend the cervical spine to the left and rotate *left* about 40 degrees (half rotation) and to then slowly flex their neck towards their chest. The therapist applies a gliding pressure through the tissues with their fingers laterally and inferiorly towards the superior angle of the scapula for the levator scapulae (figure 16.29).

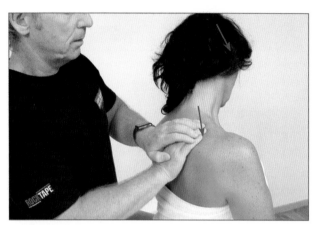

Figure 16.29: *Levator scapulae (right). The patient is asked to side bend their cervical spine to the left and also rotate left and then to flex towards their chest*

I have a tendency to use a fanning type in at least three specific motions (figure 16.30), as this will cover all the necessary muscles.

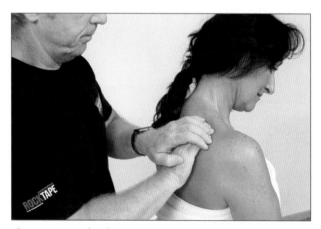

Figure 16.30: *The therapist applies a fanning motion across the neck and shoulder to cover all muscles*

Note: It is very common for the patient to have rotated and flexed the neck all of the way; however, the therapist might have only treated half of the soft tissue area. If that is the case the patient is asked to return to neutral and the therapist continues with the treatment from the midpoint to finish the second half of the muscles.

Technique 2 – MET active gliding

The patient is asked to push their head back to the right for 10 seconds to initiate a PIR effect (figure 16.31a). After the relaxation phase the therapist continues with the same gliding techniques as were shown earlier (figure 16.31b).

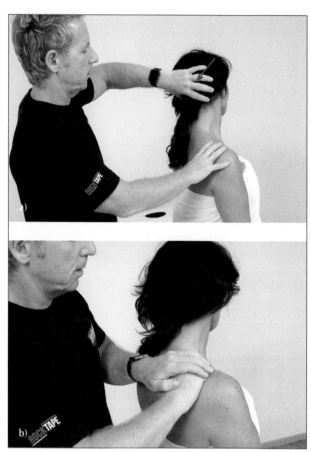

Figure 16.31a & b: *a: PIR contraction for 10 seconds. b: The therapist repeats active gliding*

Note: I am hoping that by now what I have taught you has given you enough knowledge, especially from the above two techniques, to effectively treat the upper trapezius and levator scapulae. I have only shown you a small part of a repertoire of techniques I know and of course you can add in other ways to treat these muscles. I have also demonstrated a multitude of techniques on the previously mentioned muscles – for example, the passive gliding and the lock and so on – and there is no reason why these cannot be included as well.

■ Sternocleidomastoid (SCM) and scalenes

I tend to treat these muscles with a lot of respect compared to all other muscles as I find them generally sensitive on most patients, even with light contact, and also their relationship and proximity to the delicate thoracic outlet (brachial plexus and subclavian artery) structures has to be considered when conducting the treatments. I normally treat these muscles passively, with myself as the controller, rather than actively by the patient, as I like to control all of the passive movements under my fingertips.

Technique 1 – passive gliding

Like most of the techniques shown the patient is sitting with the head in a neutral position. The therapist's left knee is placed onto the couch and the left hand is cradled across the top of the cranium with the elbow resting on top of the patient's shoulder. The left hand is now able to rotate the cervical spine to the right through use of the cranium (figure 16.32).

The therapist contacts the origin of the sternocleidomastoid (SCM) at the mastoid process with their fingers (figure 16.33).

Next the therapist passively controls and induces left rotation of the cervical spine with their left hand while the right hand is slowly gliding inferiorly down the SCM muscle (figure 16.34).

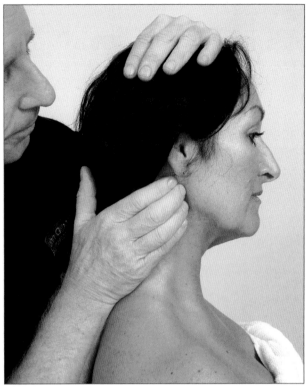

Figure 16.33: *The therapist contacts the origin of the SCM at the mastoid process*

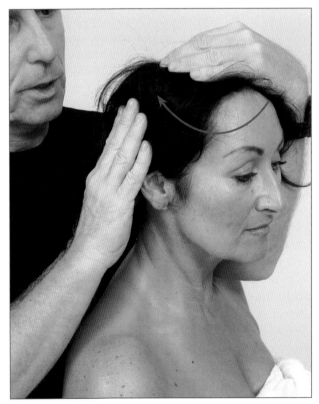

Figure 16.32: *The therapist cradles the cranium and rotates the cervical spine to the right*

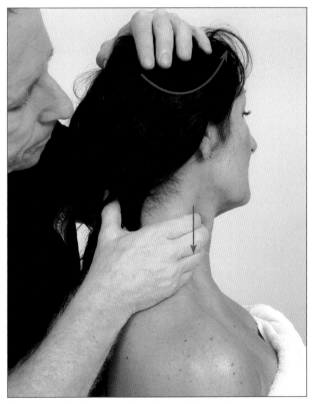

Figure 16.34: *The therapist controls left rotation of the cervical spine at the same time gliding down the SCM*

Note: It is a true saying that right rotation of the cervical spine will *lengthen* the right SCM and left rotation of the cervical spine will *shorten* the right SCM because the muscle is responsible for rotation to the *opposite* side. So the LEFT SCM will rotate the cervical spine to the right. The reason I mention this is because I rotate the cervical spine to the left but I am in theory *shortening* the muscle and the whole objective of these techniques is to *lengthen* the muscle. However, because I am treating these muscles passively, it means the patient is not responsible for the motion; hence the muscle is not in a true state of contraction and this way of treating works very well for me in practice. I also consider that because I am taking the cervical spine *away* it allows me to open up the area as compared to the opposite motion of moving *towards* where I feel the space would be compromised and so would the treatment (that is my opinion only!).

Technique 2 – passive gliding (scalenes)

The scalenes (anterior, medial, and posterior) attach to C2–7 and the thoracic outlet structures exit between the scalene anterior and medial fibers. Out of all the muscles I have taught how to assess and treat in this book, one has to be very careful with these particular muscles, especially the techniques I demonstrate below. On occasion a number of patients will mention altered sensations such as tingling in their shoulder, arms or hand, or a localized shooting pain from the pressure being applied too firmly. This indicates that a neurological structure must have been contacted, so please be very careful where and what you are pressing – a light touch is recommended.

The technique is almost identical to the treatment of the SCM muscle described above. The only difference is that when you are gliding down the SCM muscle, it is quite normal for the fingers to *slip off* the muscle posteriorly and that will be fine, as the fingers will now be in contact with the scalene muscles (figure 16.35). You will probably notice that the cervical spine is also in some flexion, as well as left rotation. I believe this is a better way of treating these delicate structures.

Note: As with the trapezius treatment, I use a fanning type of motion but on a smaller scale to treat the individual fibers of the scalenes.

■ Mid/lower trapezius and rhomboids

In reality it is very therapeutic for the patient to have soft tissue work performed to some of the scapular muscles,

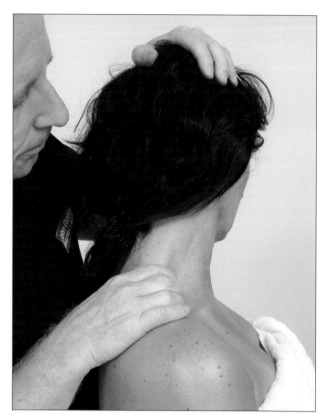

Figure 16.35: *The therapist contacts the scalenes and applies an inferior gliding technique as the cervical spine is rotated to the left and flexed*

especially the retractor muscles located between the shoulder blades, even though this might go against some of my teachings regarding treating symptoms and do not chase pain, chase dysfunction, etc. What I mean by that statement is that many patients present with symptoms/pain to the mid scapular region of the body and one reason could be from tight short antagonistic muscles, which in this case are the pectoral muscles. These tight facilitated muscles of the pecs might be the underlying reason why the rhomboids and mid trapezius are held in a lengthened, weakened or inhibited position. It makes perfect sense (if that is the case) to lengthen the pectoral muscles prior to treating/strengthening the weakened mid scapular muscles, and I have already shown you how to achieve this.

Technique 1 – active gliding

The patient adopts a sitting position and is asked to slightly retract the scapula, so that the muscles are in a shortened position and the therapist applies contact to the patient's mid scapular region using the knuckles of their hand and with a straight arm (figure 16.36).

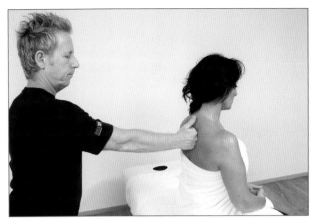

Figure 16.36: *The patient is asked to slightly retract the scapula and the therapist applies pressure to the mid scapular region using the knuckles of their straight arm*

The patient is now asked to either protract (ideally one side at a time even though bilateral protraction is easier) their scapula and/or flex their cervical spine at the same time (figure 16.37) as the therapist is applying an inferior gliding technique to the soft tissues.

Alternative technique

The patient is asked to place their arm into 90 degrees of abduction and elbow flexion (figure 16.38a). The therapist glides using their straight arm inferiorly over the rhomboids and lower trapezius muscles as the patient continues the horizontal flexion motion (figure 16.38b).

The patient (if they prefer) can horizontally flex their arm and rotate their trunk at the same time. This allows the thoracic erector spinae to be treated from this position using a straight arm, as demonstrated by the therapist,

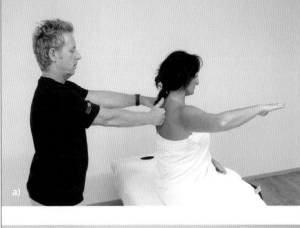

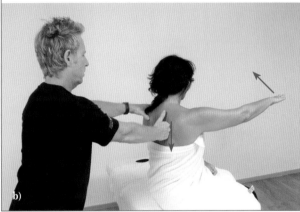

Figure 16.38a & b: *a: The therapist applies inferior gliding pressure to the mid scapular region. b: The patient is horizontally flexing their shoulder as the therapist applies an inferior gliding motion*

especially if the pressure is directed closer to the spine (figure 16.39), or the rhomboids and mid/lower trapezius can be treated if the pressure is directed closer to the scapula.

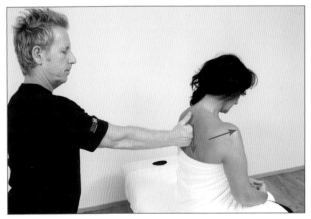

Figure 16.37: *The therapist applies inferior gliding pressure to the mid scapular region while the patient is protracting their scapula and/or flexing their neck*

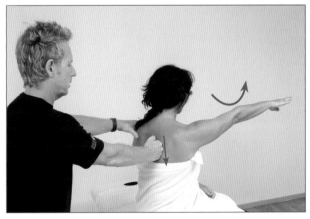

Figure 16.39: *The therapist applies inferior gliding pressure to the thoracic erector spinae and rhomboid muscles while the patient is rotating their thoracic spine*

17

Athletic and kinesiology taping techniques for the shoulder and cervical spine

Some of this chapter is taken from my book *A Practical guide to Kinesiology Taping*. My aim here is to describe and encourage the use of athletic taping techniques, as this is a skill that is becoming almost extinct. It is my opinion that every therapist should be taught these skills early on in their therapy careers and I hope this small chapter may inspire some therapists to become more knowledgeable in the use of both athletic and kinesiology tape and perhaps find a training course so they can become certified.

This skill is particularly necessary when it comes to sports-related injuries to the shoulder complex and cervical spine. I have completed a very long apprenticeship in this field, from my first introduction to athletic taping as a physical training instructor in the British Army, and I am truly thankful to the skilled military physiotherapists who taught me those skills.

Initially I used only athletic tape, employing a variety of rigid and elastic type of tapes for many years. However, I have also been taught the classical McConnell taping techniques (named after an Australian physiotherapist by the name of Jenny McConnell) for the knee, shoulder and spine as well as the power flex and power taping system; these techniques were taught to me by an American athletic trainer called Ron O'Neil, who for many years had looked after the well-being of the Super Bowl teams.

Not that long ago I was teaching athletic taping courses on a monthly basis; however, jump ahead a few years

and now I only teach kinesiology taping courses because the demand for standard athletic taping has diminished tremendously in last few years. My sincere hope is that the 'old school' methods of athletic taping are not forgotten as I consider they will always have a place in sports medicine (and my heart).

A true professional operating within the physical therapy sector should be knowledgeable in all aspects of taping techniques. I am therefore a little disappointed by how many of my manual therapy students have never seen any of the typical white athletic tapes, only the colored tape that I lift out of my training boxes.

This chapter describes the standard way of taping the shoulder complex using materials such as Leukotape, zinc oxide (Z/O) and microporous tape; however, most of the taping techniques described use a relatively new system of taping employing kinesiology tape.

Kinesiology taping is currently the most frequently employed taping method in the field of sports medicine and has been for some years. The brightly colored tape is now a very common sight at all major sporting events throughout the world and is even seen at some recreational activities. Therefore, therapists need to master the techniques, which are relatively simple to learn and once applied in a specific way can potentially improve the performance of an athlete as well as reducing any pain and swelling.

■ A brief history of kinesiology taping

In the 1970s, a Japanese chiropractor, Dr Kenzo Kase, started using a unique type of taping method that led to the development of a new form of sports tape. He was keen to develop a new style of taping compared to the standard form of athletic strapping and taping, such as the zinc oxide (Z/O) technique. He felt that the conventional methods provided support to the muscles and joints but would sometimes restrict the range of motion (ROM), and in certain applications could limit, and potentially inhibit, the natural healing process. After extensive research, Dr Kase developed the Kinesio Taping® technique: a taping system that naturally assists in the healing of damaged tissue by encouraging lymphatic drainage and provides support to the joints and muscles without causing restriction to the ROM. This form of kinesiology taping was widely seen at the 1988 Seoul Olympics as 50,000 rolls of kinesiology tape were donated to 58 countries, which gave the taping product great exposure throughout the athletic world.

■ Kinesiology taping method (KTM)

The KTM is simply another 'tool' for the toolbox that can be used effectively in any sports- or non-sports-related setting. It is not a 'stand-alone' treatment for the shoulder complex as it is normally used in combination with other manual therapies such as soft tissue treatments, including muscle energy techniques (METs), myofascial techniques and joint mobilizations. Once this taping system has been thoroughly understood and practically applied, then, and only then, will it provide an adjunct to any treatment protocol to assist the overall well-being of patients and sporting athletes.

■ Kinesiology tape vs conventional athletic tape

Most types of athletic tape, especially the ones I will demonstrate in this chapter, have very little or no stretch because a lot of the taping techniques that are currently used on athletes are designed as a 'preventative' or even a 'true stability' measure: this method simply aims to limit specific injuries that are sustained in sport and to provide the necessary support and stability to the area it is applied to. In contrast, kinesiology tape is very elastic and can be stretched longitudinally up to 120–180% of its original

size. In addition, the thickness of kinesiology tape and its elasticity are considered similar to that of human skin.

When non-elastic athletic tape is applied to an injury, the rigidity of the tape can cause a restriction or it can even prevent movement of the taped area. This is desirable for moderate to severe injuries where immobilization is particularly necessary to prevent further damage. Most injuries, however, do not require full immobilization and this is where the flexibility of kinesiology tape comes into its own. Unlike conventional taping, KTM can therefore provide support to injured muscles and joints while still allowing a safe and pain-free range of motion, which enables patients and athletes to continue training or competing while they are in the recovery phase.

When conventional athletic tape is applied there is the possibility that circulation can be compromised, plus there is the issue of removing the tape after every sporting event. Kinesiology tape, on the other hand, can be worn for many days, providing support and therapeutic benefits '24/7'. In addition, this tape does not cause problems to the underlying tissues or restriction to the associated joint(s). Another benefit is that once kinesiology tape is removed it does not tend to leave any glue-like residue, again unlike some conventional athletic strapping and taping products.

Kaya et al. (2011) compared Kinesio Taping to physical therapy modalities for the treatment of shoulder impingement syndrome. They concluded that Kinesio Taping could be an alternative treatment option for shoulder impingement syndrome, especially when an immediate effect is needed.

Tape adhesion

Standard athletic tapes commonly have an adhesive applied to them called zinc oxide (Z/O) and this sometimes leaves a residue on the skin after removal. In addition, some patients have had an adverse reaction to this type of taping system. However, these techniques are still a very effective way of stabilizing areas and naturally still have a place in the taping sector, as will be demonstrated later in this chapter.

Most of the currently available kinesiology taping products have an acrylic-based adhesive that is normally latex free and hypoallergenic. The acrylic adhesive is much gentler on the skin than conventional athletic tape adhesive and seldom causes skin irritation or breakdown. It does not require the use of a protective under- or pre-wrap to prevent skin damage, and can be applied directly to the skin on any area of the body.

The acrylic adhesive is generally applied to the back of the kinesiology tape in a wave- like pattern that creates alternating areas of adhesive and non-adhesive so that moisture can escape easily from the taped area. In addition, the cotton fabric dries quickly so that kinesiology tape can be worn comfortably throughout showering and even swimming.

Even more importantly, it is felt that the alternating ridges of adhesive create a pressure differential in the tissues under the tape. In theory this will allow the tape to interact with pain receptors (nociceptors), blood vessels and the lymphatic system to assist in relieving pain and reducing the inflammation.

Types of kinesiology tape

Perhaps the main difference between kinesiology tape and other athletic tapes can be seen in the specific method of application. Conventional athletic tape is sometimes typically wrapped tightly around an injured area to promote stability (these techniques are not covered in this text) and in some cases athletic tape can be applied to provide immobility. However, kinesiology tape is applied over and around the contours of the muscles and the associated joints, and the amount of stretch applied to the tape can vary depending on the purpose of the application.

How to choose the right type of kinesiology tape

The company called Rocktape (whom I personally consider to be one of the leaders in the field) mention in their literature that there are essentially two types of tape: 'cheap and good tape'. Rocktape highly recommend avoiding cheap tape, as it tends to cause a skin reaction, often peels, and frays much faster than high-quality tape. As Rocktape suggests, I would avoid the cheaper and less known or tested products.

Personal recommendations

Rocktape® as you can probably guess is a company that I recommend highly and I use their products on all of my kinesiology courses as well as in the clinic at Oxford

and on all of the athletes and patients I treat for whom taping is appropriate. They have various kinesiology taping products on the market and I am a huge fan of their alternative designs and funky colors, and all without compromising the effectiveness of the tape.

Rocktape brand will be used throughout all of the kinesiology taping demonstrations within this chapter and it is possible to buy the tape directly from the company (www.rocktape.net).

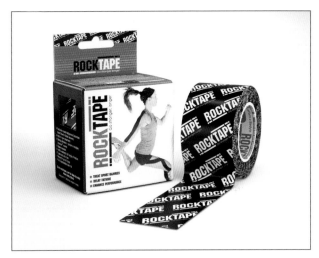

Figure 17.1: *Rocktape® brand*

Some features of Rocktape® (5m × 5cm)

- 180% stretch
- latex free and hypoallergenic
- water-resistant, especially the H20 version
- allows the skin to breathe
- ultra flexible and moldable to the body's contours
- thickness and weight of the tape is similar to that of human skin
- allows the natural joint and muscle ROM and does not restrict motion
- elastic properties to help support and reduce muscle fatigue
- helps assist the flow of lymphatic drainage
- can be worn for 3–5 days without re-application.

■ So how does kinesiology taping work?

Any type of injury or trauma to the body will set off the body's natural protective mechanism known as the inflammatory response (figure 17.2). The main identifiable signs of this response are: pain, swelling, heat and redness as well as restriction to the ROM.

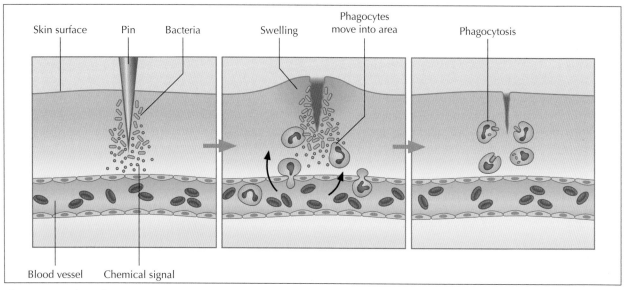

Figure 17.2: *The inflammatory process*

Kinesiology taping has been clinically shown to help with the natural response to inflammation as it targets different receptors within the somatosensory system. Correct application of KTMs helps alleviate pain and encourages the facilitation of lymphatic drainage by microscopically lifting the skin. This lifting effect helps create distortions in the skin, thus increasing interstitial space and allowing a decrease in the inflammatory process for affected areas (figure 17.3a&b).

As shown in figure 17.3, the underlying nerve endings, lymphatic vessels and blood vessels are in a state of 'compression' due to an injury. Any type of injury will cause an inflammation, as explained earlier, and this natural process will produce some form of swelling. One common type of swelling is a hematoma, and subsequent pressure will build up within the tissue. This naturally occurring process, with the increased pressure that is building up within the soft tissues, will start to irritate the nociceptors (pain receptors) and pain will be perceived. As I often quote during any of my taping courses, 'swelling causes pressure and pressure causes pain. To reduce the pain we have to reduce the pressure, and this is where specific kinesiology taping procedures can be utilized to assist in the reduction of the pressure that has built up within the soft tissues.' Other treatment methods can also be used at the same time as kinesiology taping, for example, ice packs and nonsteroidal anti-inflammatory drugs (NSAIDs).

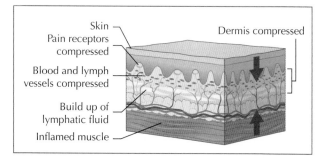

Figure 17.3a: *Cross-section of skin without tape applied*

As mentioned earlier, when kinesiology tape is applied to the skin it causes a 'lifting' or 'convolution' of the epidermis. This process is discussed by Capobianco and van den Dries (2009) in their book *Power Taping*, where the 'lifting' of the skin is referred to as the biomechanical lifting mechanism (BLM). They state that 'The BLM lifts the skin microscopically, which allows fluid to move more

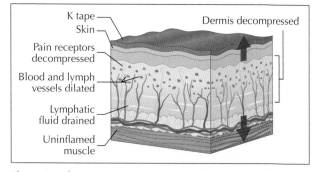

Figure 17.3b: *Cross-section of skin with tape applied*

freely. This allows more blood to flow into the injured area, thereby accelerating recovery and repair and also allows lymph fluid to more easily drain from the area, thus decreasing inflammation.' (See figure 17.3b for an example of this process.)

■ How to use and apply kinesiology tape

Kinesiology taping products tend to come in a standard size and length (normally 5cm × 5m). The therapist then decides on how and when to use this standard taping product as they will need to pre-cut the tape for the individual patient or athlete that visits the clinic. However, some kinesiology taping products come in an already pre-cut form, which in theory makes life a little bit easier. My preference is to pre-cut the size and shape of the tape myself at the time of the application.

A number of unique taping designs can be created from a single piece of tape (figure 17.4). It is very common, in all methods of kinesiology taping, to start with a single 'I' strip; for this the therapist will have decided on the specific length to use depending on the height, size and area of the athlete/patient. The standard sized 'I' strip can then be modified into a smaller version of the same strip or made into the shape of an 'X' by crossing over two smaller 'I' strips. The standard 'I' strip can also be made into a 'Y' shape or another specialized shape like a 'fan'. The 'fan' technique is generally used to help control lymphatic drainage. The direction and the amount of stretch applied to the kinesiology tape can also be changed at the time of application as this will be determined by the individual needs of the athlete/patient.

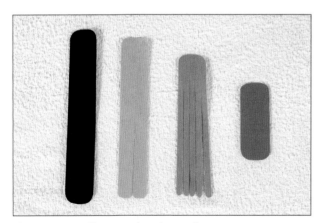

Figure 17.4: *Different styles of tape designs*

How much stretch to apply to the tape?

How much stretch should be applied to the kinesiology tape? This is a commonly asked question and there are some simple rules to follow:

Method 1: When applying the kinesiology tape to the patient, there is usually little to no stretch on the tape as the tissue of the patient has already been guided into a pre-stretched position prior to the application.

Method 2: Think of this as the 'decompression' strip or, in simpler terms, the 'pain relieving' strip. This tape can be applied with a range of 25–100% stretch, as this will help offload the specific area of pain.

The taping techniques described in this chapter show the variations in the amount of stretch that can be applied to the tape, i.e., ranging from 0% to 100%. However, there are many ways to apply kinesiology tape and I have had the good fortune of being able to modify some of the methods I was taught. In this chapter I will be demonstrating the techniques that currently work for me, based on my athletes and patients.

Rocktape have another saying: 'we believe there is no "right way" to tape for any given problem.' I am certain this is true. If you would like to see this in action you can watch, on YouTube, 15 different ways to apply kinesiology tape to the rotator cuff muscles and you will naturally wonder which technique of the 15 demonstrated is the correct one. Well, in theory, they all are correct, as the therapist that is applying the technique to the patient on the video is showing the technique that works for them in their clinic. I try to emphasize the following: it is the patient that will decide if the taping technique applied is working or not. The therapist will apply the kinesiology tape to patients in the way they were taught. However, you will need the necessary experience and underlying knowledge of functional anatomy to have the ability to change the technique to meet the individual demands of your athlete/patient.

Benefits of kinesiology taping

- Provides support for weak or injured muscles without affecting the normal ROM. This allows full participation in therapeutic exercises and/or sports training and minimizes the risk of developing compensatory imbalances or injuries.

- Can potentially activate muscles that have been weakened after injury or surgery, improving the quality of contractions and speeding up the recovery process.
- Stabilizes the area without restricting the movement like conventional athletic tape. The athlete and patient can remain active during the sport/ activity.
- Relaxes, and can offload, overused and overstrained muscles.
- Helps to reduce pain and edema by removal of lymphatic fluid.
- Helps correct postural imbalance and improves the ROM.
- Psychological benefits as well as a placebo effect.

Benefits of the uses for athletic taping

- Provides support to restrict the motion of an injured joint to provide a healing platform.
- Stabilizes joint ligaments and capsule by limiting excessive range of motion.
- Proven to be a preventative measure to reduce injuries in sport.
- Reduces the severity of injuries involved with most sports.
- Helps to manage chronic injuries.
- Helps to reduce swelling.
- Protects the injury from re-injury.

- Provides support for weak or injured muscles without affecting the range of motion in certain ranges.
- Helps to reduce pain and edema by assisting the removal of lymphatic fluid.

The two athletic taping products I have used consistently over many years (both in my practice at Oxford and for training purposes on my Bodymaster Method Masterclass) comes in a specially designed taping pack called *Tiger Tan Taping Kit* (figure 17.5). Within the kit you get one roll of Tiger Tan Tape (3.8cm × 13.7m) and one roll of Tiger Tape Fix (5cm × 10m). These can be purchased from a company called Physique Management (www.physique.co.uk).

I have used these particular tapes throughout each of the demonstrations in this book, as well as all the individual videos that are shown on YouTube.

Athletic taping helps correct postural imbalance and improves the ROM as discussed by Lewis et al. (2005), who used taping techniques to change the position of the scapula and thoracic spine and demonstrated an increase in shoulder motion in patients with or without shoulder symptoms.

Precautions/contraindications for all types of taping

Both kinesiology taping and standard athletic taping are generally safe for everyone, from the very young to the very old and from the very fit to the not so fit. It is a therapeutic taping technique not only offering athletes

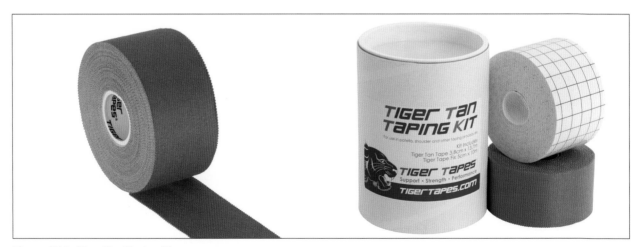

Figure 17.5: *Tiger Tan Taping Kit*

and patients the support they are looking for, but also enabling rehabilitation from their condition. Hence the athlete/patient can remain active throughout their sport or even their day-to-day activities. As with all types of taping methods, there are some precautions and potential contraindications you need to check before the application of the tape.

Precautions:
- allergic reactions to tape
- deep vein thrombosis and phlebitis
- axillary and popliteal areas as these body regions are sensitive
- local or distant sites of cancer
- fragile skin, e.g., in the elderly or with specific medical conditions
- skin healing in early phase.

Contraindications:
- infected areas of the skin
- dermatological conditions such as eczema and dermatitis
- cellulitis
- broken skin and wounds
- skin reactions to kinesiology or athletic tape.

■ Kinesiology and athletic taping applications

There are many different ways of applying kinesiology and athletic tape. I think it is best to stick to some simple rules and once one process has been learned it can then be adapted according to the needs of the athlete/patient.

General rules before application
- Always check for a history of allergies to tape adhesives.
- Cleanse the skin of any oil, cream or massage wax and trim hair if needed (especially if applying athletic tape).
- Measure and cut the tape into the size and shape required.
- Round off the corners at the end of each tape (kinesiology tape only) to prevent it from lifting/peeling.

With kinesiology tape, never stretch the ends of the tape and leave between 2 and 3 cm of tape at each end that will remain unstretched. Leaving no stretch at the ends of the kinesiology tape will avoid a 'shearing' type of tension to

the skin and will limit any potential for irritation, as the tape is normally kept on for at least a few days.

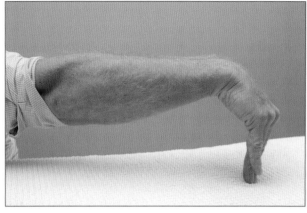

Figure 17.6: *Forearm extensors in a 'pre-stretch' position*

During application pre-stretch (K-tape)
Before the kinesiology tape is applied to the area that is injured, guide and place the soft tissue of your athlete/patient, e.g., the muscle, into a position that will cause the tissue to be naturally stretched (figure 17.6). Please bear in mind that the patient is normally presenting with some type of pain or swelling, so only go as far as required until the patient is aware of the stretch and not to the point of discomfort.

Tape application/stabilizing technique
Before applying the kinesiology tape, expose the adhesive side of the tape so that it can be attached to the specific body area. It is natural to want to 'peel off' the backing from the tape; however, this process is not needed as the tape can simply be 'torn' across one of the squares. This tearing will not damage the kinesiology tape as only the backing will be removed.

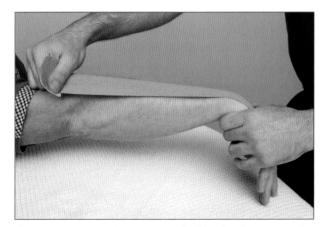

Figure 17.7: *Kinesiology tape applied by the therapist to the forearm, with little to no stretch of the tape*

Apply a prepared 'I' or 'Y' strip to the pre-stretched tissue of the body, with little to no stretch of the tape on first application. This technique will help stabilize the area (figure 17.7).

Pain offload application/decompression strip

- The kinesiology tape (normally an 'X', 'Y' or a smaller 'I' strip) can be stretched between 25% and 100% of its original length. This type of application is commonly known as the *pain relieving strip* or *decompression strip* and is applied directly over the presenting area of pain.

- If using a small 'I' strip or a small 'X' strip then it is easier to rip the backing off the tape by starting from the center of the tape, rather than starting from one end as would be the case for a longer 'I' strip. Once the center has been split, peel back each end of the backing strip from the tape, and fold over the ends that have no stretch (similar to applying a plaster for a cut on the skin) (figure 17.8).

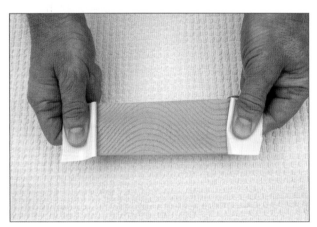

Figure 17.8: *A stretch of 50% is applied to the center of the kinesiology tape by using the thumbs*

- Once the ends have been folded over each other, the appropriate stretch is then applied to the center of the kinesiology tape.

- The decompression strip of kinesiology tape, with the appropriate stretch added, is then applied to the specific area of pain (figure 17.9).

Once the kinesiology tape has been applied to the area, it then needs to be heat activated to stimulate the acrylic adhesive on the back of the tape that adheres to the skin. Do this not with artificial heat but by rubbing the tape either with your hand or with a piece of the backing tape that was removed from the kinesiology tape (figure 17.10).

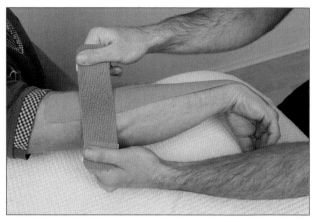

Figure 17.9: *The decompression strip is applied to the area of pain*

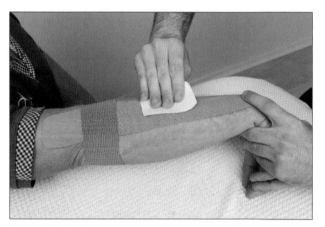

Figure 17.10: *Kinesiology tape applied by rubbing the area to generate heat and activate the glue*

The colored 'stars' and letters

For each of the individual kinesiology taping demonstrations I have placed some colored stars on specific areas of the body that relate directly to the pain that a patient might present with. I find this extremely beneficial, especially while lecturing to manual therapy students about the skills of kinesiology taping, as the application of a sticker enables accurate kinesiology taping.

Regarding the letters, S and F, they relate to the following; S = start; F = finish; and the directional arrow indicates the direction of the tape.

Once the area of presenting pain has been located, then simply apply a sticker or mark the area as an exact guide as to where the kinesiology tape should be applied (figure 17.11). Once the area is identified, preparation of the kinesiology tape can commence and the tape applied accordingly.

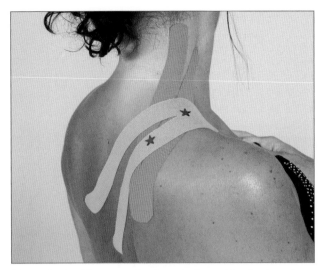

Figure 17.11: *The area of pain as indicated by the 'stars'*

■ Kinesiology taping techniques

Technique 1

Rotator cuff tendinopathy: supraspinatus, bursitis and infraspinatus pain

Hsu et al. (2009) investigated the effect of Kinesio Taping on shoulder impingement syndrome in baseball players. They found that the activation of the lower fibers of the trapezius, when returning the arm from a scapulohumeral rhythm, increased during the 60–30 degree lowering phase of the arm.

The following taping techniques can be modified depending on the soft tissue that is presenting the pain. As

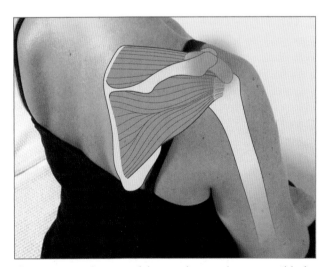

Figure 17.12: *Three painful areas that can be responsible for a patient's pain*

an example, if the patient has localized pain to the anterior aspect of the shoulder then it might be a supraspinatus tendinopathy that is the problem. Pain inferior to the acromion could well be a subacromial bursa, and pain posterior to the greater tubercle of the humerus might indicate an issue with the infraspinatus muscle, especially if this patient is a swimmer. Figure 17.12 shows the three potential areas of pain that relate to the shoulder as mentioned above.

The first technique is applied to help offload the deltoid muscle. If any shoulder issues are present then this technique is generally done first. Apply a 'Y' strip from the deltoid tuberosity, place the anterior deltoid into a stretched position and apply one tail of the tape to the anterior deltoid. Then place the posterior deltoid into a stretch and apply the second tail of the tape to the posterior deltoid, with little to no stretch (figure 17.13).

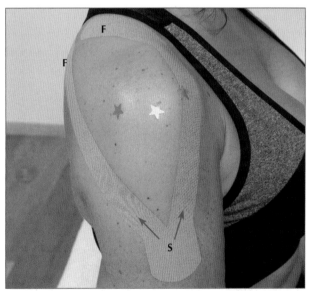

Figure 17.13: *First application is used to offload the deltoid muscle*

Ask the patient to place their hand onto their lower back, as this will stretch the supraspinatus and the infraspinatus muscles. Apply a 'Y' strip from the area of pain: start at the anterior aspect of the shoulder to cover the supraspinatus, the inferior aspect of the acromion for the bursa, and the posterior aspect of the greater tubercle of the humerus for the infraspinatus (figure 17.14). Each tail of the tape is applied with 50–75% stretch. You can also ask the patient to retract their shoulder slightly as this will enhance its position prior to the application of the tape.

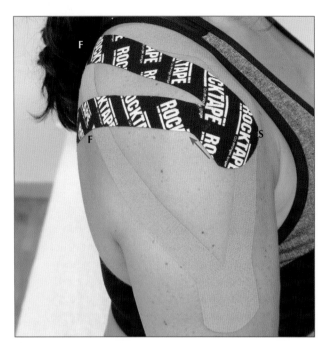

Figure 17.14: *Second application to cover the specific area of pain*

Heat activate the tape.

Technique 2

Acromioclavicular joint (ACJ) sprain

When I was a physical therapist working with a rugby team, sprains of the acromioclavicular joint (ACJ) were a regular occurrence, almost to the point that I would

see some type of injury to this joint at almost every training session and game. As rugby is a contact game, subluxations/sprains from this sport are regularly seen by physical therapists (figure 17.15). However, ACJ sprains are not exclusive to rugby as most sports can, at some point, involve this joint.

This area is tricky to treat as the patient finds it difficult to rest the shoulder – even getting dressed requires movement from this part of the body, not to mention the

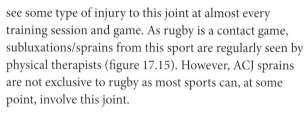

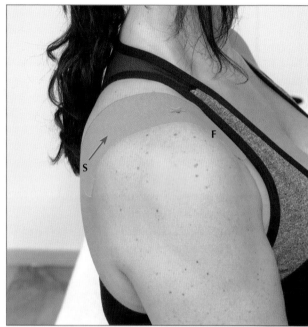

Figure 17.16: *First application of an 'I' strip across the ACJ*

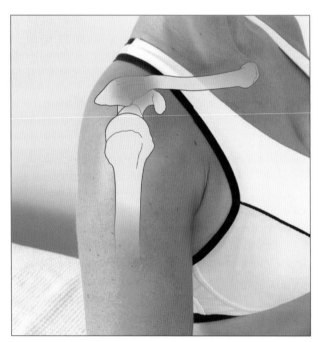

Figure 17.15: *ACJ sprain*

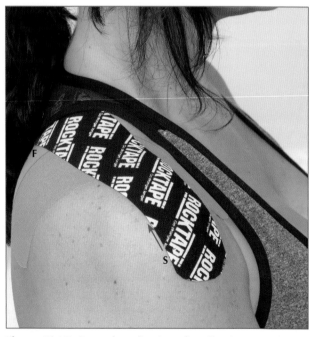

Figure 17.17: *Second application of an 'I' strip across the ACJ*

fact that athletes like to keep active. Hence, the following kinesiology taping technique is a perfect option as it assists the healing mechanism.

Place the patient's arm by their side so that there is no stretch applied to the ACJ. Apply a standard 'I' strip across the ACJ with 75–100% stretch of the tape (figure 17.16).

Apply a second standard 'I' strip with 75–100% stretch (figure 17.17).

Apply a third standard 'I' strip with 75–100% stretch (figure 17.18).

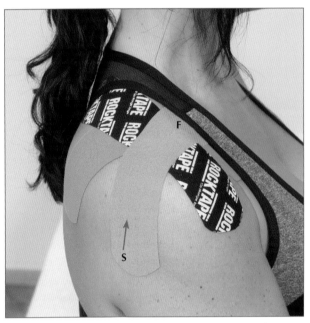

Figure 17.18: *Third application of an 'I' strip across the ACJ*

Heat activate the tape.

Technique 3

Biceps: long head

Fratocchi et al. (2012) conducted a study to see if Kinesio Taping applied over the biceps brachii influenced isokinetic elbow peak torque. They concluded that there was indeed an increase in the concentric elbow peak torque for a group of healthy subjects.

Pain at the anterior aspect of the shoulder, as mentioned earlier, could be coming from the supraspinatus tendon. However, it could also be a tendinopathy of the long head of the biceps as this structure originates from the supraglenoid tubercle, penetrates through the shoulder structures, continues through the bicipital groove, and

finally attaches to the radius and the bicipital aponeurosis (figure 17.19). Ruptures of the long head are relatively common in men over 45 years. This is known as a 'Popeye' arm as the rupture causes recoil and subsequently gives the appearance of an increased lump when the biceps is contracted.

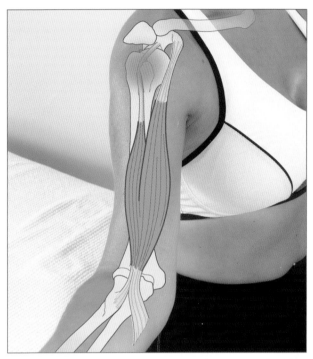

Figure 17.19: *Bicipital tendinopathy of the long head of the biceps*

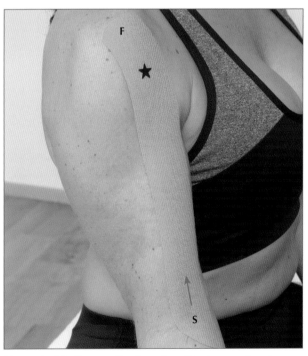

Figure 17.20: *First application of an 'I' strip covering the long head of the biceps*

Place the biceps muscle into a stretched position and apply an 'I' strip, with little to no stretch, starting from the insertion point on the radius. The tape is applied towards the origin of the long head of biceps (figure 17.20).

Apply a smaller than standard 'I' strip with 50–75% stretch across the area of pain (figure 17.21).

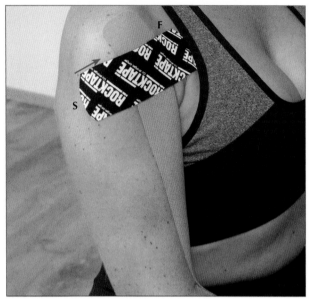

Figure 17.21: *Second application of a small 'I' strip across the area of pain*

Heat activate the tape.

Technique 4

Mid-thoracic and rhomboid pain
Karatas et al. (2011) found, through their study of surgeons presenting with musculoskeletal pain, that Kinesio Taping made a significant improvement to the range of motion (ROM) of the cervical spine as well as providing a reduction in pain. They concluded that Kinesio Taping would be an effective method for reducing neck and lower back pain and improving cervical and lumbar ROM and functional performance.

Pain that presents itself to the mid-thoracic region between the shoulder blades (scapulae) is possibly due to a strain of either the rhomboid or the lower trapezius muscle (figure 17.22). The pain may also be referred and potentially coming from the lower cervical spine. It is also essential to consider a rib or the thoracic spine dysfunction as part of the differential diagnosis. Rarely, the symptoms might also suggest an issue from the lungs and the intercostal muscles.

Many patients that come to the clinic have postural issues so that the mid-thoracic muscles are continually on stretch; this could be due to the shortened and tight antagonistic (opposite) muscles of the pectoralis major and minor. Treatment should include some muscle lengthening techniques of the pectorals rather than just treating where it hurts – remember 'where the pain is the problem is not' (Ida Rolf).

Kinesiology taping for this type of condition is an excellent adjunct to the treatment program as it makes the patient aware of their posture and more inclined to do the recommended exercises.

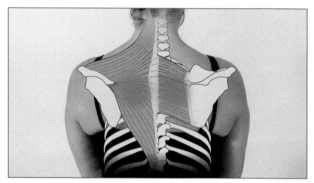

Figure 17.22: *Mid-thoracic muscles (rhomboids and trapezius)*

Place the mid-trunk into flexion and ask the patient to protract their shoulders so that the mid-thoracic muscles are on stretch. Apply two standard 'I' strips, starting one at a time, from the upper trapezius. Continue caudally along the erector spinae muscles with 50–75% stretch to each strip (figure 17.23).

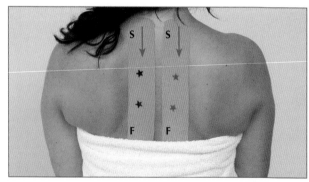

Figure 17.23: *First application of two 'I' strips lengthways between the shoulder blades*

Apply two standard 'I' strips across the mid-thoracic region between the shoulder blades and with 50–75% stretch to each strip (figure 17.24).

Heat activate the tape.

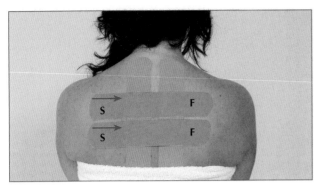

Figure 17.24: *Second application of two 'I' strips between the shoulder blades*

Technique 5

Levator scapulae/upper trapezius strain

González-Iglesias et al. (2009) conducted the study 'Short-term effects of cervical Kinesio Taping on pain and cervical ROM in patients with acute whiplash injury'. They concluded that when patients presented with acute whiplash-associated conditions, kinesiology taping exhibited statistically significant improvements immediately following application and at a 24-hour follow-up period.

At the superior angle of the scapula is the attachment of the levator scapulae muscle; therefore, one might presume

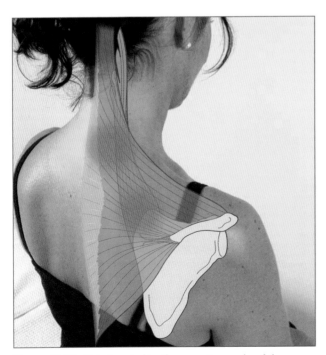

Figure 17.25: *Pain located to the superior angle of the scapulae and a strain of the upper trapezius muscle*

when a patient presents with pain to this area that the muscle is the problem. I agree that this muscle might be part of the whole picture of the patient's symptoms, but one must also consider what other structures may be involved; these have already been covered in earlier chapters (figure 17.25).

Place the levator scapulae on stretch by lateral flexion and rotating the neck to the opposite side from the pain. Apply one 'I' strip from the origin of the levator scapulae (C1–4), inferiorly towards the superior scapula, with little to no stretch of the tape (figure 17.26).

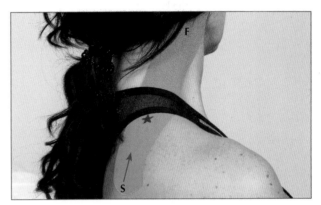

Figure 17.26: *First application to the levator scapulae muscle*

For the upper trapezius, ask the patient to laterally flex their cervical spine to the opposite side of the pain. Apply the second 'I' strip starting from the base of the occipital bone and continue to the insertion point onto the clavicle with little to no stretch (figure 17.27).

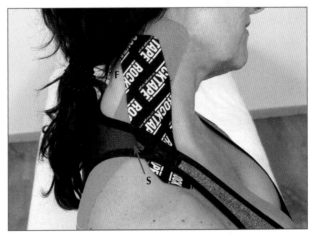

Figure 17.27: *Second application to the trapezius muscle*

Heat activate the tape.

Technique 6

Postural taping

This technique probably goes against the kinesiology philosophy because we are asking the patient to shorten the muscles rather than placing them on a pre-stretch position; however, I think it is justified, as it seems to provide better control for the patient's posture.

Ask the patient to sit on a couch and then to slightly retract and depress the scapula. Apply one piece of K-tape with 50–75% stretch from just above the right supraclavicular fossa to the left side of the trunk and repeat the same process to the opposite side (figure 17.28) so that they cross in the midline of the body.

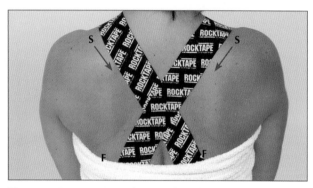

Figure 17.28: *K-tape application from left and right supraclavicular fossa to the lower trunk with 50–75% stretch*

An alternative technique, rather than tape left to right (opposite) and vice versa, is to actually tape the same side, from the trapezius to the lower back (figure 17.29). Some patients prefer this method of postural taping.

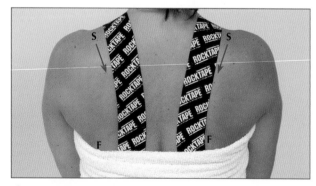

Figure 17.29: *K-tape application from same side trapezius to the lower back (same side) 50–75% stretch*

■ Athletic taping techniques for the shoulder and cervical complex

For the demonstrations outlined below it is very common to use using two taping products, one is a zinc oxide-based tape called Leukotape, or in this case I will be using a similar product called Tiger Tan Tape, and the other is a micropore type called Fixomull or Hypafix, and again for these demonstrations it is called Tiger Tape Fix. The idea of the two taping product system is that the white porous tape acts as a barrier to protect the skin and the brown tape is applied directly over the white porous tape because if the brown zinc oxide tape is applied and left on the skin for many hours, or sometimes even days, this this can cause a skin reaction.

Before we apply tape to the patient we can *test-tape-retest*. I am sure you can work out what I mean by that statement. We simply ask the patient to abduct and/or flex their shoulder as far as they comfortably can and we observe the range of motion that is possible. We also ask our patient to inform us when they feel any pain during the movement. The therapist then applies the tape as outlined below and retests the specific motion to see if the range of motion has improved and the perception of pain has reduced.

The following athletic taping techniques are very different from the previous kinesiology taping techniques, even though they might be considered related in one respect because they are treating the same presenting shoulder pathology. However, kinesiology taping generally allows motion, while athletic taping, due to its limited stretch capabilities, will naturally feel more restrictive to the patient in terms of joint motion. However, the patient will probably mention that the joint feels more stable than with the kinesiology taping method.

Pain off-load techniques

I consider the following athletic taping demonstrations will help re-position some of the components of the shoulder complex to assist in 'off-loading' the presenting pain, which then potentially allows the patient to perform their normal daily tasks within a pain free zone. These techniques can also be though of as 'stabilizing' techniques.

Technique 1 – shoulder impingement syndrome

The patient is normally sitting and they are asked to place their painful arm in a position of external rotation. Apply one micropore strip from the anterior inferior aspect of the humeral head to the midpoint of the scapula (figure 17.30).

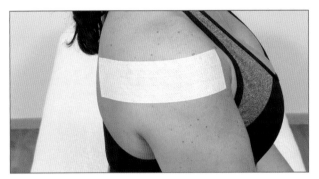

Figure 17.30: *Micropore application from anterior humerus to mid scapula*

Ask the patient to maintain this position of external rotation and then apply the second strip, in this case the brown Tiger Tan Tape, and apply the tape with tension directly over the first piece of white tape, with no direct contact to the skin. If the tape has been applied correctly you will notice a puckering of the white tape that is lying underneath (figure 17.31).

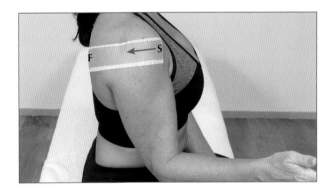

Figure 17.31: *Application of the Tiger Tan Tape*

Technique 2 – glenohumeral multidirectional instability

Ask the patient to stand or sit and place the right arm in a relaxed position. Apply one micropore strip from the anterior inferior aspect of the humeral head to the superior part of the scapula as shown. Apply the second micropore strip from the posterior inferior aspect of the humeral head to superior part of the clavicle. Apply the

third micropore strip from the lateral inferior aspect of the humeral head (near the deltoid tuberosity) and finish just above the AC joint (figure 17.32).

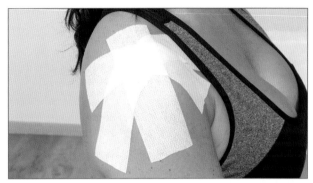

Figure 17.32: *Three applications of the micropore to the glenohumeral joint*

Ask the patient to maintain this position and now the therapist has to gently control the position of the humerus with their right hand and stabilize the acromion with their

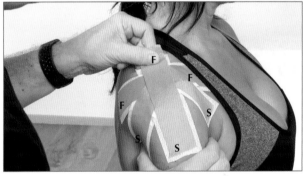

Figure 17.33: *The therapist controls the humeral position, while applying the Tiger Tan Tape*

left hand (figure 17.33). From this position, the therapist glides the humerus superiorly into the glenoid fossa and applies each strip of the Tiger Tan Tape in turn over the three white micropore tapes with no direct contact to the skin. If the tape has been applied correctly you will notice

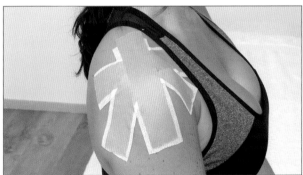

Figure 17.34: *Three applications of the Tiger Tan Tape*

a puckering of the white tape that is lying underneath (figure 17.34).

Technique 3 – acromioclavicular (AC) joint sprain

Ask the patient to stand or sit and place the right arm in a relaxed position. Apply one micropore strip from the anterior inferior aspect of the humeral head and across the AC joint to finish at the superior part of the scapula. Apply the second micropore strip from the posterior inferior aspect of the humeral head and across the AC joint and finish at the superior part of the clavicle. Apply the third micropore strip from the lateral inferior aspect of the humeral head (near the deltoid tuberosity), again crossing the AC joint, and finish just above the joint (figure 17.35).

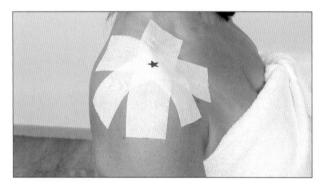

Figure 17.35: *Three applications of the micropore to the acromioclavicular joint*

Ask the patient to maintain this position and now the therapist has to gently control the position of the humerus and stabilize the clavicle and AC joint. From this position, the therapist glides the humerus superiorly as this motion will encourage a closing of the right AC joint. The therapist then applies each strip of the Tiger Tan Tape in turn over the three white micropore tapes with no direct contact to the skin. If the tape has been applied correctly

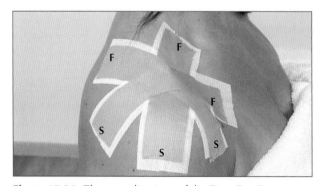

Figure 17.36: *Three applications of the Tiger Tan Tape*

you will notice a puckering of the white tape that is lying underneath (figure 17.36).

Technique 4 – postural taping

Ask the patient to slightly retract and depress the scapula. Apply one micropore strip from just above the right supraclavicular fossa to the lower thoracic spine and repeat the same process to the left side (figure 17.37).

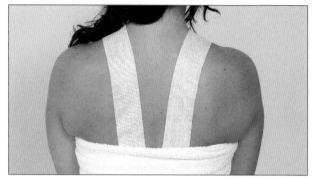

Figure 17.37: *Micropore application from left and right supraclavicular fossa to the lower thoracic spine*

Ask the patient to maintain this position of scapula retraction and depression and then apply the Tiger Tan Tape with tension directly over the two pieces of white micropore tape, with no direct contact to the skin. Again, if the tape has been applied correctly you will notice a puckering of the white tape that is lying underneath (figure 17.38).

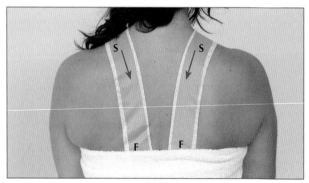

Figure 17.38: *Two applications of the Tiger Tan Tape*

18

Rehabilitation and exercise protocols for the shoulder complex

This final chapter examines various options for rehabilitative exercises for the upper limb and specifies exercises that focus on the shoulder complex; however, as you continue reading it will become obvious that some of the exercises I have included are related to the inner and outer core, which, in the grand scheme, helps the overall function and stability of the shoulder complex, which in reality is a bonus.

When I teach exercise concepts to students of physical therapy, I discuss with them many examples of patients who have visited my clinic. I ask students to look at whatever the problem is as simply as they can, rather than making it complex, and to ask themselves 'what is the primary goal or objective for the patient with this type of presentation?' Often within a few seconds, someone will say something like 'to improve the patient's mobility', and someone else will say 'to reduce their pain.' We, as therapists, try our best to improve the function of the shoulder joint by focusing on mobility exercises (as well as other protocols), either active by the patient or passive by the therapist, or a combination of both, and this in turn will hopefully have the desired effect of reducing any painful symptoms.

In this chapter we will partly be discussing mobility exercises as well as a multitude of other rehabilitation protocols. But let us look at another aim: if, say, a patient has dislocated their shoulder a few weeks ago, perhaps while playing rugby, and they are nervous or apprehensive about participating in their chosen sport, then the simple

primary goal is to stabilize. We can do this by focusing on specific strengthening protocols. Again, in this chapter we will look at stability with the use of strengthening exercises.

Think back to the earlier chapter on METs in which I discuss in some detail that one should lengthen the short and tight agonist muscles before considering strengthening the lengthened and weak antagonistic muscles. That needs to be remembered because if you only focus on strengthening the weak muscles then I can assure you that the weak muscles of the shoulder *will not* improve their strength until the short antagonistic (opposite) muscles have been lengthened. The METs (if performed correctly) will enable this lengthening process to occur. They have already been covered in a previous chapter but this chapter includes some self-help MET lengthening exercises that one can do anytime of the day (see the end of the chapter). These can be used prior to strengthening, as the specific movements will encourage normal length of the soft tissues of the shoulder complex. Because you are actively contracting the muscles and then moving the limb, these techniques can act as part of the warm-up prior to your normal exercise routines. So basically, in this chapter, I will be focusing on *functional* protocols that will include *mobility, stability, strengthening* as well as some exercises for *self-lengthening*.

These concepts naturally overlap, of course. If we are focusing on a particular exercise motion of the shoulder, let's say a standing push (see below), then this movement will be activating the anterior oblique sling musculature, but obviously we will also use the following muscles: pectoralis major, anterior deltoid, and triceps, as this movement of the push is similar to a single arm bench press motion and will be *strengthening* the muscles that have been mentioned. And because the motion is *functional* and is related to day-to-day activities, then the overall *stability* of the shoulder complex will greatly improve. The antagonistic muscles to the push motion (posterior deltoid and infraspinatus) will naturally be going through a lengthening phase to allow the push motion because another of the primary rehabilitation goals will be trying to achieve a full range of motion. At the same time the thoracic spine is rotating as part of the exercise, because of the combined movements, we will be improving the overall *mobility* of not just the shoulder complex but other areas of the body as well. By giving you an example of one functional movement pattern exercise (standing push), we can see that this one specific motion can almost fulfil all the necessary requirements of the rehabilitation program, we are achieving all of that through one simple exercise, without us actually realizing it.

Many people attend a gym to exercise, and that can be for many reasons, for example, weight loss or to strengthen and tone their bodies. Some might exercise to promote healing and speed up the recovery of a specific injury. However, the exercises I have observed in gyms around the world are frequently non-functional as they are biased towards frontal-plane or sagittal-plane types of exercise: people either lift a weight to the sides (frontal plane) of their body or to the front (sagittal plane) of their body. For the region of the shoulder complex, there is nothing wrong at all with these types of exercises, because they will strengthen certain muscle groups; however, it would make more sense to try and make the exercises more functional to daily activities and also movements relating to sports-specific activities such as tennis, golf or running.

Let me give you an example. If one were to ask these individuals to demonstrate an exercise to train their *core*, and also to perform that specific exercise in the transverse plane (rotation), I am sure that after some thought they would probably lie on their back and perform an abdominal crunch type of motion with a rotation; in other words, their elbow would be directed toward their opposite knee while performing the crunch movement, as shown in figure 18.1.

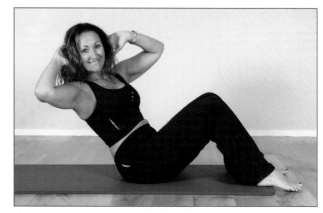

Figure 18.1: *Abdominal curl in the transverse plane*

Just think about this motion for a minute and let us be a little realistic here, because, apart from when we get out of bed in the morning, when do we ever perform that type of motion on a daily basis? When do we ever lie on our back and rotate the elbow toward the opposite knee? I remember doing these exercises every day as a young man in basic training in the military and even then I did not think they were very relevant to, say, shooting a rifle; then again, we didn't have a choice so we just did whatever we were told to do. If the sergeant major said *jump*, our answer was to simply say *how high* and nothing else!

The abdominal exercise demonstrated above is what I would call *non-functional*, even though the majority of gym users routinely perform this exercise for their *core* muscles every day in their personal exercise routines.

If you think about it, most sporting movements, or simply walking and running come to that, involve some type of action through the shoulder complex and especially in the *transverse plane* (movement across the body) of motion. Does it not make perfect sense, therefore, to train specifically within the parameters of the transverse plane, in combination with training in the sagittal (coronal) and frontal planes?

■ Movement-based exercise

To have a strong, stable and effective functional shoulder complex we need to have a strong inner and outer core unit. The inner core unit musculature is generally made up of postural (tonic) muscle types that function mainly as stabilizers. These inner core muscles effectively stabilize the spine and sacroiliac joint at low levels of muscular contraction, with a low susceptibility to fatigue. Coordination of the inner core is critical for proper stabilization, especially for the shoulder complex, which then allows a coordinated recruitment of the muscles of the outer core unit. The ability of the inner core unit muscles to contract prior to force production by the phasic muscles (biased toward movements) is actually considered more important than their inherent strength.

The outer core unit is mainly a phasic system, with large muscles that have the ability, because of the fact that they are very well orientated, to produce enough force to subsequently propel the body forward. The outer core, consisting of the four myofascial slings, also plays a very important role in stabilization of the pelvis, as all of the four individual sling systems mentioned earlier cross and naturally assist in force closure of the sacroiliac joint (SIJ), which then ultimately provides a stable base for the shoulder complex.

We need the inner and outer core units to function synergistically to: (1) stabilize the body; and (2) create powerful and economic movement. Without efficient functioning of the inner unit there is no stability of the spine and SIJs and this will have a direct influence to the upper limb and more importantly the shoulder complex. Moreover, the core will not be able to provide a stable base of contraction for the phasic muscles (outer core) to contract, which can result in a loss of upper limb power and a reduced economy of movement patterns, as well as an increased susceptibility to musculoskeletal overuse injuries.

A well-conditioned inner core unit is very dependent on strong outer core unit systems, and vice versa, in order to protect the smaller inner unit muscles, the spinal ligaments, and the associated joints of the spine and pelvis.

Let me try to explain this concept with the following example. I have been fortunate to work with the Oxford University rowing teams for many years. The motion of rowing is very much biased towards specific movements from the shoulder complex as well as other areas of the body. When the crew have been rowing on very flat and calm lakes and rivers, the outer core unit (i.e., the phasic muscles) is doing most of the work to propel the boat through the water, and the inner core unit is relatively relaxed in comparison. When they finish rowing, I always ask them how they feel (in terms of their shoulders, lower back and pelvis, etc.). Most of the time there are no reports of musculoskeletal issues. However, it is a different story when they row on the River Thames in London. This river can be very unpredictable – one minute the water is particularly choppy and the next it is calm. The Thames is tidal fed from the sea, which alters

the tone of the water; in addition, passing motorboats produce waves that can also affect the flow and manner of the water. Because of these variable circumstances, if the river appears rougher than usual, then I consider the inner core unit to be working a lot harder than normal, because it has to stabilize each of the individual rowers in their seats. Moreover, the inner core unit is trying to stabilize the rowing boat to prevent it from tilting from side to side, while at the same time the outer core unit is still being utilized to propel the boat forward. At the end of the training session, probably around half of them need to see me for treatment to help reduce the musculoskeletal symptoms that they are experiencing.

In order to have a strong outer core unit, and subsequent shoulder complex, it is paramount that the inner core unit be stabilized first. Most of the rowers know a bit about core stability training, and some have done one or two exercises before, mainly abdominal trunk curls and planks (two exercises that I typically classify as *non-functional* and definitely not effective for the inner core – hence not recommended). During the times I have been involved in their training, I have tried to make the inner core training fun, as these exercises are generally not appealing to a bunch of young rowers who are used to doing only bench presses, squats and lunges.

For example, I would get all the team (eight in this case, or nine including the cox) to sit on gym balls in a straight line, one behind the other, facing the same way – except for the cox at the end, who would sit facing them. While sitting on the ball, they would then place their feet on the ball in front and try to maintain stability by using their inner core muscles, which is especially challenging, as the feet are now lifted off the floor.

The idea of this exercise was to mimic sitting in a boat on water. From this position, each team member had to keep the line of eight rowers (nine including cox) stable by activating his or her inner core muscles. Once this had been achieved, we would then try to mimic the motion of rowing and focus on good technique while still sitting on the gym balls. Apart from being fun, this is a great way of activating the inner core muscles without having to think about the processes involved.

This exercise is just one example that emphasizes to the team *why* training the inner core unit is every bit as important as training the outer core unit. The mentality of many athletes I have come into contact with is to train only the muscles they can see and not the ones that they cannot.

Note: For this text, I have not included many inner core exercise explanations or demonstrations, as I feel it is not within the scope of this book. The reason for this is mainly that I wanted to focus my attention on training and stabilizing the shoulder complex. There are numerous books available that offer specific inner core activation exercises, so I would suggest that you consult one of them. I have discussed here only briefly some of the inner core exercises that I have incorporated into the rowing training program – my current strategy is to train the rowers' inner core muscles without them actually being aware that they are training them!

With regards to functional types of exercise, movement patterns must be identified and resistance applied to those patterns in a specific way. This is what resistance training is all about – resisting movements but trying to do it in a functional way.

If specific movements performed by patients and athletes on a daily basis can be identified, these can be replicated by using some form of resistance training, thereby creating a stability protocol. This stability protocol will be further enhanced if these movements can be performed at a speed of contraction that mimics their daily functions. This will not only improve levels of overall fitness but will also promote force closure of the pelvis, and subsequently promote a stable foundation for the shoulder complex. Each exercise will now have a direct purpose and function, instead of just increasing the size of the cross-sectional area of a particular muscle.

Before embarking on any training program, especially for the shoulder complex (and this is also true for the outer and inner core), it is important to understand the meanings of the words 'rep' and 'set.'

Repetitions and sets

Definition: A *repetition* (or *rep*) is one complete motion of an exercise. A *set* is a group of consecutive repetitions.

You may have heard someone comment that they performed, for example, three sets of 10 reps on the shoulder press machine. This means that they did 10 consecutive shoulder presses, had a break (rest), and then repeated the process a further two times.

There is no simple answer to the question of how many repetitions and sets should be performed, as the number of repetitions required depends on many factors, including where the patient/athlete is in their current training and what their individual goals are. Remember, the purpose of

this book/chapter is to improve the optimum functionality and stability of the shoulder complex through activation of the outer core unit so that your patient/athlete can perform the activities needed for everyday life, as well as participate in any sports-related activities. I suggest we aim for between 10 and 12 reps and between one and two sets of each exercise, at least to start with.

Please also remember that, as with any training program, the workouts will need to be progressive. For example, let us say the patient/athlete starts with two or three exercises that I have chosen from the primary movement patterns, and they perform two sets of 10 reps for each exercise; when the patient gets to the stage where they find these exercises to be relatively easy, it is then time to progress. This might happen after one week or it might take longer, perhaps three or four weeks. The exercise can be made more difficult by simply changing the number of repetitions, reducing the rest period between sets, adding in another exercise, or changing the resistance of the band (another color), as shown in figure 18.2. For example, the green band is level 1 (easy), the blue band is level 2 (moderate), and the black band is level 3 (hard).

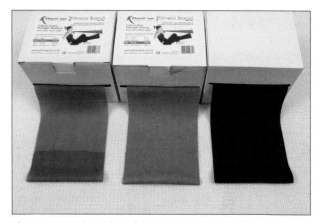

Figure 18.2: *The color of the exercise band indicates the level of resistance*

To progress in the program, you could, for example, ask the patient to either increase the number of repetitions, i.e., perform two sets of 12 reps (instead of 10 reps), or rest for only 30 seconds (instead of 45 seconds) between the sets. I highly recommend that everything be written down, as it is very easy to forget what was done in the previous training session – trust me on this! I can guarantee that within a few weeks the patient/athlete will easily be doing three sets of 12–15 reps for six or seven different types of the functional exercises.

The following exercises do not specify the number of repetitions and sets next to the exercise diagram, as I want to demonstrate how to perform the individual exercises correctly. Refer to Appendix 2 at the end of the book for an 'Exercise Stabilization Sheet' for the shoulder complex; it has been designed specifically for you to photocopy and give out to your athletes and patients (or even for your own personal use). The blank boxes allow you to record the number of repetitions and sets for your patient's rehabilitation program for the pelvis.

Unfortunately, there are a multitude (indeed, an almost infinite number) of movements that are performed in everyday life, making it near impossible to ensure that they are all included in every gym-based training program. However, I have selected the following seven exercises, which can be incorporated into any strength and stability training regime and not just for the shoulder complex but for all areas of the body, as they will specifically target the global muscles of the outer core sling system.

■ Primary movement patterns for the shoulder complex

The following exercises are what I consider to be the primary movement patterns, especially for the shoulder complex, and one or more of these demonstrated exercises could be included in any functional, strength, or stability-training program, especially for functionality of the upper limb. The therapist/trainer should nevertheless be able to modify and adapt these primary movement exercise patterns accordingly (I will explain later in this chapter). This adaptability protocol will make the exercises far more functional, as well as being more interesting and specific to the needs and demands of your athletes and patients.

Through experience you will find that certain patients and even athletes will be unable to start at this point in the chapter of the primary movements. That can be for many reasons, mainly pain and restriction, so you will need to understand the needs and requirements for every person that presents with shoulder pain. We are all different in one way or another so each exercise program has to be tailored individually. The therapist will need to look at other rehabilitative protocols first, such as the exercises on mobility as a starting point. I always say that we are all on a 'ladder' system and some of us, in terms of say strength, stability or flexibility, are near the top while others are near the bottom. This is unimportant as long as the exercises are designed to allow the person to continue reaching up and to naturally progress rather than reaching

down and regressing. If they can do this then it is a win–win situation.

Some of the exercises I mention will activate one particular outer core sling more than another and this also applies to certain musculature; remember, however, that there is a natural crossover on each of the movement patterns, so it is difficult to exercise and target only one specific sling or muscle group at a time. This is because all of the four slings I have mentioned have to be involved in one way or another, depending on the particular movement one is performing. For example, the anterior (standing push) and posterior (standing pull) oblique sling will be classified as agonist and antagonist (opposite to each other); however, I consider them to be also synergists (helpers to each other), because when you throw a ball, walk or run in a forward direction, the right arm moves in a forward motion, subsequently activating the anterior oblique sling, but at the same time the left arm moves in a backward type of motion, activating the posterior oblique sling. Hence the opposite and synergistic theory!

I believe the theory above is explained very well by the following:

> *'When walking, running or throwing, every forward motion of the right limb elicits an automatic backward motion of the left limb, and vice versa. You cannot have one movement without the other.'*

The seven primary movement pattern exercises are:

1. standing push
2. standing pull
3. curl with press
4. horizontal press
5. shoulder rotation – internal/external
6. overhead press
7. overhead pull

Each of these primary movement patterns can be reproduced in a gym environment using specific exercise machines (e.g., cable machine) or resistance bands; they can also be performed practically anywhere, as the majority of the exercises that I demonstrate in this chapter simply involve using a single piece of resistance exercise band, a core ball, Bosu (unstable base) foam roller, TRX (suspension exercises) and some dumbbells. Example movement/exercises for incorporating sling patterns are presented in the following sections.

It is considered nearly impossible to isolate one single muscle to one single joint motion. Why? Because muscles naturally work in harmony with each other and do not function very well on their own: they work as a team rather than as a solo entity. We naturally talk about muscles individually, but in reality they work collectively to allow certain movements of the joints in which they attach. So how does that affect the rehabilitation program? Quite simply in one respect, as we will look at the specific *movement patterns*, rather than looking at the individual muscles.

1. Standing push

The first exercise I propose is very effective at utilizing the *anterior oblique* sling as this will naturally integrate and augment the musculature of the anterior shoulder complex. If you look at the start position in figure 18.3a, you will notice that the exercise band (alternatively a cable machine can be used) is held with the athlete's right hand at shoulder height, and their left arm and left leg are placed in a forward position. The exercise motion is shown in figure 18.3b: the athlete pushes the band forward across their body, using their stance leg adductors, internal oblique, and contralateral external oblique, as well as the muscles of the serratus anterior, pectoralis major, anterior

deltoid and triceps. At the same time, the left arm comes backward, as this induces a rotation of the trunk to the left side, subsequently working the anterior oblique sling in the transverse plane of motion.

All day-to-day movements will work this muscle sling, but particularly good examples are the actions of walking, running, and especially any types of throwing motion.

Note: It is very important that the athlete controls the horizontal motion of the standing push in both phases, i.e., the concentric (shortening) phase and the eccentric (lengthening) phase, and does not let the band control the movement. Moreover, one has to be very aware of the activation of the inner core musculature in order to provide the necessary stability to perform all of these exercises I describe. If you are unsure about performing these exercises please seek professional advice before you begin them, or any type of resistance training.

The following statement is relevant to all of the sling exercises:

> *'You control the movement – never let the movement control you.'*

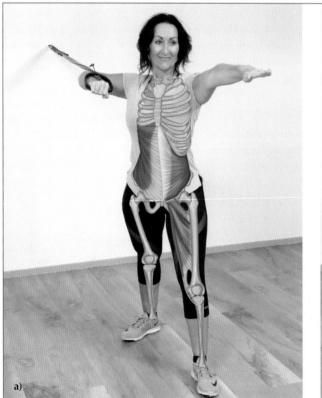 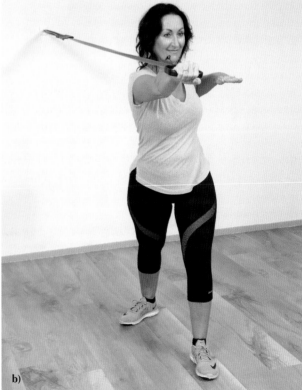

Figure 18.3a & b: *Anterior oblique sling. a: Start position; b: finish position*

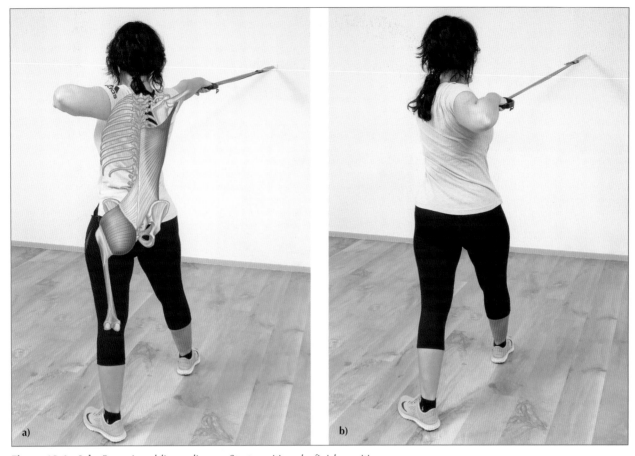

Figure 18.4a & b: *Posterior oblique sling. a: Start position; b: finish position*

2. Standing pull

This particular exercise is one of my personal favorites, as it is very effective in utilizing the *posterior oblique* sling. If you look at the start position in figure 18.4a you will see that the exercise band/cable is held with the athlete's right hand at shoulder height, and their left leg and left arm are placed in a backward position. The exercise motion is shown in figure 18.4b, using the latissimus dorsi, thoracolumbar fascia and contralateral Gmax, as well as the musculature of the posterior shoulder complex. The athlete pulls the band backward across their body with their right arm. At the same time, the left arm comes forward, as this induces a rotation of the trunk to the right side, subsequently working the posterior oblique sling in the transverse plane of motion.

I often say the following to my patients and athletes, as it reinforces perfectly the motion in the two exercises outlined above:

> *'Every pull is a push and every push is a pull – you cannot have one without the other.'*

3. Curl with press
Exercise 1 – Sitting curl with press

This exercise – another of my personal favorites – is a very functional motion for the shoulder complex as it complements motion from the wrist, elbow, glenohumeral and scapulothoracic, as well as the SC and AC joints all in one continual motion.

If you look at the start position in figure 18.5a you will see that the patient is sitting with the dumbbells held in both hands, their arms internally rotated and their forearm pronated. The patient is asked supinate their forearm, as this initiates the activation of the biceps brachii muscle, and to continue the motion by flexing the elbow until the dumbbells reaches the height of the shoulder (figure 18.5b). The patient is asked to continue and press or push the weight towards the ceiling (figure 18.5c).

Exercise 2 – Standing curl with press

The alternative exercise from the above sitting position is that the patient is asked to adopt a standing position and holds the dumbbell as shown in figure 18.6a and

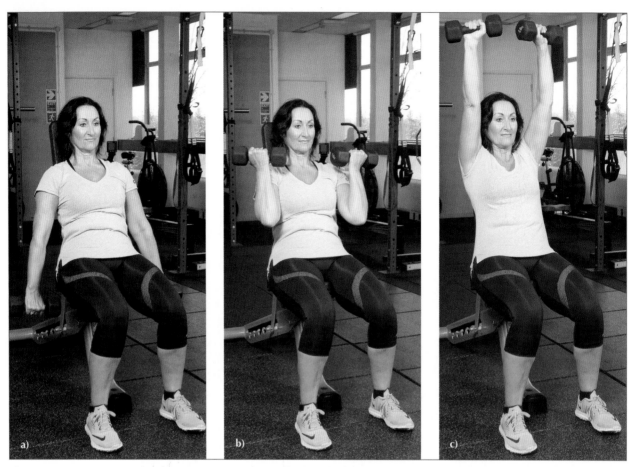

Figure 18.5a–c: *Sitting curl with press. a: Start position; b: dumbbell at shoulder height; c: finish position*

then is asked to curl the weight to the midway position (figure 18.6b), then continue to press the weight above their head (figure 18.6c).

Exercise 3 – Alternate curl with press

As in exercise 1 or 2, the patient adopts either a sitting or a standing position and grasps a dumbbell with each hand (figure 18.7a); this time they are asked to curl the weight in their right arm towards the end position of the shoulder press (figure 18.7b). On the return phase of the right arm the patient is also asked to lift the weight in their left arm towards the end range (figure 18.7c, half way point) of the shoulder press position (figure 18.7d).

4. Horizontal press
Push-up

The push-up motion is probably considered to be one of the best horizontal exercises one can perform for the shoulder complex as it incorporates motion from the glenohumeral joint as well as the scapulothoracic joint. Not only is the push-up a great strength exercise for the musculature of the upper limb, thorax and lumbopelvic-hip region but it is a very functional movement as well.

The push-up can also be used as an evaluation exercise of movement to assess the athlete's inner and outer control mechanisms to see how stable they are when performing the motion, as well as using the movement as part of any strength/rehabilitation training program.

The following exercises are progressive and most patients and athletes should be able to perform a push-up just by simply changing the angle of the body.

Exercise 1 – Kneeling push-up

The patient is asked to kneel on the mat and adopt a neutral position for the head, thorax and lumbar spine (figure 18.8a). The patient is instructed to slowly lower their trunk towards the mat, while maintaining their posture as they perform the motion (figure 18.8b). From the finish position, they are instructed to push back slowly to the start position without compromising their position of neutral.

Exercise 2 – Push-up

This exercise is similar to the one above; however, the patient is asked to lift their knees off the mat and to adopt a push-up position while maintaining a neutral position

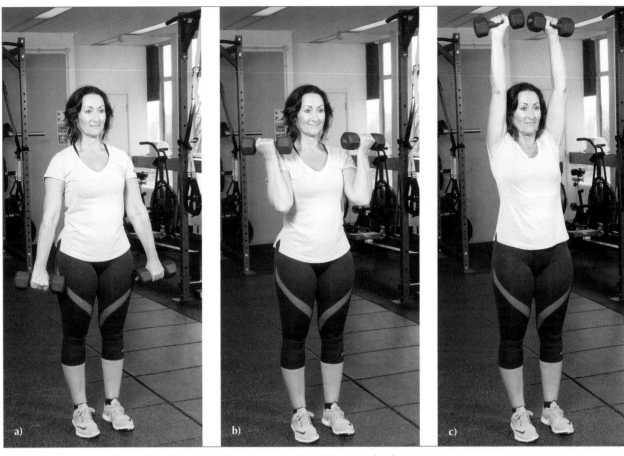

Figure 18.6a–c: *Standing curl with press. a: Start position; b: mid way; c: finish position*

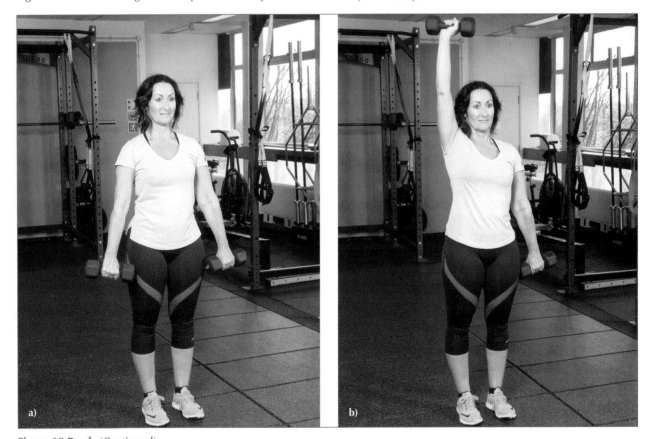

Figure 18.7a–d: *(Continued)*

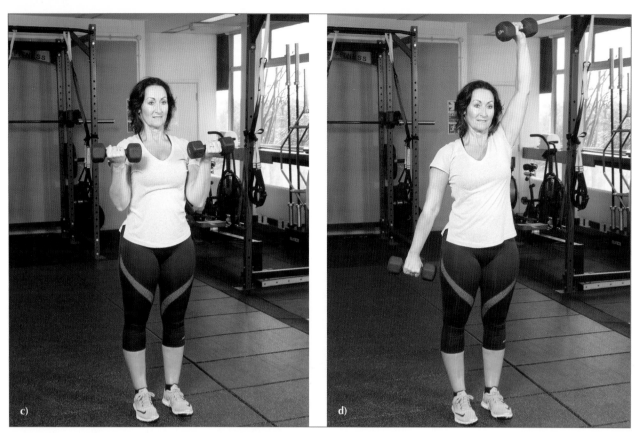

Figure 18.7a–d: *Alternate curl with press. a: Start position; b: right arm at end range; c: half way point; d: left arm at end range*

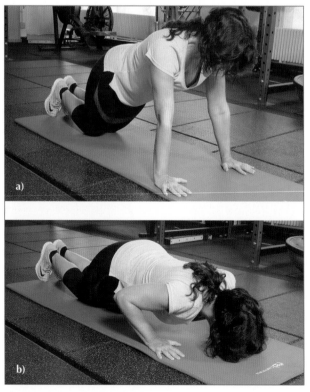

Figure 18.8a & b: *a: Start position; b: finish position*

for the head, thorax and lumbar spine (figure 18.9a). The patient is instructed to slowly lower their trunk towards the mat, while maintaining their posture as they perform the motion (figure 18.9b). From the finish position, they are instructed to push back slowly to the start position without compromising their position of neutral.

Exercise 3 – Push-up with use of ball
Progression 1 – Kneeling push-up-ball
The patient is kneeling on the mat and places both hands shoulder-width apart onto the exercise ball. The patient adopts a push-up position while maintaining a neutral position for the head, thorax and lumbar spine (figure 18.10a). The patient is instructed to slowly lower their trunk towards the ball, while maintaining their posture as they perform the motion (figure 18.10b). From the finish position, they are instructed to push back slowly to the start position without compromising their position of neutral.

Note: Please make sure there is no moisture present on the ball or your hands as you will have a natural tendency to slip and an injury might occur.

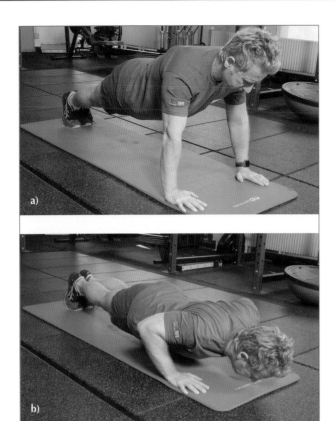

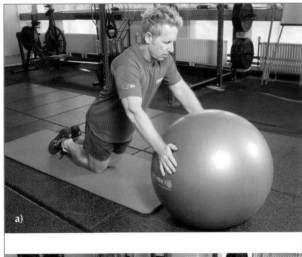

Figure 18.9a & b: *a: Start position; b: finish position*

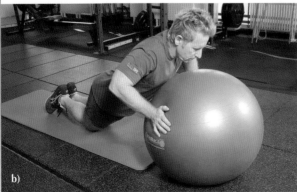

Figure 18.10a & b: *Kneeling push-up using ball. a: Start position; b: finish position*

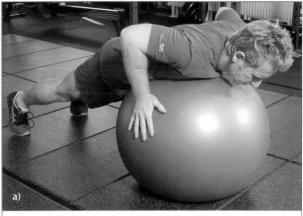

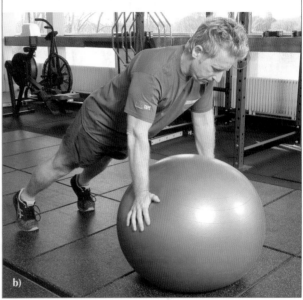

Figure 18.11a & b: *Push-up using ball. a: Start position; b: finish position*

Progression 2 – Push-up-ball

The patient is initially kneeling on the mat and places their chest and both hands shoulder-width apart onto the exercise ball. The patient is then instructed to lift their knees off the mat and adopt a neutral position for the head, thorax and lumbar spine (figure 18.11a). The patient is instructed to slowly push their trunk off the ball, while maintaining their posture as they perform the motion (figure 18.11b). From the finish position, they are instructed to slowly lower their trunk towards the ball to the start position without compromising their position of neutral.

Progression 3 – Push-up-ball-arms lift

This is exactly the same exercise as above, but after the eccentric lowering phase of the exercise has been completed the patient is instructed to maintain stability through their chest a16nd legs and perform the following motions: slowly horizontally extend their arms to

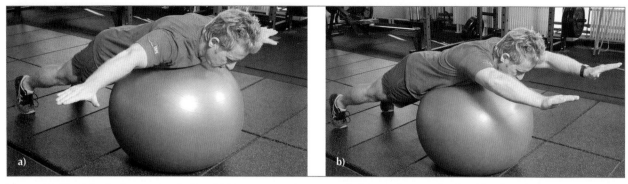

Figure 18.12a & b: *Push-up using ball and lifting arms. a: Arm extended to 90 degrees; b: shoulder flexed to 180 degrees*

90 degrees (figure 18.12a); bring their arms back to the ball and then flex their shoulders to 180 degrees (figure 18.12b). After these motions the patient is asked to bring their arms back to the side of the ball and then to repeat the concentric phase of the push-up.

These two extra movements of the arms will utilize more of the scapula-stabilizing muscles such as the rhomboids as well as the middle and lower fibers of the trapezius.

Progression 4 – Push-up-ball-single leg lift

This is exactly the same exercise as the push-up off ball in progression 2, but this time the patient is asked to lift one leg a few inches off the floor (figure 18.13a) and then to perform the concentric phase of the push-up with the leg still lifted off the floor. After the lowering phase of the exercise has been completed the patient is then instructed to horizontally extend their arms to 90 degrees and then to flex their arms to 180 degrees (figures 18.13b and c) with one leg still lifted off the floor.

Progression 5 – Push-up-step

The patient adopts a push-up position, this time with their feet on a step (figure 18.14a), and is asked to lower towards the floor (figure 18.14b). To progress the patient is asked to lift one leg a few inches off the floor (figure 18.14c) and then to perform the concentric phase of the push-up with the leg still lifted off the floor.

Progression 6 – Push-up-feet on ball

The patient adopts a push-up position and as a starting point can place their mid thigh (figure 18.15a), then progress to shins (figure 18.15b) and eventually to using their feet (figure 18.15c) on the ball, both hands shoulder-width apart on the mat, and adopts a neutral position for the head, thorax and lumbar spine. The patient is instructed to slowly perform a push-up motion by

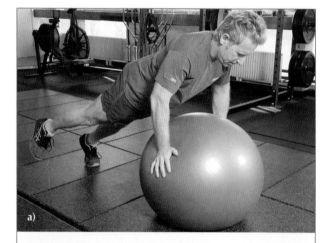

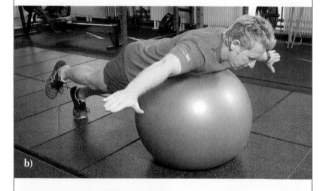

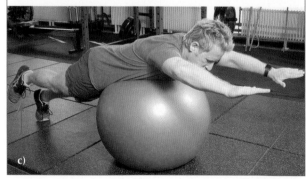

Figure 18.13a–c: *a: Push-up position with one leg off the floor; b: arm abducted; c: flexed to 180 degrees with leg lifted*

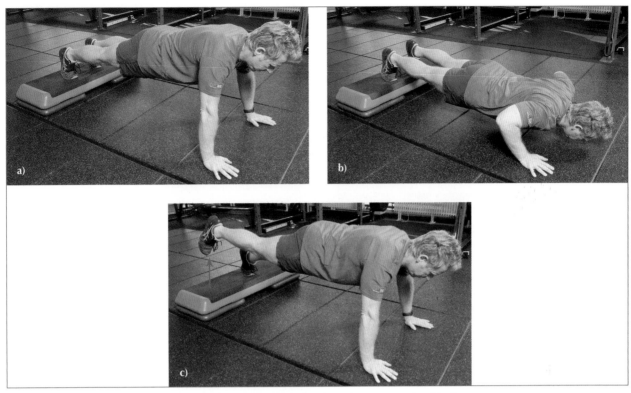

Figure 18.14a–c: *Push-up using a step. a: Start position; b: finish position; c: one leg lifted*

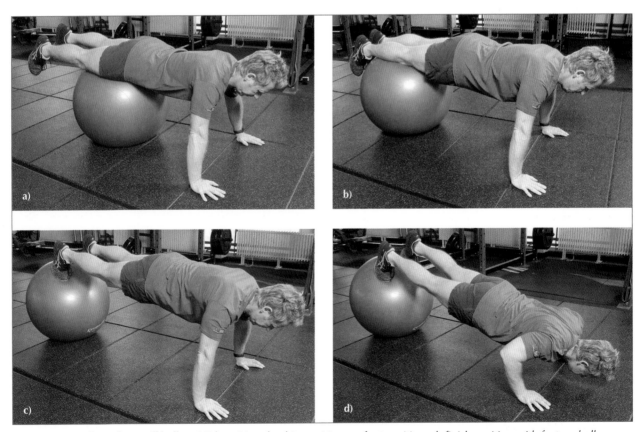

Figure 18.15a–d: *Push-up off ball. a: Mid position; b: shin position; c: foot position; d: finish position with feet on ball*

lowering their trunk towards the mat (figure 18.15d) and then to return to the starting position.

Progression and variation

Figures 18.15e–l are examples of other exercises that can be used.

Note: Please be very careful if you decide to try the last few exercises where I demonstrate the push-up on two balls (figures 18.15j–l) – they are very difficult to perform

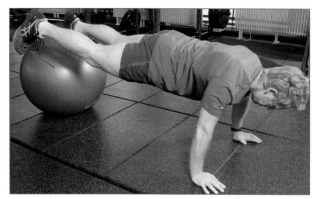

Figure 18.15e: *Shows progression by lifting one leg off the ball and performing the push-up motion*

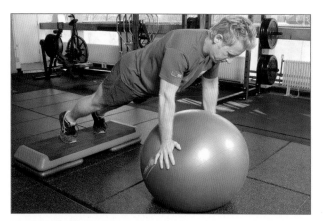

Figure 18.15f: *Push-up using a ball and a step*

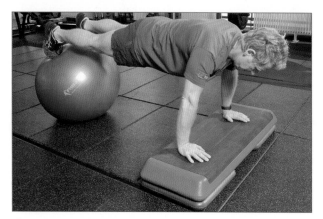

Figure 18.15g: *Opposite motion of push-up using a ball and a step*

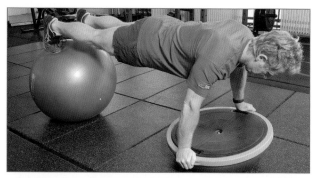

Figure 18.15h: *Push-up using a ball and a Bosu (using feet)*

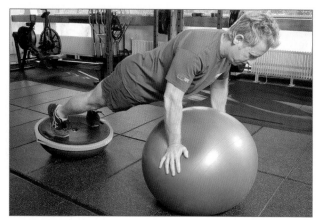

Figure 18.15i: *Opposite motion of push-up using a ball and a Bosu (using feet)*

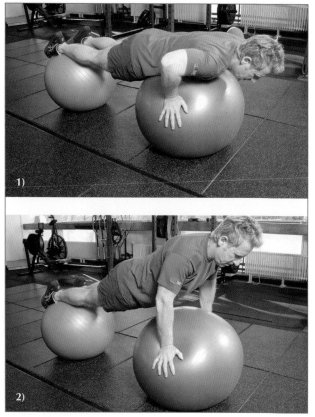

Figure 18.15j: *Push-up using two balls (using shins). 1: Start position; 2: finish position*

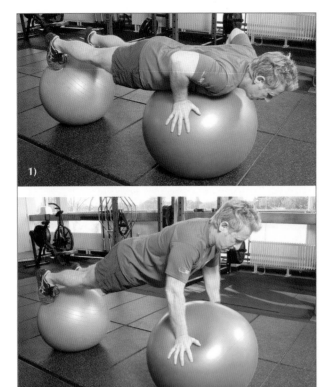

Figure 18.15k: *Push-up on two balls using feet. 1: Start position; 2: finish position*

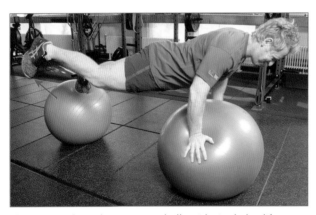

Figure 18.15l: *Push-up on two balls with single leg lift*

correctly, even for strong athletes. It is not recommended to even try these movements unless/until you are near the top of the strength ladder and you are under the supervision of someone who is trained in rehabilitation therapy.

TRX press-up
The TRX suspension system is a great tool one can use for a multitude of functional movements and not only for the shoulder complex as the whole body can be incorporated.

The following push motion using the TRX is very good because it will target the strength components of the shoulder complex as well as activating the stabilizing and inner core systems.

The patient is asked to place the feet into the straps of the TRX and adopt a push-up position (figure 18.16a). The patient is then asked to perform a push-up (figure 18.16b). The variation from this position is that the patient can bring their knees towards their chest (figure 18.16c) as this promotes shoulder stability while activating the core muscles. Figures 18.16d–e show single hip and knee flexion exercises.

TRX – Standing push
The patient stands with their feet shoulder-width apart, takes hold of each of the TRX grips with both their hands and then takes a step backwards and is asked to lean forwards, maintaining the grip on the bands (the patient controls their position by varying how far they step back and lean forward) (figure 18.17a). The patient is next instructed to push their arms until they are almost straight (figure 18.17b) and then return slowly to the starting position. Figure 18.17c shows a variation by lifting one leg.

5. Rotation – Internal and external
Many authors and trainers consider exercises that include internal and external rotation as the gold standard of all the exercises they can offer for shoulder complex pathologies. Most texts on shoulder rehabilitation will include these two motions. I do the same; however, once the typical movements have been learned, I would like to vary them in a more functional way that relates to the patient or athlete that is visiting your clinic.

Internal rotation
The patient is typically standing with their elbow at 90 degrees and their shoulder externally rotated. They are instructed to grasp the exercise band (figure 18.18a) and to slowly internally rotate their shoulder as far as the abdomen (figure 18.18b). This will activate the 'SALT' and 'Pepper' muscles. (SALT stands for subscapularis, anterior deltoid, latissimus dorsi and teres major and pepper relates to the pectoralis major.)

We can vary the internal rotation by placing the arm in 90 degrees of abduction and elbow flexion (figure 18.18c). The patient is asked to internally rotate the arm to 90 degrees (figure 18.18d).

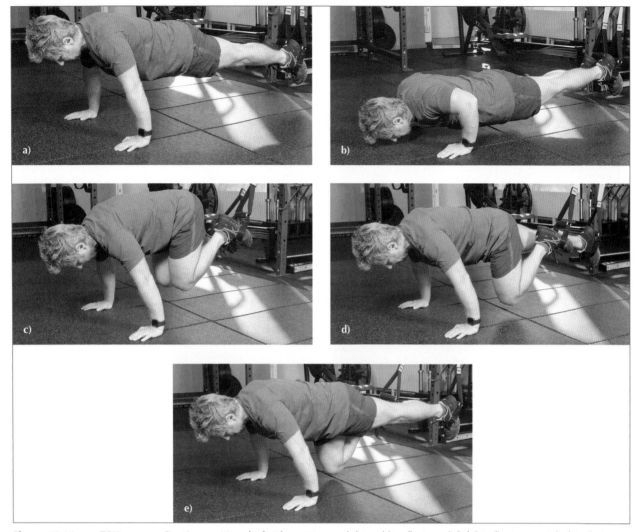

Figure 18.16a–e: *TRX press. a: Starting position; b: finish position; c: bilateral hip flexion; d: left hip flexion; e: right hip flexion*

External rotation

The patient is standing with their elbow at 90 degrees and their shoulder internally rotated and is instructed to grasp the band (figure 18.19a) and to slowly externally rotate their shoulder as far as possible (figure 18.19b). This will activate the infraspinatus, teres minor and posterior deltoid muscles.

Functional external/internal rotation in abduction (throwing)

Think of the throwing action described earlier in the book as the following exercises are designed to mimic this specific throwing motion and it makes perfect sense to try and promote functional stability within the clinical setting. We can also modify some of the exercises towards the requirements of the sporting athlete.

Exercise 1

The patient is standing and is instructed to grasp the exercise band. The movement starts with their arm in

abduction to 90 degrees and full external rotation and their weight on the back leg, as if to mimic the wind-up phase of throwing (figure 18.20a).

From this position the patient is instructed to reproduce the throwing action (acceleration) by slowly resisting against the exercise band so that the arm now extends and internally rotates as the weight is transferred to the front leg (figures 18.20b). The patient is instructed to control both phases of motion, that is, the concentric and eccentric phases of the movement.

Exercise 2

This movement is basically the reverse of Exercise 1, so we start where the arm finished in the last exercise. The patient now starts as shown in figure 18.21a and is then asked to resist the wind-up phase of the throwing action. However, the emphasis in this exercise is not only about the concentric (shortening) phase of the posterior shoulder muscles; the focus will be on the eccentric

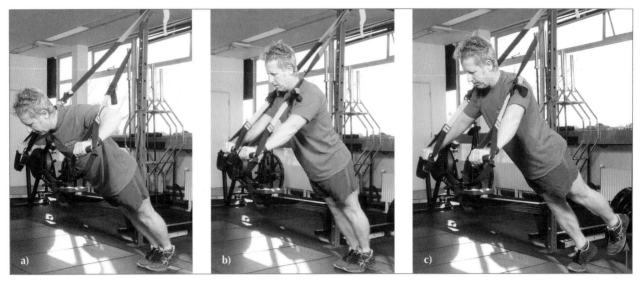

Figure 18.17a–c: *Standing TRX push. a: Start position; b: finish position; c: one leg lifted*

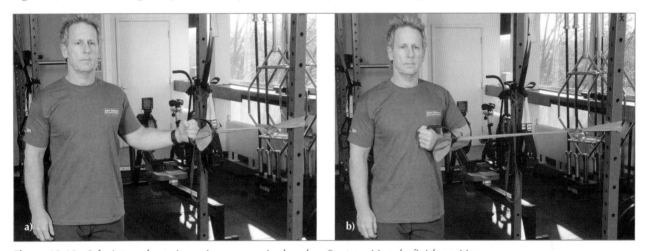

Figure 18.18a & b: *Internal rotation using an exercise band. a: Start position; b: finish position*

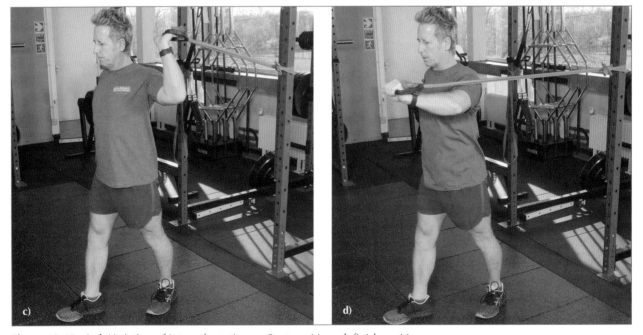

Figure 18.18c & d: *Variation of internal rotation. c: Start position; d: finish position*

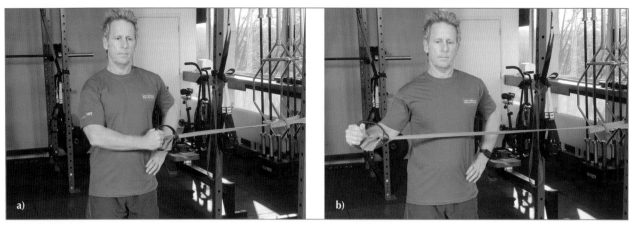

Figure 18.19a & b: *External rotation using an exercise band. a: Start position; b: finish position*

(lengthening) phase as this helps the deceleration phase of the throwing action (figures 18.21b and c). I suggest 1–2 seconds for the concentric phase and 3–4 seconds for the eccentric phase.

6. Overhead – Vertical push

In terms of function, overhead motion has to be one of the most common of the movements that are performed regularly throughout the day. It is a great exercise overall as it will improve strength and stability of the shoulder and thoracic complex and, depending on how this motion is performed, it will incorporate many other components of the musculoskeletal system. Typically, the usual way

is for the patient to sit with their back against the bench and then to lift the dumbbells over their head. In this chapter I want to demonstrate a variety of overhead press movements that I consider are more functional.

Exercise 1 – Overhead push – standing – band

The patient is standing in a neutral position, and placing their feet on each of exercise bands, grasps the bands with their hands and brings them up until they are level with the shoulder (figure 18.22a). The patient is then instructed to slowly push the bands towards the ceiling (figure 18.22b) and to then return slowly to the starting position.

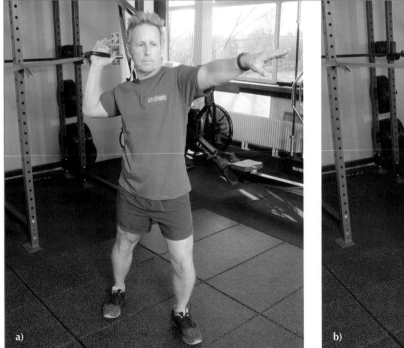
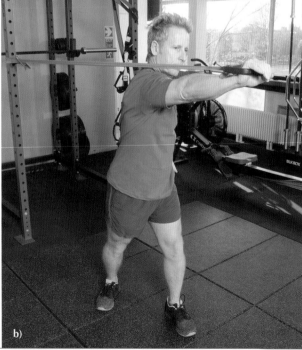

Figure 18.20a & b: *The patient reproduces a throwing action using the exercise band as a resistance. a: Start position; b: finish position*

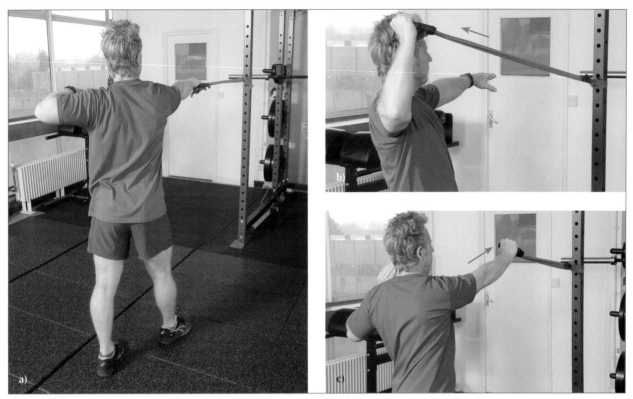

Figure 18.21a–c: *The patient reproduces the wind-up phase using the exercise band as a resistance. a: Start position; b: mid way; c: eccentric phase*

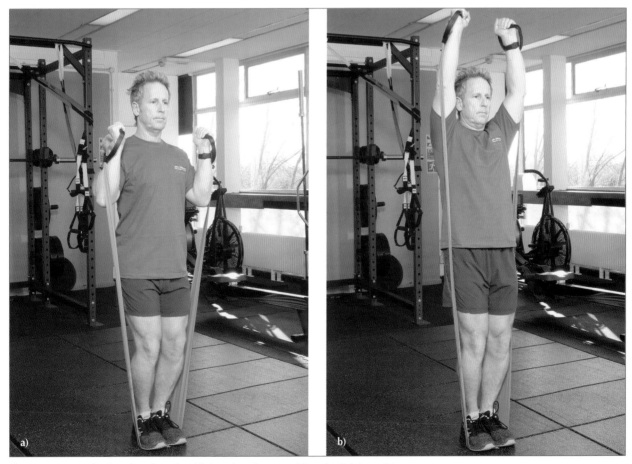

Figure 18.22a & b: *Overhead push with band. a: Start position; b: finish position*

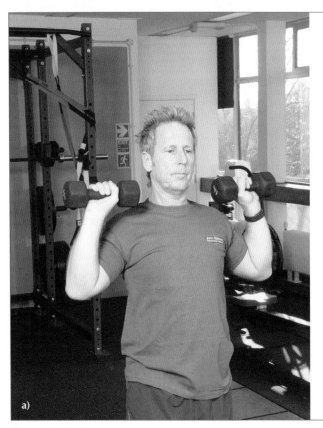
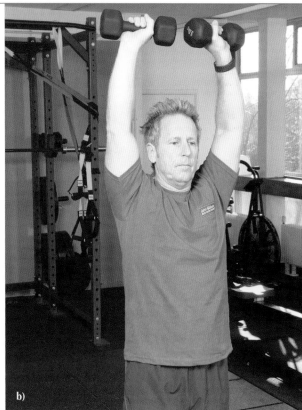

Figure 18.23a & b: *Overhead push with weights. a: Start position; b: finish position*

Exercise 2 – Overhead push – standing – dumbbells

This is the same as the exercise above but this time, instead of using a band, the patient uses a set of dumbbells. The patient takes the weights and places them level with the shoulder (figure 18.23a) and is then instructed to slowly push the weights towards the ceiling (figure 18.23b) before returning slowly to the starting position.

A progression from the standard standing dumbbell press can easily be made by changing the angle of the press to a 'V' shape (figure 18.23c) and also a 'Y' shape (figure 18.23d); these two progressions will naturally make the exercise harder to perform. Another simple progressive exercise is to do the motion of the press alternately, by pushing one arm at a time towards the ceiling (figure 18.23e). The most difficult of all in this progressive sequence is if we perform the motion of the press and instruct the patient to lift one leg as they are pressing both the weights (figure 18.23f) and to lift alternately (figure 18.23g).

Exercise 3 – Overhead push – ball – exercise band

The patient is sitting on an exercise ball with their spine in a neutral position and their knees below the level of the

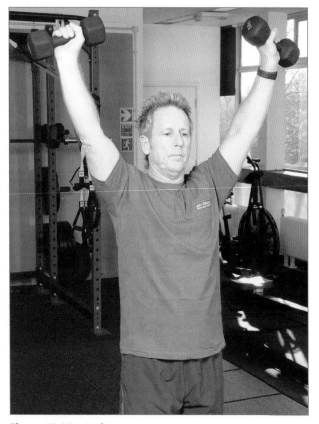

Figure 18.23c: *V shape*

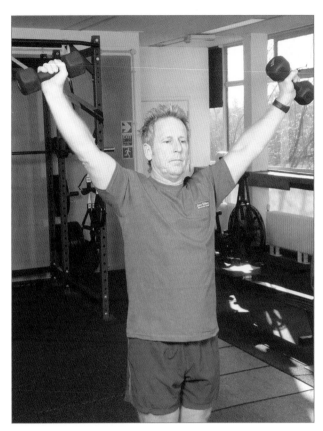

Figure 18.23d: *Y shape*

hips; they place a foot on each of the exercise bands, grasp the bands with their hands and raise them level with the shoulders (figure 18.24a). The patient is then instructed to slowly push the bands towards the ceiling (figure 18.24b) and then return to the starting position. Figures 18.24c and d show single arm movements.

Exercise 4 – Overhead push – ball – dumbbells
Same as above with the patient sitting on an exercise ball and placing the weights level with the shoulders (figure 18.25a). The patient is instructed to slowly push the weights towards the ceiling (figure 18.25b) and then return slowly to the starting position. Figures 18.25c and d show the same exercise using single arms.

7. Overhead – Vertical pull
This specific type of motion is another functional movement that is similar to a vertical press/push, but obviously going in the opposite direction. In the gym environment a latissimus pull-down exercise is one of the most commonly performed movements; however, I want to show variations on this motion. It is a great exercise overall as it will improve strength, stability and even mobility in one respect for the shoulder and thoracic complex as well as other musculoskeletal components.

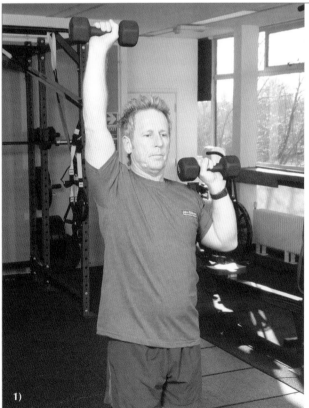

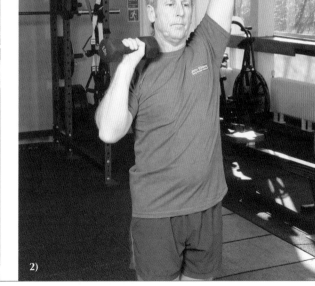

Figure 18.23e: *Single arm press. 1: Right arm; 2: left arm*

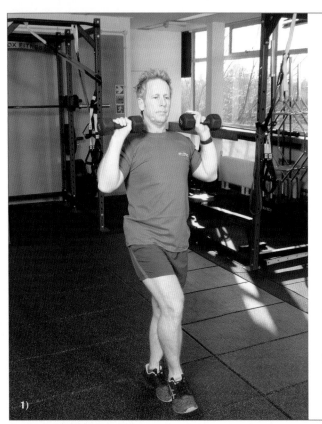
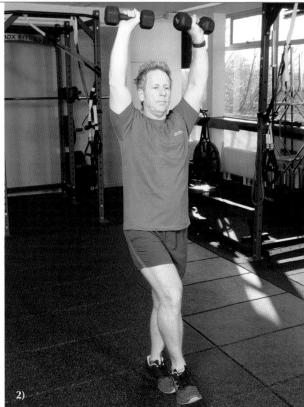

Figure 18.23f: *Bilateral press with one leg lifted. 1: Start position; 2: finish position*

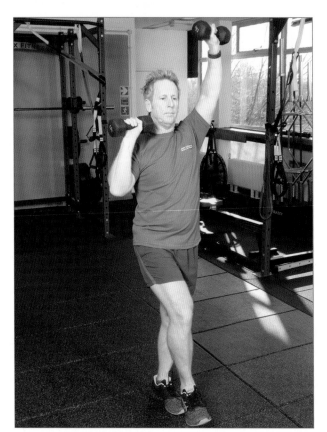

Figure 18.23g: *Unilateral press with one leg lifted*

Exercise 1 – TRX standing pull

The patient is standing with their feet shoulder-width apart and takes hold the TRX grips with their hands, and then walks forward a step and is asked to lean backwards, maintaining the grip on the bands (the patient controls their position by varying how far they step forward and lean back) (figure 18.26a). The patient is then instructed to slowly pull the bands towards them (horizontal extension) (figure 18.26b) and then return slowly to the starting position.

The patient is able to vary this exercise by leaning back a bit further (figure 18.26c), as this will increase the resistance of the exercise, and also the position of the arms can be changed to extension (figure 18.26d).

Exercise 2 – Exercise band vertical pull

The patient sits on a bench with their feet shoulder-width apart and takes hold of the exercise bands with their hands (figure 18.27a). They are then asked to slowly pull downwards, maintaining the grip on the bands (figure 18.27b). The patient is then instructed to eccentrically control each of the bands slowly back to the starting position. Figures 18.27c and d show the patient using alternate arms.

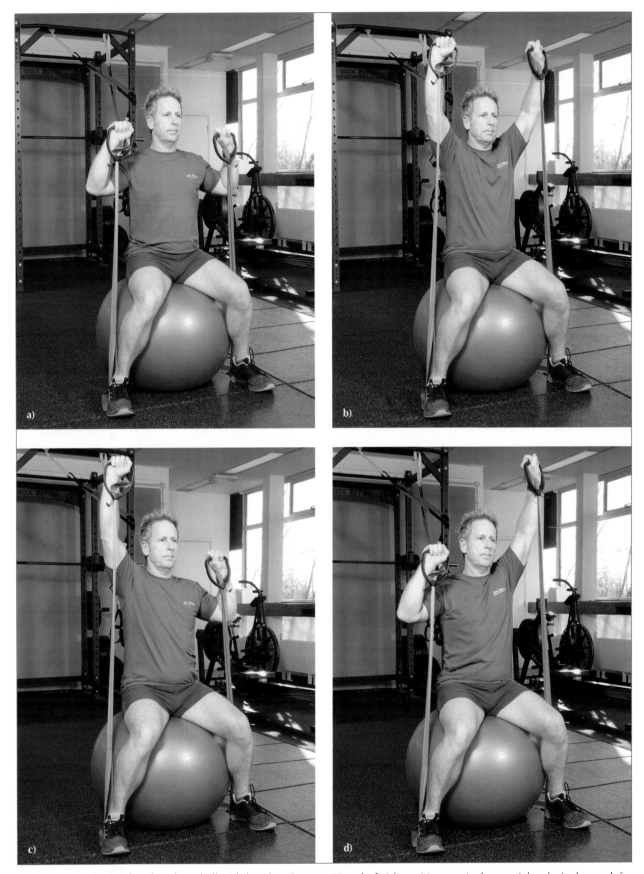

Figure 18.24a–d: *Overhead push on ball with band. a: Start position; b: finish position; c: single arm right; d: single arm left*

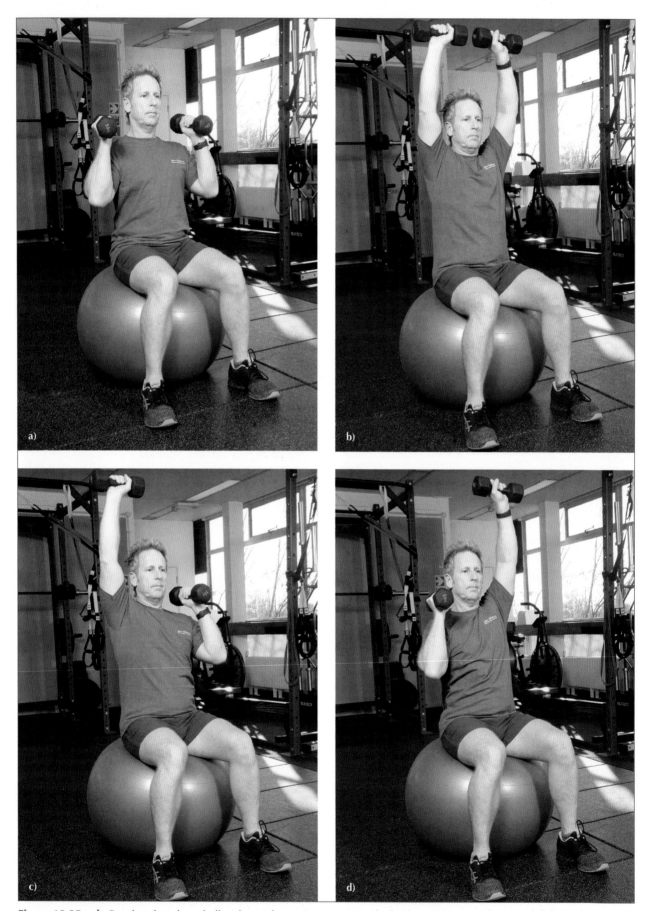

Figure 18.25a–d: *Overhead push on ball with weights. a: Start position; b: finish position; c: right arm; d: left arm*

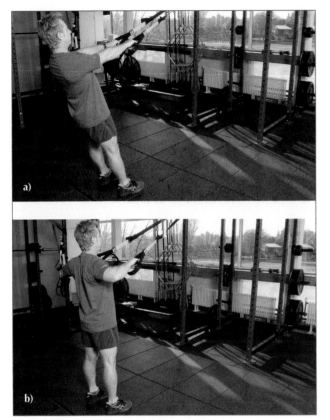

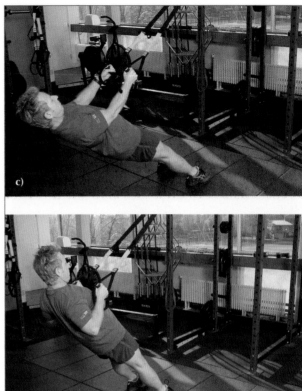

Figure 18.26a & b: *Standing TRX pull. a: Start position; b: finish position*

Figure 18.26c & d: *c: The patient is leaning back further; d: the patient extends the shoulder*

The following exercises are exactly the same but this time the patient is facing forward with both arms grasping the exercise band above their head (figure 18.28a); the movement is directed towards the chest (figure 18.28b) as this will target the back and shoulder muscles in an alternative way to the exercise above.

Exercise 3 – Pull-up

Pull-ups are a great exercise; however, to perform it in the normal way (i.e., unassisted) a natural amount of strength, coordination and stability is required. You will sometimes hear friends saying how many pull-ups they can do, or the more common scenario, perhaps, 'I can't actually do any'!

If you are one of those individuals that struggle to do a single pull-up correctly then it is probably a good idea to start with some form of assistance, whether from a machine, a partner to hold your legs, or an exercise band.

Mobility exercise protocol

If a patient presents with a restrictive and painful shoulder then some of the following exercises will be difficult and

too painful for them to achieve. However, the long-term goal has to be to try and improve full range of motion. Is the restriction of the movement due to a tight muscle or a stiff joint, or both? If it is both then all the components causing the restriction have to be treated. As I often say to my students and even to patients:

> 'A stiff joint can cause a tight muscle and a tight muscle can cause a stiff joint.'

I believe that if you have a problem with the joint then it will naturally affect the muscle and vice versa; hence the term musculoskeletal restriction.

When I see patients with a stiff/painful shoulder I generally use a numerical pain scale that has '10' on the scale being the most pain and '0' on the scale being no pain at all. I say that you need to be below a '5' on the pain scale for every exercise that you do, because if you are performing the movement and you are at an '8' or a '9', then when you are exercising the shoulder it will probably react to the increased pain and start to compensate. The *old school* credo of exercising was '*no pain, no gain*', but when exercising the shoulder, the idea that no pain equals no gain should definitely not be used to improve function.

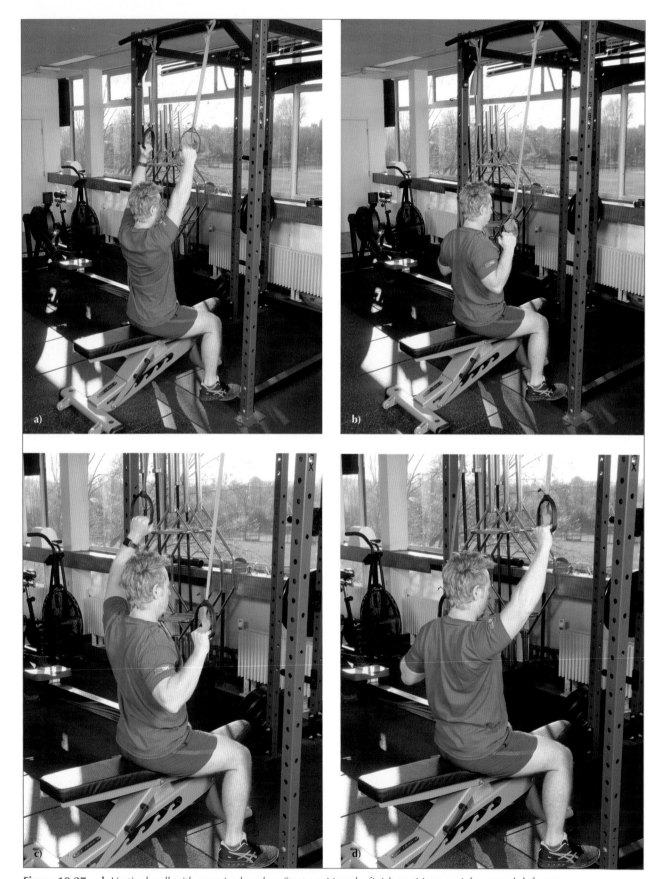

Figure 18.27a–d: *Vertical pull with exercise band. a: Start position; b: finish position; c: right arm; d: left arm*

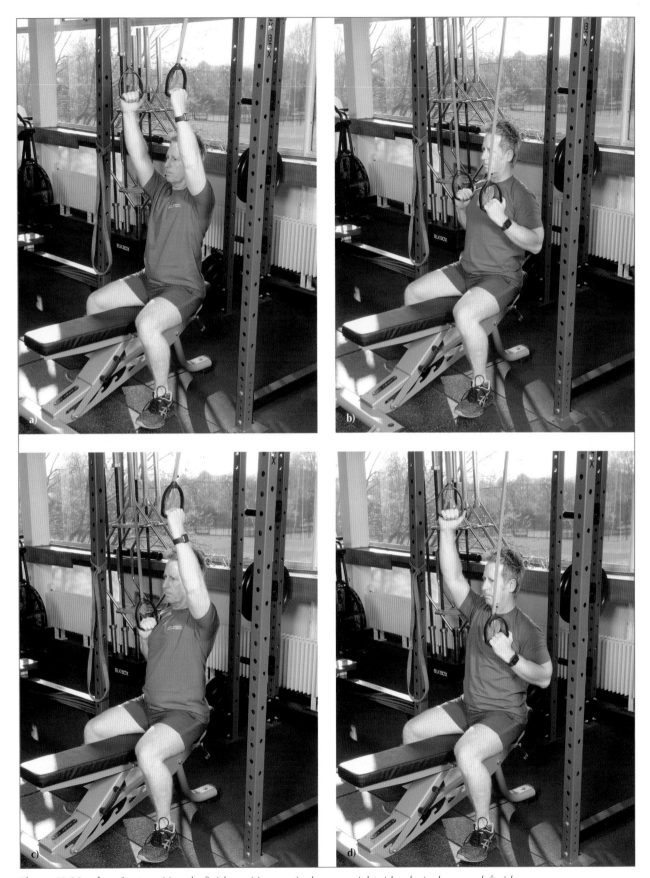

Figure 18.28a–d: *a: Start position; b: finish position; c: single arm – right side; d: single arm – left side*

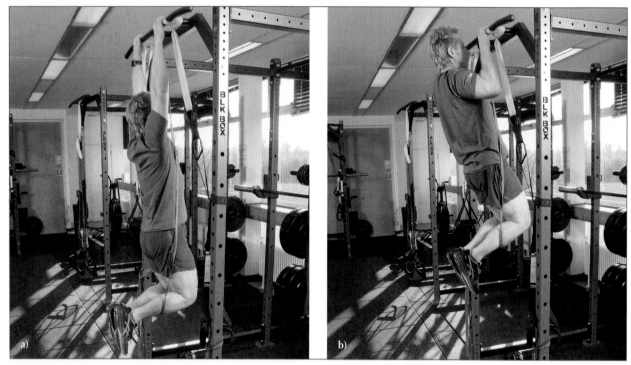

Figure 18.29a & b: *Pull up. a: Start position with assistance from a band; b: finish position*

Mobility exercises using a core-ball
Progression 1 – Standing press – ball

The patient adopts a standing position and gently holds onto a core-ball that is placed against the wall at shoulder height (figure 18.30a). The patient is asked to apply light pressure to the ball and then to perform a sequence of set exercises; they start with rolling the ball towards the ceiling (flexion) and then towards the floor (extension) (figure 18.30b). Next, the patient glides the ball from side to side into horizontal abduction and adduction (figure 18.30c). Next they are asked to circle the ball in a clockwise direction, then an anticlockwise direction (figure 18.30d). Lastly the patient is asked to guide the ball obliquely to the right and then obliquely to the left (figure 18.30e).

Progression 2 – Supine – ball

The patient adopts a supine position and is instructed to take hold of the ball at the level of their thighs (figure 18.31a). From this position the patient can take the ball into shoulder flexion to 90 degrees (figure 18.31b) then continue as far as comfortable (figure 18.31c). From the position of 90 degrees, the patient can circle the ball clockwise and anticlockwise as (figure 18.31d) and also horizontally flex and extend or go into an oblique direction (figure 18.31e).

Progression 3 – Kneeling press – ball

The idea of this exercise is similar to the standing press; however, by kneeling on the floor you can lean onto the ball to increase the resistance. Basically you are able to change the angle of how much you are leaning, and the more you lean the more the resistance increases.

The patient is kneeling on a mat and then takes control of the core-ball and gradually leans onto the ball (figure 18.32a). From here they can repeat some of the exercises from the standing press, e.g., forwards and backwards (figure 18.32b), side to side (figure 18.32c) and circular motions (figure 18.32d).

Mobility exercises using a foam roller
Progression 1 – Sitting to roll

The patient adopts a sitting position and places their hand on top of the foam roller (figure 18.33a). The patient is asked to roll the foam roller along the top of the table as far as is comfortable (figure 18.33b), as this will improve flexion of the shoulder, and then to roll the foam roller back to the starting position.

Progression 2 – Standing to roll

The patient adopts a standing position and places their hand on top of the foam roller at shoulder height

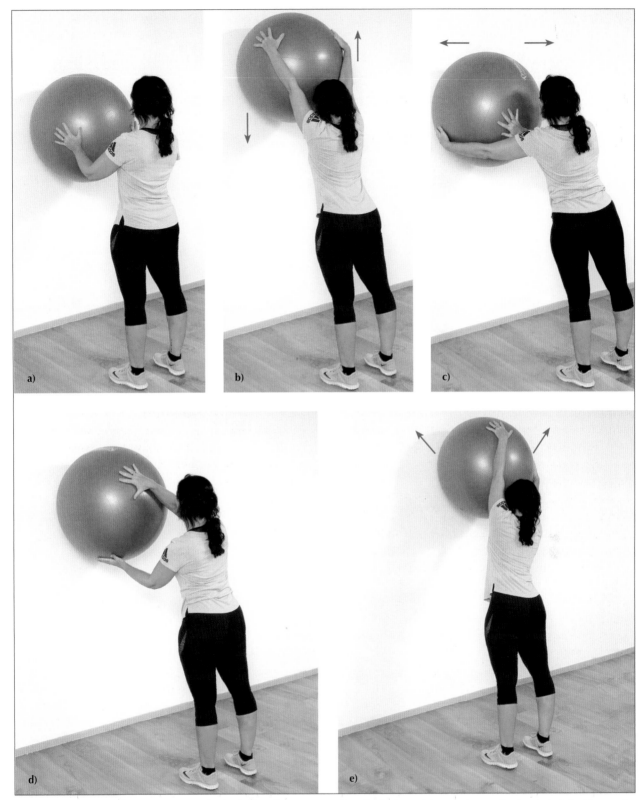

Figure 18.30a–e: *a: The patient controls the ball and then moves into b: flexion and extension; c: horizontal abduction and adduction; d: clockwise and anticlockwise; e: oblique right and oblique left*

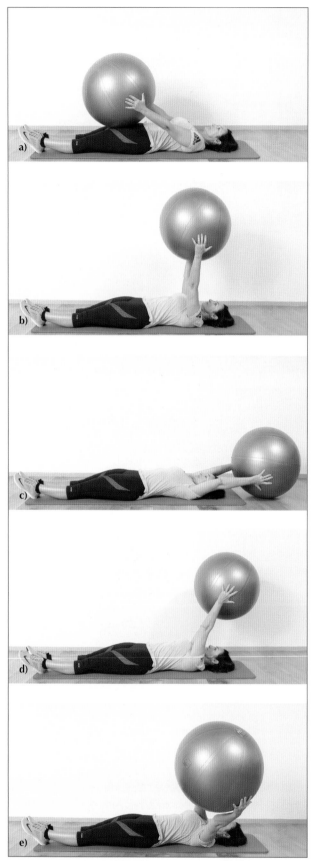

Figure 18.31a–e: *a: The patient holds the ball at the level of their thigh; b: flexion 90 degrees; c: 180 degrees; d: circular motion; e: horizontal flexion and extension*

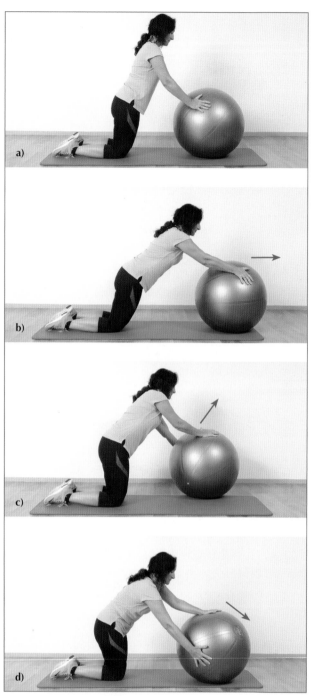

Figure 18.32a–d: *a: The patient kneels and controls the ball into: b: flexing and extension; c: horizontal abduction and adduction; d: clockwise and anticlockwise*

(figure 18.34a). The patient is asked to roll the foam roller up the wall as far as is comfortable, as this will improve flexion of the shoulder (figure 18.34b), and then roll the foam roller back to the starting position. The technique can be modified by a change of position of the hand, from palms down (pronation), as per the figure, to palms up (supination), as this will assist the external rotation of the shoulder (figure18.34c).

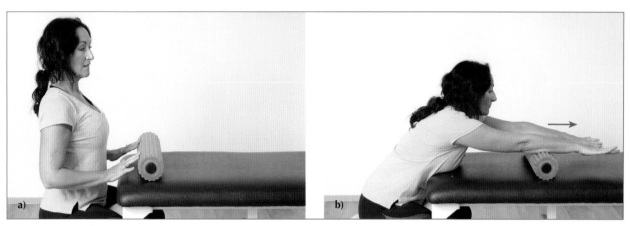

Figure 18.33a & b: *Patient rolls the foam roller along the tabletop. a: Start position; b: finish position*

Progression 3 – Kneeling to roll

The patient adopts a kneeling position and places their hand on top of the foam roller (figure 18.35a). The patient is asked to roll the foam roller along the exercise mat as far as is comfortable, as this will improve flexion of the shoulder (figure 18.35b), and then roll the foam roller back to the starting position.

The exercise demonstrated above is potentially more difficult than it looks because it is designed as a mobility exercise; however, depending on how far you lean forward with your body, the change of position will suddenly change the exercise to a stability and strength component rather than being a primary mobility exercise.

Thoracic mobility

I have already mentioned the importance of mobility in the thoracic spine and shoulder complex – if this part of the spine is restricted then the end range movements of the shoulder complex will also be affected, so it goes

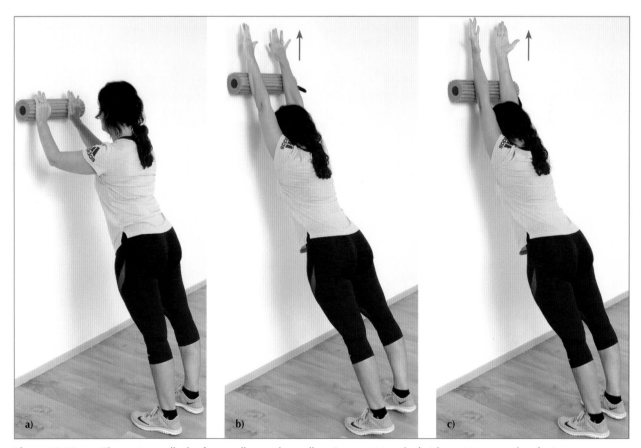

Figure 18.34a–c: *The patient rolls the foam roller up the wall. a: Start position; b: finish position; c: palms facing up*

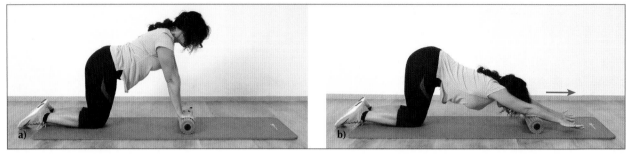

Figure 18.35a & b: *The patient rolls the foam roller along the exercise mat. a: Start position; b: finish position*

without saying that we need to try and maintain good flexibility within the thoracic spine. In reality this is not a straightforward process because for most of us (including myself) this is a relatively rigid structure, especially if we have developed an increased flexion curvature (kyphosis). Trying to improve the motion into extension is therefore not an easy task, to say the least.

One way that might be of value is through the use of a foam or rigid roller.

The patient adopts a supine position on an exercise mat and the roller is placed horizontally between their shoulder blades (figure 18.36a). The patient places their hands across their chest and is asked to slowly extend their thoracic spine over the roller (figure 18.36b). The patient can roll down or up the roller to target other thoracic segments and also place their fingers by their ears (figure 18.36c); or the arms can be flexed (figure 18.36d), which will increase the lever and can promote further mobility to the thorax.

Mobility exercises using a wooden pole

A simple broom handle (without the brush) can be very useful when it comes to advising mobility exercises for your patients. These exercises can be done at home, on the floor or even on top of a bed.

The patient is supine and they are asked to grab hold of the pole with both hands and to place it across their thighs. The first movement is to simply bring the handle to 90 degrees (figure 18.37a). If this motion is initially painful then the patient should bring the stick as far as is comfortable. The patient can repeat this motion of flexion to 90 degrees for approximately 5×. From here the patient can continue flexion to a level that is still comfortable (figure 18.37b) as 180 degrees will be the maximum range, and repeat for approximately 5×.

From the position of 90 degrees the patient is asked to make small circles clockwise (×5) and then to make small circles counterclockwise (×5) (figure 18.37c). The patient

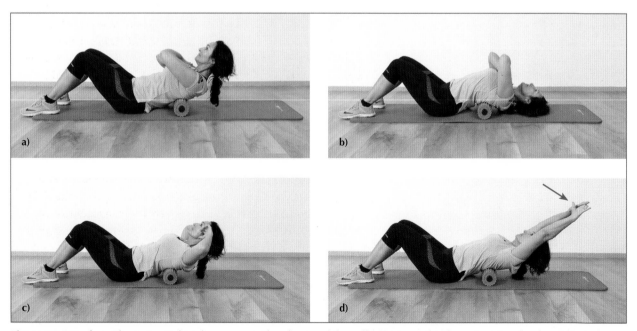

Figure 18.36a–d: *a: The patient's hands are across the chest and the roller is across the thoracic spine. b: The patient mobilizes the thoracic spine over the roller. c: The fingers are placed by the ears. d: The arms are flexed to increase leverage*

(if no pain present) can now make larger circles (×5) in both directions.

Progression – Horizontal/scapula plane motion

The patient can now perform horizontal adduction and abduction from the position of 90 degrees (figure 18.38a). Next the patient is asked to obliquely take the pole into the right and left scapula plane motion (scaption) (figure 18.38b).

The mobility exercises using a pole can also be advised with the patient standing, as shown in figure 18.39. The patient is asked to take hold of the pole and start at the level of the mid thigh (figure 18.39a) and then flex their shoulder to 90 degrees (figure 18.39b). Next the patient is asked to continue to 180 degrees (figure 18.39c). From this position the patient can side bend left and side bend right (figures 18.39d and e). Figures 18.39f and g show the patient holding the pole at 90 degrees and then making circles clockwise and circles counterclockwise.

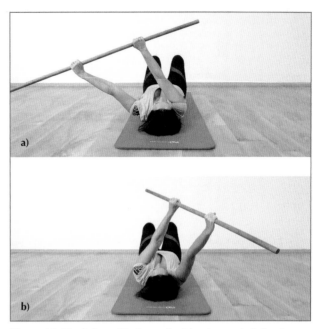

Figure 18.38a & b: *a: Horizontal adduction and abduction at 90 degrees; b: scapula plane/oblique motion right and left*

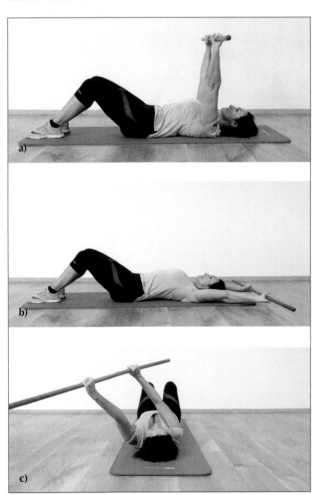

Figure 18.37a–c: *a: Arms at 90 degrees; b: flexion 90 degrees to 180 degrees; c: circles clockwise and counterclockwise – start small and increase to larger circles*

Advanced training and sports-specific protocol

When considering what are the best exercises to give your athletes it is worth thinking about the sport they participate in. This should influence your choice of exercise recommendations, rather than just suggesting the standard strengthening exercises. However, there will come a time in your career when you will have not heard of the sport the athlete participates in. Let me give you an example: when I first started my work as a sports osteopath at the University of Oxford many years ago, I had never heard of sports like *Real Tennis* or *Rugby Fives*. I therefore had to make sure that I understood the biomechanics of these sports and also the potential for injuries for the competing athletes.

CASE STUDY

A 32-year-old professional boxer came to see me with pain between his shoulder blades, especially to the right side. This pain had been present for many months. The pain originally came on after an intensive sparring session during which he felt he over-reached his right arm and felt a sudden pain, mainly to right side of his rhomboids. He took some medication and iced the area, then rested for five days. He then tried to box again but could not, due to the intensity of the pain. He saw another osteopath,

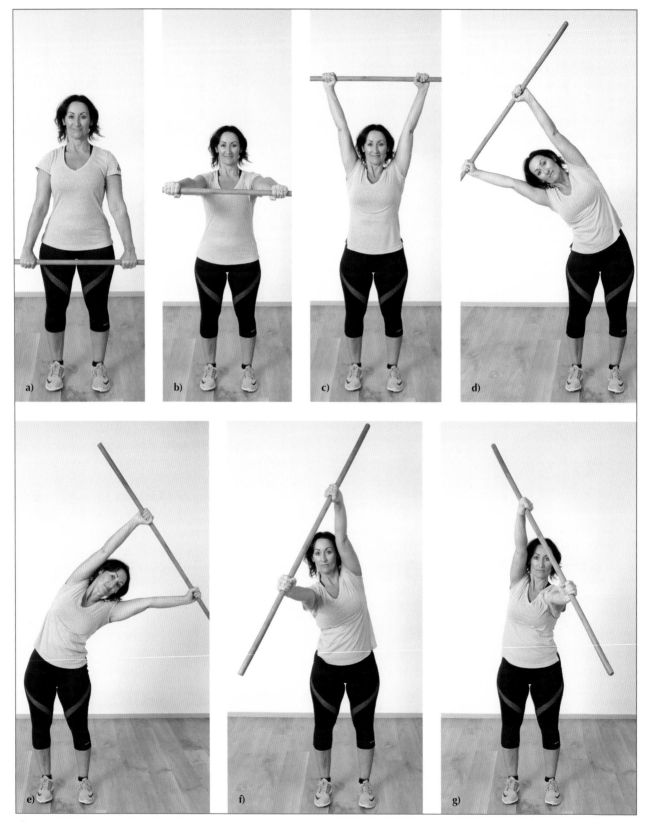

Figure 18.39a–g: *a: The patient holds the pole; b: 90 degrees; c: flexion to 180 degrees; d: side bending right; e: side bending left; f: circle clockwise; g: circle counterclockwise*

who said he had strained his rhomboid muscle and proceeded to give him strengthening exercises using an exercise band to retract his shoulder blades. The patient performed these exercises conscientiously every day for the next two weeks then tried to box/spar again; however, within a few minutes the pain had come back. So he rested again for another few days, did the rhomboid retraction exercises again, and tried to box again, but as soon as he reached with his right arm the pain came back. Why do you think that this pain keeps coming back? The problem is that he was given *standard* and basically *non-functional* exercises to strengthen the rhomboids. This patient needed to be given *functional* exercises that related to his sport. I proceeded to give him exercises with an exercise band that related to his movements during his sport. The main exercise was the standing press, which we modified slightly to replicate his motion in boxing. We also worked on the reverse motion, the standing pull, with the focus not on the shortening concentric phase for the rhomboids but the eccentric contraction (lengthening phase while the muscle is still contracting) of the rhomboid muscle. Within two weeks he was training normally and fought in a professional fight one month later – more importantly, with no recurrence of the original injury. I am very pleased to say that he won the contest.

Below are a few examples of some of the advanced training and sports-specific exercises you can include for the sporting patient. These are especially good for athletes that participate in any throwing type of events, swimming, tennis and golf and they can also be recommended for running events. You can even advise the non-sporting patient to participate in these exercises because they are functional not only to athletes but to all, as they can improve the performance of many daily activities.

Note: Please remember the exercises that have already been described in earlier chapters of this book. Some of the techniques I demonstrated can be classified as sports-specific or even advanced training and some of them are not particularly easy to perform with good technique, especially if you are a beginner to exercising and/or have some underlying restriction or weakness. I hope I have discussed the exercises with an emphasis on the idea of their being progressive in one way or another – we start on the lower part of the ladder with the easier exercises and we slowly make our way up the ladder with the more difficult ones. We are only allowed to move forward when we can correctly do the easier exercises.

Siff (2003) states:

> 'The strength exercise should not only reproduce the full amplitude of the movement but also the specific direction of resistance to the pull of the muscles.'

Once all of the seven primary exercises have been incorporated into their exercise regimen, we can then start to add a bit of variety and adapt the exercises accordingly to make them more specific and tailored to the athlete, depending on their individual sporting requirements. Although the following exercises are explained and generally demonstrated for only one side of the body, they would of course be incorporated in a program for both sides (an exercise performed on the right is repeated on the left, and so on).

1. Combined push–pull
The athlete in figure 18.40a holds a piece of exercise band with their left hand and another piece of exercise band with their right hand. They are asked to combine the motion of a push from the right arm and a pull from the left arm, as indicated in figure 18.40b. It is recommended that the inner core muscles are activated, to make sure that they are stable while performing this motion.

2. Standing push on unstable base
In the start position shown in figure 18.41a, the exercise band is held in the right hand at shoulder height and the left arm is placed in a forward position. The exercise motion is shown in figure 18.41b: the athlete pushes the band forward across their body, and at the same time the left arm moves backward while maintaining stability on the unstable base.

3. Standing pull on unstable base
In the start position shown in figure 18.42a, the athlete holds the exercise band in the right hand at shoulder height, and the left arm is placed in a backward position. The exercise motion is shown in figure 18.42b: the athlete pulls the band backward across their body, and at the same time the left arm moves forward while maintaining stability on the unstable base.

4. Bend to extend with rotation on unstable base
In the start position shown in figure 18.43a, the athlete holds the exercise band with their right hand at shoulder height and places their left arm in a backward position, while adopting a squat position on the unstable base. The exercise motion is shown in figure 18.43b: the athlete pulls

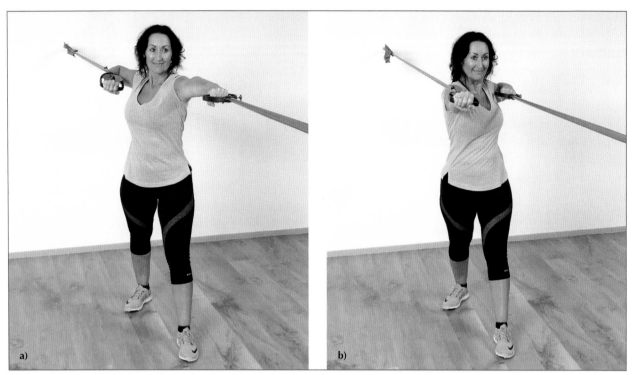

Figure 18.40a & b: *Combined push–pull. a: Start position; b: finish position*

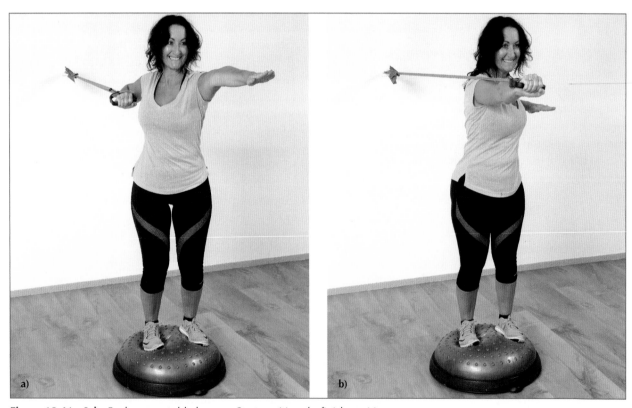

Figure 18.41a & b: *Push on unstable base. a: Start position; b: finish position*

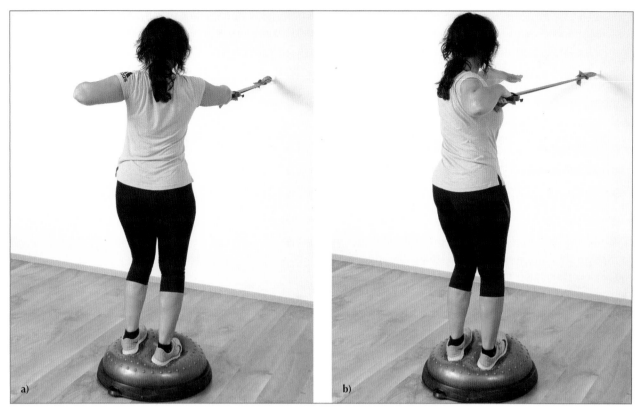

Figure 18.42a & b: *Pull on unstable base. a: Start position; b: finish position*

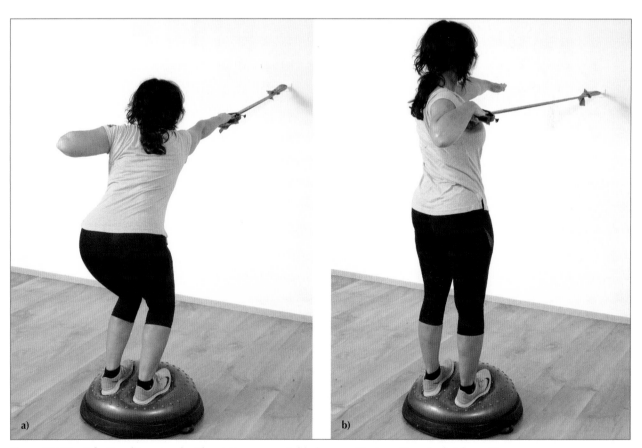

Figure 18.43a & b: *Bend to extend with rotation on unstable base. a: Start position; b: finish position*

the band backward across their body, and at the same time the left arm moves forward as they return to the erect position while maintaining stability on the unstable base.

5. Bend high to low (wood chop)

In the start position shown in figure 18.44a, the athlete holds the band simultaneously with their right and left hands at a point above shoulder height. The exercise motion is shown in figure 18.44b: the athlete pulls the band across their body to a low position, while at the same time performing a squatting motion. This movement is similar to chopping wood.

6. Bend low to high (reverse wood chop)

In the start position shown in figure 18.45a, the athlete squats down and holds the band simultaneously in the right and left hands at a point below shoulder height. The exercise motion is shown in Figure 18.45b: the athlete pulls the band across their body to a high position, while at the same time rising from the squat to an erect position.

7. Medicine ball push-up

The patient is asked to adopt a typical push-up position (if they wish they can start with their knees in contact with the mat). They place a medicine ball under one of their hands (figure 18.46a) and then they are asked to perform

a push-up motion (figure 18.46b). After one repetition the ball is transferred to the other hand and the exercise is repeated (figure 18.46c).

Stability exercise protocol

The following examples for glenohumeral and scapula stabilization can be used in combination with strength protocols. In reality there is no doubt that stabilization protocols and strength protocols naturally overlap, so it is very difficult just to focus on shoulder stability without incorporating some components of strength, and you will need to be relatively strong in one respect to perform the following stability exercises.

The glenohumeral joint and the humeral bone are basically suspended from the scapula, so wouldn't it make perfect sense to stabilize the position of the scapula to the thoracic cage prior to advising stabilization exercises for the glenohumeral joint? I guess one could debate this protocol; however, it is thought that the majority of impingement type syndromes – especially to the rotator cuff muscle group – could be caused and exacerbated by a relatively unstable scapula position, termed scapula dyskinesis. This is typically due to weakness of the scapula

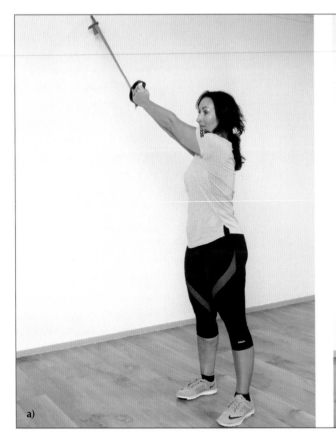
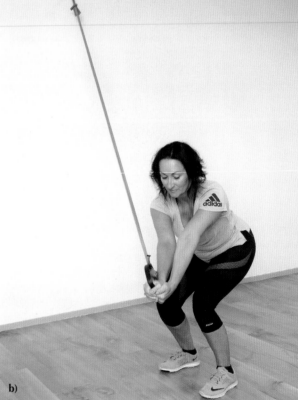

Figure 18.44a & b: *Bend high to low. a: Start position; b: finish position*

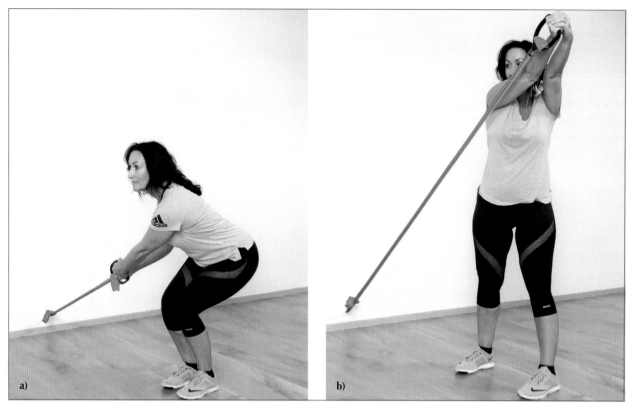

Figure 18.45a & b: *Bend low to high. a: Start position; b: finish position*

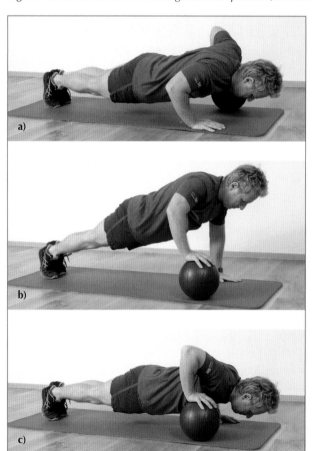

Figure 18.46a–c: *Medicine ball push-up. a: Start position; b: finish position; c: opposite hand*

stabilizing muscles. Think about that statement just for a moment. The scapula is what I think of as being the *upper limb pelvis*. The area of the normal pelvis and SIJ needs to be in a relatively stable and level position before exercises (inner and outer core) and functional movement patterns are implemented into the treatment plan. The position and function of the scapula should also provide a stable platform to allow the normal mobility of the glenohumeral, AC and SC joints. If the scapula is similar in one respect to the pelvis then this area also needs to be stable and level before glenohumeral exercises are advised, especially if the scapula fails to provide its stabilization role. That is my personal opinion but I have not so far had reason to doubt it.

The main scapula stabilization muscles are the serratus anterior, rhomboid major and minor, pectoralis minor, trapezius and levator scapulae. It is, however, poor activation (weakness) of the serratus anterior and the lower trapezius muscles with overstimulation and contraction of the scapula protractors (pectoralis minor) that can place the scapula into an anterior tilted position, commonly called 'winging'. If that is the case and one performs the scapula stabilization exercises then it can exacerbate the situation so the overactive protractors would need to be addressed initially; this has already been discussed in earlier chapters. One other thing to mention is that the scapula has a tendency to *wing* on the downward phase (eccentric) of overhead movements and unfortunately, some of the typical exercises that are recommended (Y, T and W) for the scapula are designed to work concentrically (shorten), so these will not improve the scapula dyskinesis (overhead concentric and eccentric exercises to promote scapula rotation have already been covered in this chapter).

However, the following exercises still have a role in the rehabilitative protocol as they can make the patient very aware of their scapula position, especially in the short term prior to progressing to more functional movements.

Paine and Voight (2013) mention that an effective scapular strengthening program is especially important for the overhead athlete or swimmer where normal scapular firing and control may have an effect on performance and may also relate to injury prevention. Implementation of the scapular program can begin early in the rehabilitation protocol and progress to more aggressive strengthening approaches and should be a part of all rehabilitation programs relating to the shoulder complex.

Before one begins a corrective strengthening program for the scapula musculature, it is important that the therapist regain normal flexibility of the muscles as well as functional mobility of all the joints associated with the scapula, as it is a common finding to identify tightness or adaptive shortening of the pectoralis major and minor and these muscles can inhibit activation of the opposite (antagonist) muscle groups.

Ys, Ts and Ws

The names of these scapula exercises refer to the shape of certain letters of the alphabet, Y, T and W. The following exercises are what I currently recommend to stabilize the posterior aspect of scapula, including the rhomboid and lower trapezius muscles. I teach the patient initially using the letter *T* to demonstrate specific exercises.

Technique using letter T – rhomboid/middle trapezius

The patient is asked to kneel on a mat and place their chest onto the exercise ball; they are then instructed to place their arms in 90 degrees of abduction with their elbows also bent to 90 degrees (figure 18.47a). From this position the patient is asked to focus on squeezing their scapulae together for approximately 1 or 2 seconds (figure 18.47b). Arms straight is shown in figure 18.47c.

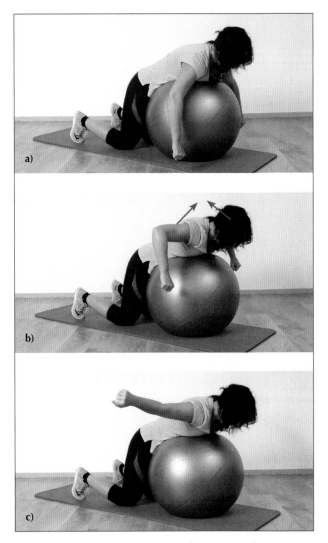

Figure 18.47a–c: *a: Start position: the patient adopts a position on an exercise ball with arms and elbows at 90 degrees. b: Finish position – the patient is asked to squeeze the scapulae together. c: The patient squeezing the scapulae with straight arms*

Progression 1

The exercises above are repeated but this time with the knees off the floor, so the patient adopts a prone position with their chest on the ball, as this will increase the difficulty of the exercises (figure 18.48).

TIP: *It is very tempting (and common) to see patients wanting to hyperextend their lumbar spine during this scapula exercise. This extra motion is not recommended because potentially the facet joints of the lumbar spine can be irritated. (This incorrect position is shown in figure 18.49.)*

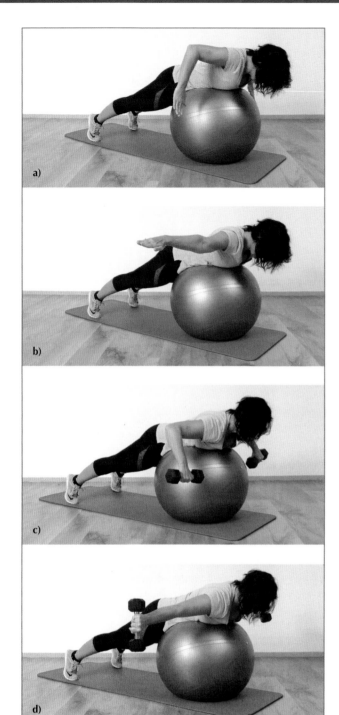

Figure 18.48a–d: *a: The patient adopts a prone position on the exercise ball and with elbows bent is asked to squeeze the scapulae together. b: The same exercise with arms extended. c: Elbows bent with a light weight. d: Arms straight with a weight*

Technique using letter *Y* – lower trapezius

This exercise is similar to the above T motion; however,

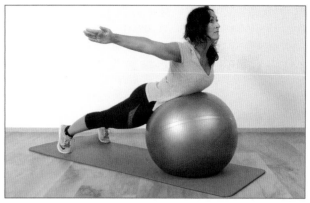

Figure 18.49: *Incorrect position with increased hyperextension to the lumbar spine*

the Y movement has more emphasis on activating the lower trapezius muscle.

The patient starts with and adopts a prone position over an exercise ball and places their chest on the ball. They are instructed to place their arms to approximately 130 degrees of abduction (this mimics a letter Y position). From this position the patient is asked to extend their shoulders backwards into the scapular plane and to focus on depressing and adducting their scapulae together for approximately 1 or 2 seconds (figure 18.50a).

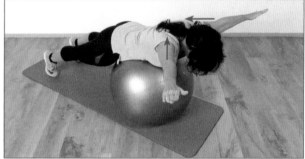

Figure 18.50a: *The patient is asked to squeeze the scapulae together in a letter 'Y' motion*

Letter *W* – lower trapezius

This technique is a variation of the start position from the exercise above: now the patient is asked to mimic bringing the hands down (adduction) like a letter W, towards their back pockets (figure 18.50b).

The above letters Y and W can be made more difficult by the use of an exercise band or a light weight

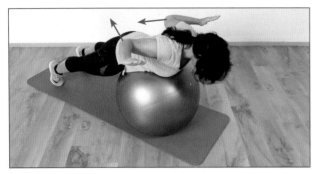

Figure 18.50b: *The patient is asked to bring the hands down towards their back pockets*

Serratus anterior

The patient is kneeling and is instructed to place their hands onto a step and keep their arms straight (figure 18.51a). From this position the patient is asked to slowly retract their shoulders (figure 18.51b) without bending their elbows and next to focus on protracting their scapulae for approximately 1 or 2 seconds as this is the action of the serratus anterior (figure 18.51c).

Progression 1
In this exercise the patient is kneeling in a push-up position with their hands placed onto an exercise ball (figure 18.52).

Progression 2
Same exercise as above but this time the patient is in a full push-up position on an exercise mat (figure 18.53).

Progression 3
In this exercise the patient is in a push-up position with their hands on an exercise ball (figure 18.54).

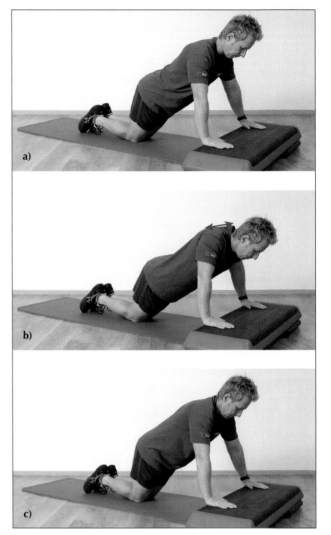

Figure 18.51a–c: *a: Start position: the patient kneels and adopts a push-up position on a step. b: The patient slowly retracts the scapula. c: Finish position – the patient is asked to protract the scapula as far as is comfortable*

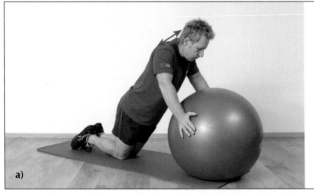
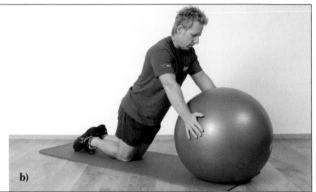

Figure 18.52a & b: *The patient kneels and adopts a push-up position on the ball. a: The patient slowly retracts the scapula. b: Finish position – the patient is asked to protract the scapula as far as is comfortable*

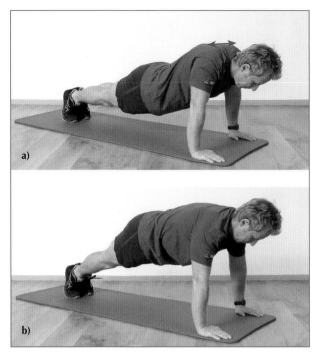

Figure 18.53a & b: *The patient adopts a push-up position on a mat. a: The patient slowly retracts the scapula. b: Finish position – the patient is asked to protract the scapula as far as is comfortable*

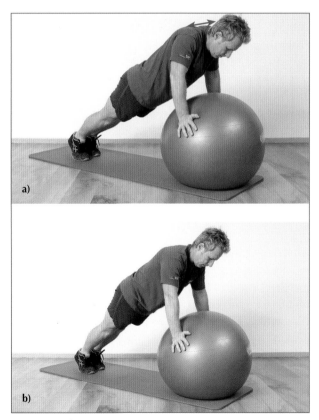

Figure 18.54a & b: *The patient is in a push-up position on the ball. a: The patient slowly retracts the scapula. b: Finish position – the patient is asked to protract the scapula as far as is comfortable*

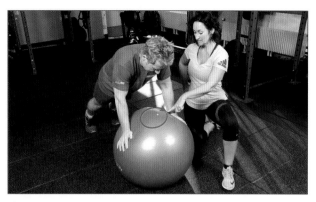

Figure 18.55: *The patient is in a push-up position on the ball. The patient follows the finger as guided by the therapist*

Progression 4

This exercise has the same start position as above; however, the patient is gripping the ball in a push-up position. The therapist indicates one of the top circles on the core ball with their finger and the patient tries to circle the ball in a clockwise and a counterclockwise direction (figure 18.55) but the patient is not allowed to bend their elbows. The therapist can now place their finger on the second circle, which is slightly larger, meaning the patient has to work harder for the circle motion.

Note: The above exercise is more difficult than it might first appear and is not recommended early into the program. That is why I have placed it here, at the end. One needs a lot of the overall stabilization mechanisms of the whole of the upper body complex to perform this exercise correctly and without the body trying to compensate.

Self-lengthening protocol

Athletes and patients generally ask me after treatment what exercises and stretches they can do, especially in the gym. In this chapter I have already covered the majority of the exercises I would recommend so for the final phase of this book I will only focus on self-stretches or self-lengthening techniques. These can be done at any time of the day and anywhere, as no equipment is required. I like to call these *active lengthening* techniques as the patient is doing all of the motion. I use a 5-5-5 methodology, which basically means they will contract the muscle for 5 seconds, then lengthen and hold for 5 seconds and repeat 5 times. These can be done before, during or even after the workout. I like this simple approach because for one it activates the muscle to contact as in a self post isometric relaxation (PIR) of the MET approach, then we use the antagonistic muscle (opposite) to activate, as in reciprocal inhibition (RI), and this will assist in strengthening, even though we are using the contraction to lengthen the antagonist muscle.

Let us look at some examples.

Technique 1 – Pectoral active lengthening

The patient is either sitting or standing and places both of the palms of their hands on the lower back (figure 18.56). The patient is then instructed to activate the pectoral muscles isometrically (no motion) for approximately 20% effort from this position for 5 seconds (figure 18.56).

After 5 seconds of contraction, the patient is then asked to squeeze the shoulder blades together (scapula adduction) using the rhomboids and middle trapezius and to hold the contraction for 5 seconds (figure 18.57). This will induce a lengthening of the pectoral muscles and subsequent strengthening of the rhomboids and middle trapezius. This is repeated approximately 5 times.

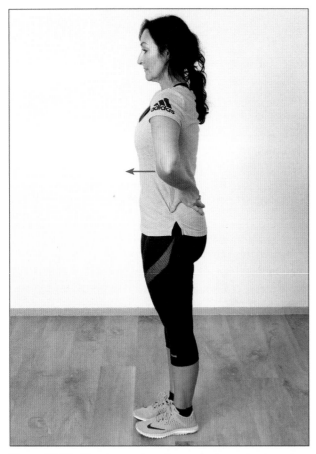

Figure 18.56: *Hands are placed onto the lower back and patient isometrically activates the pectoral muscles*

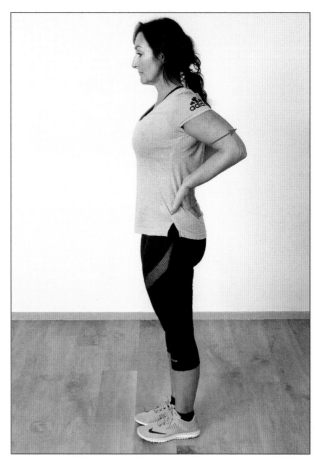

Figure 18.57: *The patient activates the scapula adductor muscles for 5 seconds as this lengthens the pectoral muscles*

Technique 2 – Pectoral active lengthening – horizontal

The patient is either sitting or standing and straightens their arms and places both of the palms of their hands together in the horizontal plane. The patient is then instructed to activate the pectoral muscles isometrically (no motion) for approximately 20% effort from this position for 5 seconds (figure 18.58).

After 5 seconds of contraction, the patient is then asked to horizontally extend and to squeeze the shoulder blades together (scapula adduction) using the rhomboids and middle trapezius and to hold the contraction for 5 seconds (figure 18.59). This will induce a lengthening of the pectoral muscles. It is repeated approximately 5 times.

Technique 3 – Shoulder adductors active lengthening

The patient is either sitting or standing and places the palms of their hands on their hips. The patient is then instructed to activate the shoulder adductor muscles

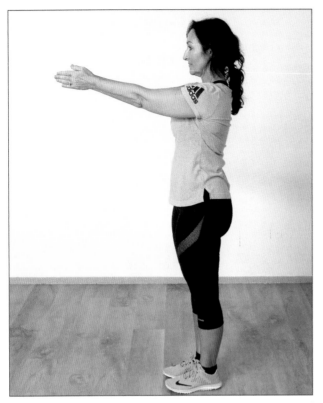

Figure 18.58: *The patient isometrically activates the pectoral muscles by squeezing the hands together*

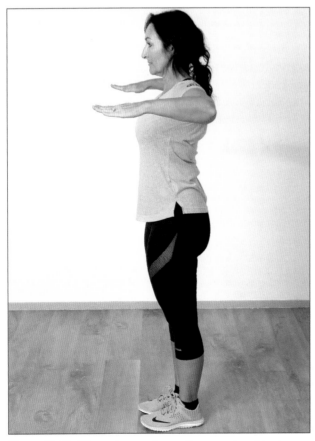

Figure 18.59: *The patient activates the scapula adductor muscles for 5 seconds by horizontally extending*

isometrically (no motion) for approximately 20% effort from this position for 5 seconds (figure 18.60a).

After 5 seconds of contraction, the patient is then asked to fully abduct their shoulders with thumbs leading the motion (external rotation) using the supraspinatus and deltoid, and to hold the contraction for 5 seconds (figure 18.60b). This will induce a lengthening of the adductor muscles and is repeated approximately 5 times.

Technique 4 – Shoulder flexors active lengthening

The patient is either sitting or standing and places each arm into a 45-degree position of flexion. The patient is then instructed to hold this position for 5 seconds (figure 18.61).

After 5 seconds of contraction, the patient is then asked to fully extend their shoulders as far as is comfortable and to hold the contraction for 5 seconds (figure 18.62). This will induce a lengthening of the flexor muscles and is repeated approximately 5 times.

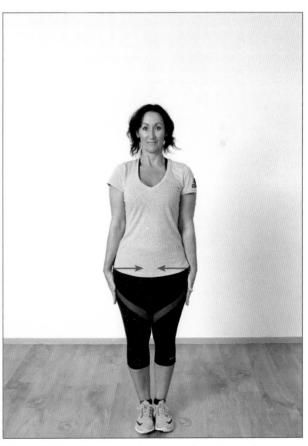

Figure 18.60a: *The patient isometrically activates the shoulder adductor muscles*

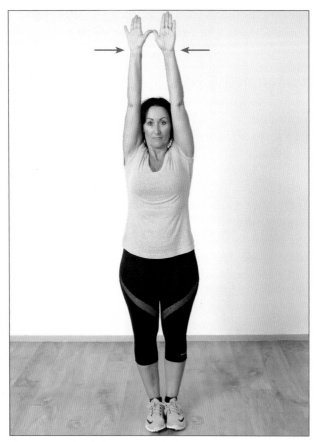

Figure 18.60b: *The patient activates the shoulder abductor muscles for 5 seconds*

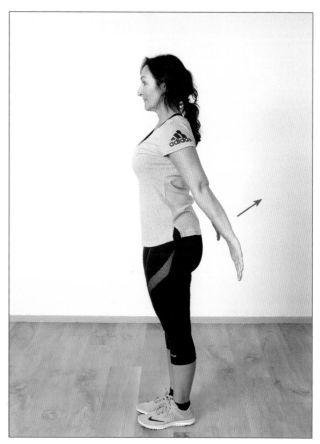

Figure 18.62: *The patient activates the shoulder extensor muscles for 5 seconds*

Technique 5 – Shoulder extensors active lengthening

The patient is either sitting or standing and places each arm into a full motion of shoulder extension. The patient is then instructed to hold this position for 5 seconds (figure 18.63).

After 5 seconds of contraction, the patient is then asked to fully flex their shoulders with the thumbs leading the motion as far as comfortable and to hold the contraction for 5 seconds (figure 18.64). This will induce a lengthening to the extensor muscles and is repeated approximately 5 times.

■ Conclusion

You have now reached the end of the book and if I have done my job well, as I truly hope, you actually enjoyed reading and hopefully understood what I have written. More importantly, I want to be able to feel deep inside myself that I have personally helped you in your quest for progressing your own knowledge of this fascinating but highly complex subject.

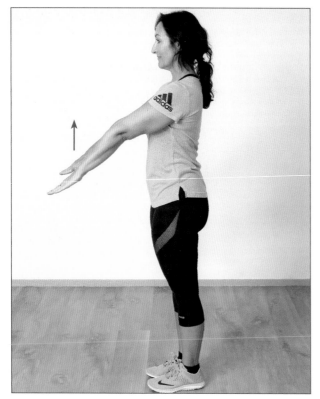

Figure 18.61: *The patient isometrically activates the shoulder flexor muscles*

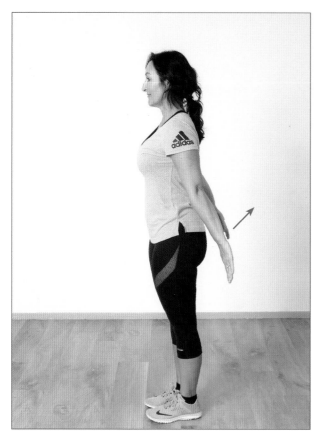

Figure 18.63: *The patient isometrically activates the shoulder extensor muscles*

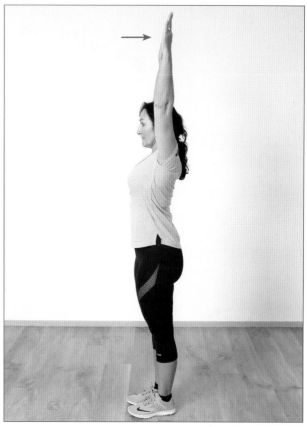

Figure 18.64: *Patient activates the shoulder flexor muscles for 5 seconds*

The first draft of this book was well over hundred thousand words on completion and I could have easily doubled the amount I wrote; however, my personal preference is for books that are not *too* thick, with plenty of color pictures, and also where the font is actually readable. I consider that all the books I have written to date fit this description. This book is no exception and I think it contains enough information to guide therapists to treat patients and athletes in a more effective way. I have mentioned previously that therapists are like *detectives* and the *clues* are there for them to find. They just have to go about finding those clues in a logical way. I hope I can make that journey a little easier for you and more importantly that you enjoy the process of assessing, treating and rehabilitating athletes and patients that present with shoulder pain and that the whole process doesn't become *a chore*. If that is the case then maybe a career in physical therapy is not for you.

I actually finished writing this book in Sri Lanka, enjoying a vacation after lecturing in Dubai, and these last words have been written in the Emirates lounge at the airport. One of the books I read while on holiday, *Fragile Lives*, was written by a cardiac surgeon called Professor Stephen Westaby, who was also based in Oxford (UK) before he retired. As soon as I started reading the introduction, it excited and inspired me so much that I couldn't put it down and literally read it in a couple of days. I hope that is the same for when you have read my book (maybe not as quickly) and it gave you as much pleasure!

Thanks again for making the effort to read this book, it means so much to me and I hope to meet you in person one day!

Till the next book … regards, JG

Appendix 1
Tables for dysfunction testing

The following tables can be used in the therapist's own clinical setting (permission to reproduce is granted).

Table A1.1: Hip extension firing pattern – left side

	1st	2nd	3rd	4th
Gluteus maximus	○	○	○	○
Hamstrings	○	○	○	○
Contralateral erector spinae	○	○	○	○
Ipsilateral erector spinae	○	○	○	○

Table A1.2: Hip extension firing pattern – right side

	1st	2nd	3rd	4th
Gluteus maximus	○	○	○	○
Hamstrings	○	○	○	○
Contralateral erector spinae	○	○	○	○
Ipsilateral erector spinae	○	○	○	○

Table A1.3: Postural assessment sheet – Upper body

Patient Name:			
Key: E = Equal in length			
L/R = Short on left or right side			
Muscles	**Date:**	**Date:**	**Date:**
Upper trapezius			
Levator scapulae			
Sternocleidomastoid			
Scalenes			
Coracoid muscles • Pectoralis minor • Biceps brachii short head • Coracobrachialis			
Latissimus dorsi			
Pectoralis major			
Subscapularis			
Infraspinatus			

Table A1.4: Anatomical landmarks checklist

Landmarks	Left side	Right side
Pelvic crest (posterior view)		
Posterior superior iliac spine (PSIS)		
Greater trochanter		
Gluteal and popliteal folds		
Leg, foot, and ankle position (anterior/posterior view)		
Lumbar and thoracic spine		
Inferior angle of scapula (T7)		
Medial border of scapula		
Superior angle of scapula		
Position of acromion (levels)		
Position of cervical spine		
Pelvic crest (anterior view)		
Anterior superior iliac spine (ASIS)		
Sternoclavicular joint		
Acromioclavicular joint		
Glenohumeral position		

Table A1.5: Normal range of motion for the glenohumeral joint

Glenohumeral joint	Left side in degrees	Right side in degrees
Flexion	180	180
Extension	60	60
Abduction	180	180
Adduction	45	45
Internal rotation	70	70
External rotation	90	90
Horizontal flexion (adduction)	130	130
Horizontal extension (abduction)	50	50

Table A1.6: Normal active range of motion (AROM) for the cervical spine

Cervical spine	Degrees
Rotation (left and right)	80
Flexion	50
Extension	60
Lateral flexion (left and right)	45

Appendix 2

Shoulder stabilization exercise sheet

The following exercises can be used in the physical therapist's own clinical setting. For each exercise there is a blank space in which a patient's repetitions and sets can be recorded.

EXERCISE	SETS	REPS
1. Standing push		
2. Standing pull		

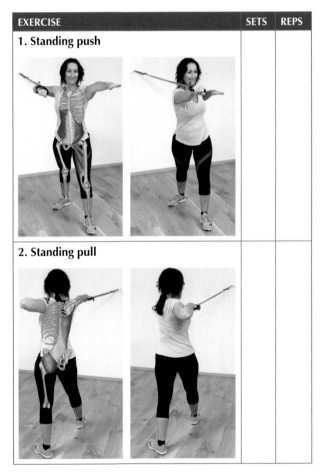

EXERCISE	SETS	REPS
3. Curl with press *Exercise 1 – Sitting curl with press*		

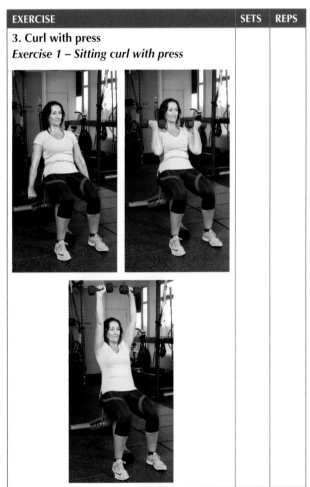

EXERCISE	SETS	REPS
Exercise 2 – Standing curl with press		
Exercise 3 – Alternate curl with press		

EXERCISE	SETS	REPS
4. Horizontal press *Exercise 1 – Kneeling push-up*		
Exercise 2 – Push-up		
Exercise 3 – Push-up with use of ball *Progression 1 – Kneeling push-up-ball*		
Progression 2 – Push-up-ball		
Progression 3 – Push-up-ball-arms lift		
Progression 4 – Push-up-ball-single leg lift		

EXERCISE	SETS	REPS
Progression 5 – Push-up-step		
Progression 6 – Push-up-feet on ball		
Progression and variation		

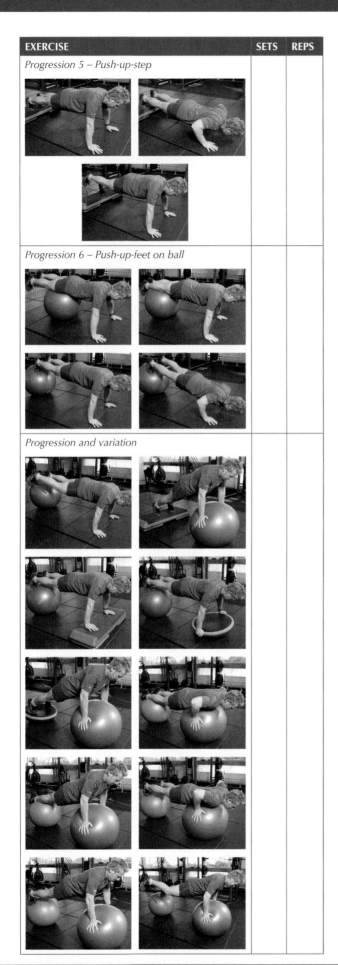

EXERCISE	SETS	REPS
TRX press-up		
TRX – Standing push		
5. Rotation – Internal and external *Internal rotation*		

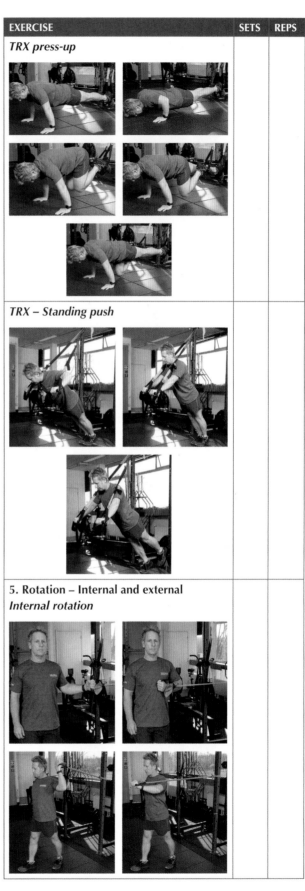

EXERCISE	SETS	REPS
External rotation		
Functional external/internal rotation in abduction (throwing) *Exercise 1*		
Exercise 2		
6. Overhead – Vertical push *Exercise 1 – Overhead push – standing – band*		

EXERCISE	SETS	REPS
Exercise 2 – Overhead push – standing – dumbbells		

EXERCISE	SETS	REPS

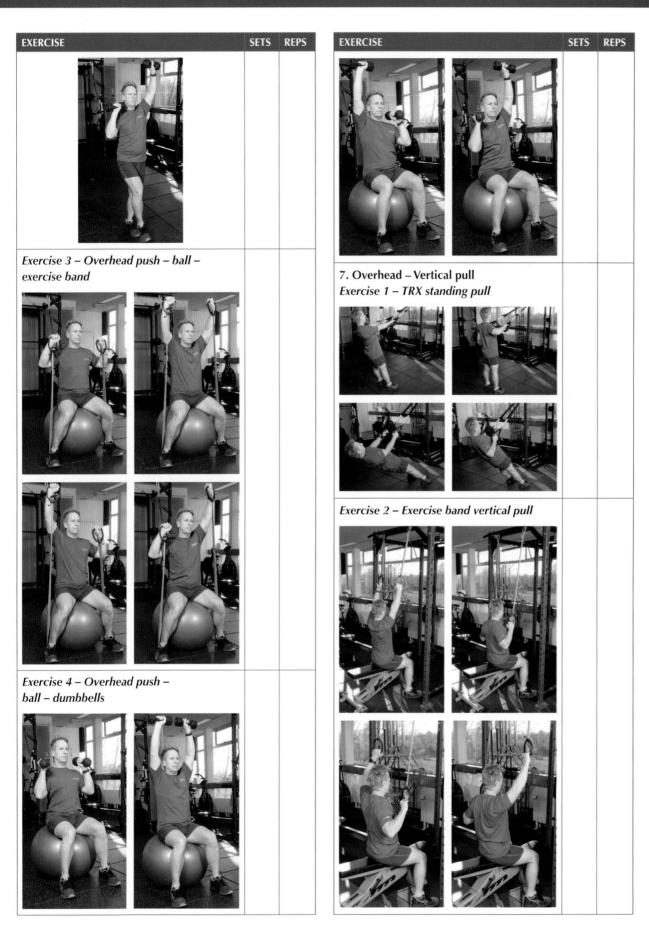

Exercise 3 – Overhead push – ball – exercise band

Exercise 4 – Overhead push – ball – dumbbells

EXERCISE	SETS	REPS

7. Overhead – Vertical pull
Exercise 1 – TRX standing pull

Exercise 2 – Exercise band vertical pull

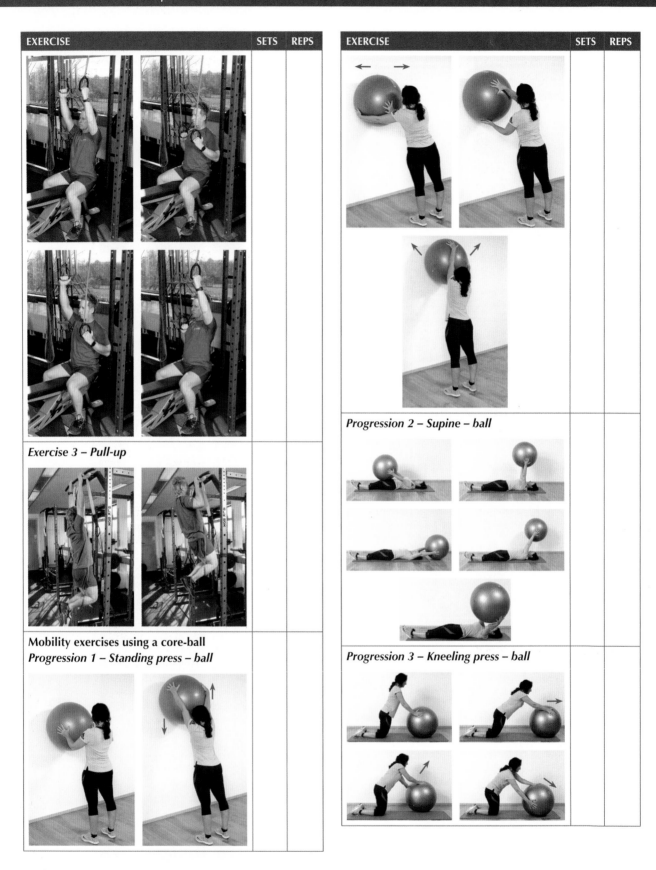

EXERCISE	SETS	REPS
Exercise 3 – Pull-up		
Mobility exercises using a core-ball *Progression 1 – Standing press – ball*		

EXERCISE	SETS	REPS
Progression 2 – Supine – ball		
Progression 3 – Kneeling press – ball		

EXERCISE	SETS	REPS
Mobility exercises using a foam roller *Progression 1 – Sitting to roll*		
Progression 2 – Standing to roll		
Progression 3 – Kneeling to roll		
Thoracic mobility		

EXERCISE	SETS	REPS
Mobility exercises using a wooden pole		
Progression – Horizontal/scapula plane motion		

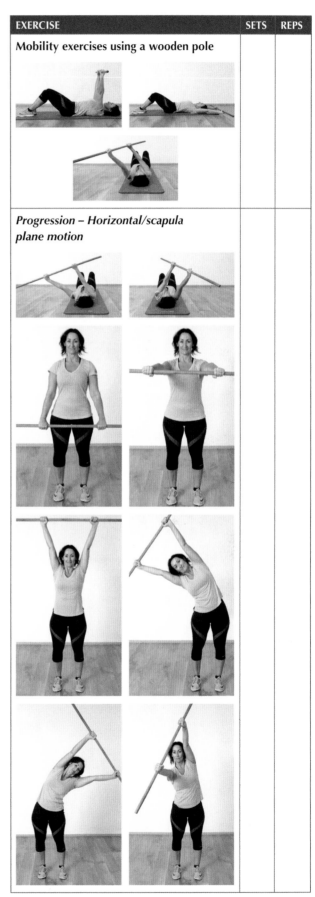

EXERCISE	SETS	REPS

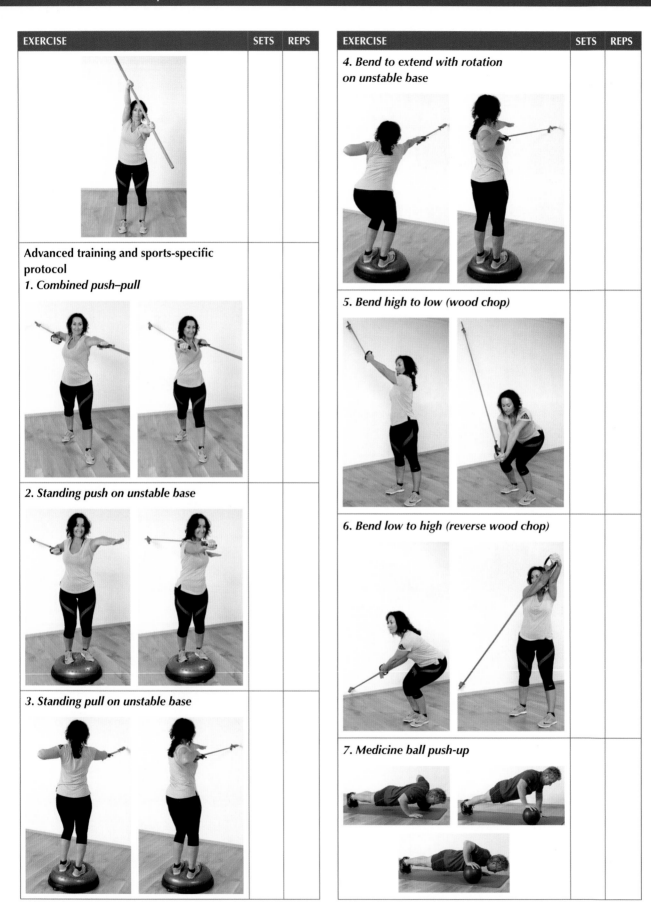

Advanced training and sports-specific protocol
1. Combined push–pull

2. Standing push on unstable base

3. Standing pull on unstable base

EXERCISE	SETS	REPS

4. Bend to extend with rotation on unstable base

5. Bend high to low (wood chop)

6. Bend low to high (reverse wood chop)

7. Medicine ball push-up

EXERCISE	SETS	REPS
Stability exercise protocol *Technique using letter T – rhomboid/ middle trapezius*		
Progression 1		
Technique using letter Y – lower trapezius		
Letter W – lower trapezius		
Serratus anterior		

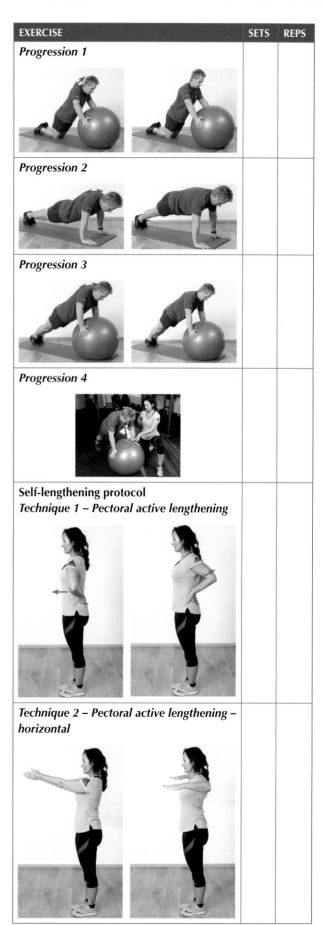

EXERCISE	SETS	REPS
Progression 1		
Progression 2		
Progression 3		
Progression 4		
Self-lengthening protocol *Technique 1 – Pectoral active lengthening*		
Technique 2 – Pectoral active lengthening – horizontal		

EXERCISE	SETS	REPS
Technique 3 – Shoulder adductors active lengthening 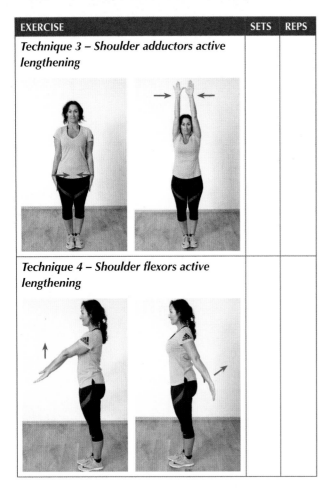		
Technique 4 – Shoulder flexors active lengthening		

EXERCISE	SETS	REPS
Technique 5 – Shoulder extensors active lengthening 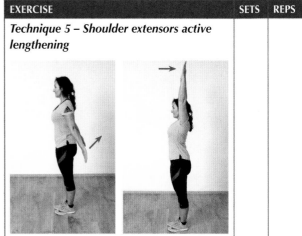		

Bibliography

Abernethy, B., Hanrahan, S., Kippers, V., et al.: 2004. *The Biophysical Foundations of Human Movement.* Human Kinetics, Champaign, IL

Adson, A.W., Coffey, J.R.: 1927. 'Cervical rib. A method of anterior approach for relief of symptoms by division of the scalenus anticus.' *Ann Surg*; 85:839–857

Anekstein, Y., Blecher, R., Smorgick, Y., Mirovsky, Y., et al.: 2012. 'What is the best way to apply the Spurling test for cervical radiculopathy.' *Clin Orthop Relat Res*; 470(9): 2566–2572

Aszmann, O.C., Dellon, A.L., Birely, B.T., et al.: 1996. 'Innervation of the human shoulder joint and its implications for surgery.' *Clin Orthop Relat Res*; 330:202–207

Basmajian, J.V., De Luca, C.J.: 1979. *Muscles Alive: Their Functions Revealed by Electromyography*, 5th edn. Williams & Wilkins, Baltimore, MD, pp. 386–387

Bigliani, L.U., Levine, W.N.: 1997. 'Subacromial impingement syndrome.' *J Bone Joint Surg Am*; 79:1854–1868

Bigliani, L.U., Morrison, D.S., April, E.W.: 1986. 'The morphology of the acromion and its relationship to rotator cuff tears.' *Ortho Trans*; 10:228

Boyle, J.J.: 1999. 'Is the pain and dysfunction of shoulder impingement lesion really second rib syndrome in disguise? Two case reports.' *Man Ther*; 4(1):44–48

Bridgman, J.F.: 1972. 'Periarthritis of the shoulder and diabetes mellitus.' *Ann Rheum Dis*; 31:69

Brossmann, J., et al.: 1996. 'Shoulder impingement syndrome: influence of shoulder position on rotator cuff impingement – an anatomic study.' *Am J Roentgenol*; 167(6):1511–1515

Calliet, R.: 1991. *Shoulder Pain*, 3rd edn. F.A. Davis Company, Philadelphia

Capobianco, S., van den Dries, G.: 2009. *Power Taping*, 2nd edn. Rocktape inc., USA

Chek, P.: 2009. *An Integrated Approach to Stretching.* C.H.E.K. Institute, Vista, CA

Codman, E.A.: 1934. *The Shoulder.* Thomas Todd, Boston

Colvin, A.C., Egorova, N., Harrison, A.K., Moskowitz, A., Flatow, E.L.: 2012. 'National trends in rotator cuff repair.' *J Bone Joint Surg Am*; 94:227–233

Duplay, S.: 1906. 'De la Peri-arthrite scapulo humerale.' *Reveue Practicien de trav de Med*; 53:226

Earl, J.E.: 2005. 'Gluteus medius activity during three variations of isometric single- leg stance.' *J Sport Rehabil*; 14:1–11

Fratocchi, G., Mattia, F.D., Rossi, R., et al.: 2012. 'Influence of Kinesio Taping applied over biceps brachii on isokinetic elbow peak torque. A placebo controlled study in a population of young healthy subjects.' *J Sci Med Sport*; 16(3):245–249

Gerber, C., Krushell, R.J.: 1991. 'Isolated rupture of the tendon of the subscapularis muscle: clinical features in 16 cases.' *J Bone Joint Surg Am*; 73:389–394

Gibbons, J.: 2008. 'Preparing for glory.' *International Therapist*; 81:14–16

Gibbons, J.: 2009. 'Putting maximus back into the gluteus.' *International Therapist*; 87:32–33

Gibbons, J.: 2011. *Muscle Energy Techniques: A Practical Guide for Physical Therapists.* Lotus Publishing, Chichester, UK

Gibbons, J.: 2014. *The Vital Glutes: Connecting the Gait Cycle to Pain and Dysfunction.* Lotus Publishing/North Atlantic Books, Chichester, UK/Berkeley, CA

Gibbons, J.: 2015. *A Practical Guide to Kinesiology Taping.* Lotus Publishing/North Atlantic Books, Chichester, UK/Berkeley, CA

Gibbons, J.: 2016. *Functional Anatomy of the Pelvis and Saroiliac Joint.* Lotus Publishing/North Atlantic Books, Chichester, UK/Berkeley, CA

Gillard, J., Perez-Cousin, M., Hachulla, E., et al.: 2001. 'Diagnosing thoracic outlet syndrome: contribution of provocation tests, ultrasonography, electrophysiology, and helical computed tomography in 48 patients.' *Joint Bone Spine*; 68:416–424

Gleason, P.D., Beall, D.P., Sanders, T.G.: 2006. 'The transverse humeral ligament: a separate anatomical structure or a continuation of the osseous attachment of the rotator cuff.' *Am J Sports Med*; 34:72–77

Gonzalez-Iglesias, J., Fernandez-de-les-Penas, C., Cleland, J., et al.: 2009. 'Short term effects of cervical kinesiology taping on pain and cervical range of motion in patients with acute whiplash injury: a randomized clinical trial.' *J Orthop Sports Phys Ther*; 39(7):515–521

Goodman, C., Snyder, T.: 2007. 'Differential diagnosis for physical therapists.' Saunders Elsevier, Pennsylvania, USA

Gracovetsky, S.: 1988. *The Spinal Engine.* Springer-Verlag, New York

Hammer, W.: 1991. *Functional Soft Tissue Examination and Treatment by Manual Methods.* Aspen Publishers, New York, USA

Hawkins, R.J., Kennedy, J.C.: 1980. 'Impingement syndrome in athletes.' *Am J Sports Med*; 8:151–158

Holtby, R., Razmjou, H.: 2004. 'Validity of the supraspinatus test as a single clinical test in diagnosing patients with rotator cuff pathology.' *J Orthop Sports Phys Ther*; 34(4):194–200

Hsu, Y.H., Chen, W.Y., Lin, H.C., et al.: 2009. 'The effects of taping on scapula kinematics and muscle performance in baseball players with shoulder impingement syndrome.' *J Electromyogr Kinesiol*; 19(6):1092–1099

Ide, K., Shirai, Y., Ito, H.: 1996. 'Sensory nerve supply in the human subacromial bursa.' *J Shoulder Elbow Surg*; 5:371–382

Inman, V.T., Saunders, M., Abbott, L.C.: 1944. 'Observations on the function of the shoulder joint.' *J Bone Joint Surg Am*; 26:1–30

Inman, V.T., Ralston, H.J., Todd, F.: 1981. *Human Walking.* Williams & Wilkins, Baltimore, MD

Ireland, M.L., Wilson, J.D., Ballantyne, B.T., Davis, I.M.: 2003. 'Hip strength in females with and without patellofemoral pain.' *J Orthop Sports Phys Ther*; 33:671–676

Janda, V.: 1983. 'On the concept of postural muscles and posture.' *Aust J Physiother*; 29: S83–S84

Janda, V.: 1987. 'Muscles and motor control in low back pain: assessment and management', in L.T. Twomey (ed.), *Physical Therapy of the Low Back.* Churchill Livingstone, New York, pp. 253–278

Janda, V.: 1988. 'Muscles and cervicogenic pain syndromes', in R. Grand (ed.), *Physical Therapy of the Cervical and Thoracic Spine.* Churchill Livingstone, New York, pp. 153–166

Janda, V.: 1992. 'Treatment of chronic low back pain.' *J Man Med*; 6:166–168

Janda, V.: 1993. 'Muscle strength in relation to muscle length, pain, and muscle imbalance', in *Muscle Strength*, vol. 8 of *International Perspectives in Physical Therapy*, ed. K. Harms-Ringdahl. Churchill Livingstone, Edinburgh, pp. 83–91

Janda, V.: 1996. 'Evaluation of muscular imbalance', in C. Liebenson (ed.), *Rehabilitation of the Spine: A Practitioner's Manual.* Lippincott, Williams & Wilkins, Baltimore, MD, pp. 97–112

Jobe, F.W., Moynes, D.R.: 1982. 'Delineation of diagnostic criteria and a rehabilitation program for rotator cuff injuries.' *Am J Sports Med*; 10(6):336–339

Jobe, F.W. et al.: 1983. 'An EMG analysis of the shoulder in throwing and pitching: a preliminary report.' *Am J Sports Med*; 2(1):3

Judge, A., Murphy, R.J., Maxwell, R., Arden, N.K., Carr, A.J.: 2014. 'Temporal trends and geographical variation in the use of subacromial decompression and rotator cuff repair of the shoulder in England.' *Bone Joint J*; 96-B:70–74

Karatas, N., Bicici, S., Baltaci, G., et al.: 2011. 'The effect of Kinesio Tape application on functional performance in surgeons who have musculo-skeletal pain after performing surgery.' *Turkish Neurosurgery*; 22(1):83–89

Kaya, E., Zinnuroglu, M., Tugcu, I.: 2011. 'Kinesio taping compared to physical therapy modalities for the treatment of shoulder impingement.' *Clin Rheumatol*; 30(2):201–207

Kelly, B.T., Kadrmas, W.R., Speer, K.P.: 1996. 'The manual muscle examination for rotator cuff strength. An electromyographic investigation.' *Am J Sports Med*; 24(5):581–588

Kendall, F.P., McCreary, E.K., Provance, P.G., et al.: 2010. *Muscle Testing and Function with Posture and Pain*, 5th edn. Lippincott, Williams & Wilkins, Baltimore, MD

Lee, D.G.: 2004. *The Pelvic Girdle: An Approach to the Examination and Treatment of the Lumbopelvic-Hip Region.* Churchill Livingstone, Edinburgh

Lewis, J.: 2009. Rotator cuff tendinopathy/subacromial impingement syndrome: is it time for a new method of assessment. *Br J Sports Med*; 43:259–264

Lewis, J.S., Tennent, T.D.: 2007. 'How effective are diagnostic tests for the assessment of rotator cuff disease of the shoulder?', in D. MacAuley, T.M. Best (eds), *Evidence-Based Sports Medicine*, 2nd edn. Blackwell Publishing, London

Lewis, J.S., Wright, C., Green, A.: 2005. 'Subacromial impingement syndrome: the effect of changing posture on shoulder range of movement.' *J Orthop Sports Phys Ther*; 35:72–87

Lollino, N., Brunocilla, P., Poglio, F., et al.: 2012. 'Non-orthopaedic causes of shoulder pain: what the shoulder expert must remember.' *Musculoskeletal Surg*; 96(Suppl 1):S63–S68

Ludewig, P.M., Cook, T.M.: 2002. 'Translations of the humerus in persons with shoulder impingement symptoms.' *J Orthop Sports Phys Ther*; 32(6):248–259

Malanga, G.A., Nadler, S.F.: 2006. *Musculoskeletal Physical Examination: An Evidence-Based Approach.* Mosby, Philadelphia, pp. 50–51

Martin, C.: 2002. *Functional Movement Development*, 2nd edn. W.B. Saunders, London

Naffziger, H.C., Grant, W.T.: 1938. 'Neuritis of the brachial plexus mechanical in origin. The scalene syndrome.' *Surg Gynecol Obstet*; 67:722

Neer, C.S., 2nd: 1972. 'Anterior acromioplasty for the chronic impingement syndrome in the shoulder: a preliminary report.' *J Bone Joint Surg Am*; 54(1):41–50

Neer, C.S., 2nd: 1983. Impingement lesions. *Clin Orthop Relat Res*; 173:70–77

Novak, C.B., Mackinnon, S.E.: 1996. 'Thoracic outlet syndrome.' *Occupational Disorder Management*; 27(4):747–762

O'Brien, S.J., Pagnani, M.J., Fealy, S., McGlynn, S.R., Wilson, J.B.: 1998. The active compression test: a new and effective test for diagnosing labral tears and acromioclavicular joint abnormality. *Am J Sports Med*; 26:610–613

Osar, E.: 2012. *Corrective Exercise Solutions to Common Hip and Shoulder Dysfunction.* Lotus Publishing, Chichester, UK

Ozaki, J., Fujimoto, S., Nakagawa, Y., Masuhara, K., Tamai, S.: 1988. 'Tears of the rotator cuff of the shoulder associated with pathological changes in the acromion. A study in cadavera.' *J Bone Joint Surg Am*; 70:1224–1230

Page, P., Frank, C.C., Lardner, R.: 2010. *Assessment and Treatment of Muscle Imbalance: The Janda Approach.* Human Kinetics, Champaign, IL

Paine, R., Voight, M.L.: 2013. 'The role of the scapula.' *Int J Sports Phys Ther*; 8:617–629

Perry, J.: 1988. 'Biomechanics of the shoulder', in C.R. Rowe (ed.), *The Shoulder*. Churchill Livingstone, New York, pp. 17–33

Plewa, M.C., Delinger, M.: 1998. 'The false positive rate of thoracic outlet syndrome shoulder maneuvers in healthy individuals.' *Acad Emerg Med*; 5:337–342

Rezzouk, J., Uzel, M., Lavignolle, B., Midy, D., Durandeau, A.: 2004. 'Does the motor branch of the long head of the triceps brachii arise from the radial nerve?' *Surg Radiol Anat*; 26(6):459–461

Richardson, C., Jull, G., Hodges, P., Hides, J.: 1999. *Therapeutic Exercise for Spinal Segmental Stabilization in Low Back Pain: Scientific Basis and Clinical Approach.* Churchill Livingstone, Edinburgh

Richardson, C.A., Snijders, C.J., Hides, J.A., et al.: 2002. 'The relationship between the transversely oriented abdominal muscles, sacroiliac joint mechanics and low back pain.' *Spine*; 27(4):399–405

Rob, C.G., Standeven, A.: 1958. 'Arterial occlusion complicating thoracic outlet compression syndrome.' *Br Med J*; 2:709–712

Roos, D.: 1996. 'Historical perspectives and anatomic considerations. Thoracic outlet syndrome.' *Semin Thorac Cardiovasc Surg*; 8(2):183–189

Rundquist, P., Anderson, D.D., Guanche, C.A., et al.: 2003. 'Shoulder kinematics in subjects with frozen shoulder.' *Arch Phys Med Rehabil*; 84:1473–1479

Sherrington, C.S.: 1907. 'On reciprocal innervation of antagonistic muscles.' *Proc R Soc Lond [Biol]*; 79B: 337

Siff, M.: 2003. *Supertraining.* 5th edn. Supertraining Institute, p. 244

Spurling, R.S., Scoville, W.B.: 1944. 'Lateral rupture of the cervical intervertebral discs: a common cause of shoulder and arm pain.' *Surg Gynecol Obstet*; 78:350–358

Thelen, M.D., Dauber, J.A., Stoneman, P.D.: 2008. 'The clinical efficacy of kinesio tape for shoulder pain: a randomized, double-blinded, clinical trial.' *J Orthop Sports Phys Ther*; 38(7):389–395

Thomas, C.L.: 1997. *Taber's Cyclopaedic Medical Dictionary*, 18th edn. F.A. Davis, Philadelphia, USA

Umphred, D.A., Byl, N., Lazaro, R.T., Roller, M.: 2001. 'Interventions for neurological disabilities', in D.A. Umphred (ed.), *Neurological Rehabilitation*, 4th edn. Mosby, St Louis, MO, pp. 56–134

Vanti, C., Natalini, L., Romeo, A., Tosarelli, D., Pillastrini, P.: 2007. 'Conservative treatment of thoracic outlet syndrome: a review of the literature.' *Eura Medicophys*; 43:55–70

Vleeming, A., Stoeckart, R.: 2007. 'The role of the pelvic girdle in coupling the spine and the legs: a clinical-anatomical perspective on pelvic stability', in Vleeming et al., *Movement, Stability and Lumbopelvic Pain: Integration of Research and Therapy*, Churchill Livingstone, Edinburgh, pp. 113–137

Vleeming, A., Stoeckart, R., Snijders, D.J.: 1989a. 'The sacrotuberous ligament: a conceptual approach to its dynamic role in stabilizing the sacroiliac joint.' *Clin Biomech*; 4, 200–203

Vleeming, A., Van Wingerden, J.P., Snijders, C.J., et al.: 1989b. 'Load application to the sacrotuberous ligament: Influences on sacroiliac joint mechanics.' *Clin Biomech*; 4, 204–209

Vleeming, A., Stoeckart, R., Volkers, A.C.W., et al.: 1990a. 'Relation between form and function in the sacroiliac joint. Part 1: Clinical anatomical aspects.' *Spine*; 15(2):130–132

Vleeming, A., Volkers, A.C.W., Snijders, C.J., Stoeckart, R.: 1990b. 'Relation between form and function in the sacroiliac joint. Part 2: Biomechanical aspects.' *Spine*; 15(2):133–136

Vleeming, A., Snijders, C.J., Stoeckart, R., et al.: 1995. 'A new light on low back pain.' *Proceedings of the Second Interdisciplinary World Congress on Low Back Pain, San Diego, CA*

Vleeming, A., Mooney, V., Dorman, T., et al. (eds): 1997. *Movement, Stability and Lower Back Pain: The Essential Role of the Pelvis.* Churchill Livingstone, Edinburgh, pp. 425–431

Vleeming, A., Mooney, V., Stoeckart, R. (eds): 2007. *Movement, Stability and Lumbopelvic Pain: Integration of Research and Therapy.* Churchill Livingstone, Edinburgh

Willard, F.H., Vleeming, A., Schuenke, M.D., et al.: 2012. 'The thoracolumbar fascia: anatomy, function and clinical considerations.' *J Anat*; 221(6):507–536

Yasojima, T., Kizuka, T., Noguchi, H., Shiraki, H., Mukai, N., Miyanaga, Y.: 2008. 'Differences in EMG activity in scapular plane abduction under variable arm positions and loading conditions.' *Med Sci Sports Exerc*; 40(4):716–721

Index